So you want to be a brain surgeon?

The essential guide to
medical careers

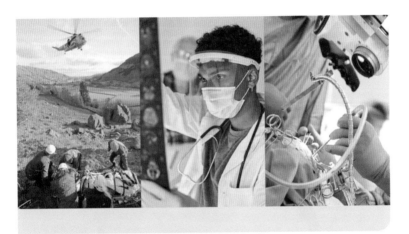

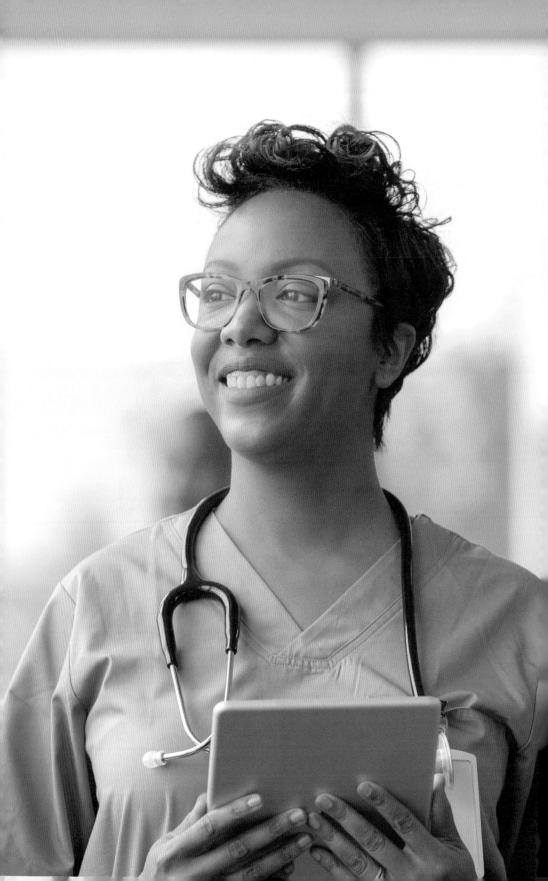

So you want to be a brain surgeon?

The essential guide to medical careers

Fourth edition

Edited by

Lydia Spurr

Clinical Research Fellow in Respiratory Medicine,
Royal Brompton Hospital, London, UK

Jessica Harris

Consultant Psychiatrist, Psychological Medicine Service,
John Radcliffe Hospital, Oxford, UK

Geoffrey Warwick

Respiratory Physician, King's College Hospital, London, UK

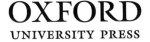

OXFORD
UNIVERSITY PRESS

OXFORD
UNIVERSITY PRESS

Great Clarendon Street, Oxford, OX2 6DP,
United Kingdom

Oxford University Press is a department of the University of Oxford.
It furthers the University's objective of excellence in research, scholarship,
and education by publishing worldwide. Oxford is a registered trade mark of
Oxford University Press in the UK and in certain other countries

First Edition published in 1997
Second Edition published in 2001
Third Edition published in 2009
Fourth Edition published in 2022

Impression: 1

Published in the United States of America by Oxford University Press
198 Madison Avenue, New York, NY 10016, United States of America

British Library Cataloguing in Publication Data
Data available

Library of Congress Control Number: 2021945144

ISBN 978–0–19–877949–0

DOI: 10.1093/med/9780198779490.001.0001

Printed in Great Britain by
Bell & Bain Ltd., Glasgow

To my family, without whom nothing would be possible (LAS)

To my parents, for paying the university fees (JH)

To my family (GW)

▌ Foreword

Choosing your specialty is always going to be a hard decision for any doctor. The ability to make this key choice is made far easier by having a really good understanding of what each possibility may mean. This excellent book brings together experts from every field to provide very clear accounts of why they chose their particular specialty. The contributors have provided frank accounts of what their job entails and what an average day is really like.

As a practising surgeon whose career now takes me all over the NHS, I have had the privilege of seeing the amazing breadth of choices that a career in medicine offers doctors. There are few other professions which offer this choice and it can be hard to truly appreciate it, even with the broader-based foundation training schemes. This book offers insights into the full range of career options, both mainstream and alternative. The editors have succeeded in including many smaller specialties to give a feel for emerging new careers as they evolve from their larger parent specialties.

This fourth edition includes timely and helpful advice on how an individual can make their CV or application forms stand out from their peers and how to ensure they always present the best of themselves. I have enjoyed reading the book and have no doubt it will prove invaluable in helping medical students and young doctors to find a career path which suits them.

Professor the Lord Darzi of Denham OM KBE PC FRS

Preface

This fourth edition of *So you want to be a brain surgeon?* has been a long time in the making, and we are very grateful for the patience of everyone who has awaited its production. Like all doctors, we have had to navigate the constantly moving goalposts of UK postgraduate medical training—we have detailed the essential ideas and key structures in this guide but are aware they will (quite rightly) continue to evolve and adapt to the needs of doctors and healthcare services. Some details and names may change, but the shape and key points along the route are pretty secure and therefore, the necessary decisions for doctors in training should remain stable for the next few years.

The biggest change from the last edition has been the change in editors. Simon Eccles has moved on to a near full-time career in management as the National Chief Clinical Information Officer for Health and Care. We thank him for his advice and support to the new team during the production of this edition. Stephan Sanders has also moved on and is now Assistant Professor studying children's neurodevelopment at the University of California, San Francisco (UCSF).

Building on the foundations of the previous three editions, further changes, including the design of the book, have been made to ensure the content is presented in a consistent and accessible format. We hope this makes it easier to find the information you want (and hopefully to encourage serendipitous discoveries of things you didn't know you wanted); the guidance on career pathways through specialty training have been updated and reorganized to sequentially build your knowledge and understanding of career pathways, and offer advice on choosing, and getting, the career you want.

Feedback from readers has helped shape this book since the first edition over 20 years ago. Please do keep sending in comments and suggestions—we remain grateful for all contributions.

Lydia Spurr
Jessica Harris
Geoffrey Warwick
2020

Acknowledgements

This book would never have been possible without the help of many kind people and organizations who gave their time and energy for our benefit. In particular:

All the authors of the individual chapters who have produced such lovely overviews of their specialties that the editors had cause to question their own career choices.

Dr Chris Ward for the original idea and the first two editions, and Dr Stephan Sanders for his work on the third edition.

Dr Simon Eccles also for his work on previous editions, and his advice and support for this edition.

Geraldine Jeffers from OUP for her continued support and dedication to this book.

Fiona Sutherland and Rachel Goldsworthy, our dedicated and patient assistant commissioning editors from OUP, for all their excellent work, support, motivation, and help coordinating author contributions.

Dr Mark Toynbee and Dr Nele Okojie for proofreading the entire manuscript.

Finally, anyone who helped us find an author for a chapter of this book.

Contents

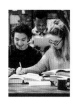

Using this book

Welcome to the fourth edition of *So you want to be a brain surgeon?*. This book is split into 6 sections, each covering a different aspect of medical careers:

Chapter 1 Career routes—the 'usual' route. These sections describe the basic career route that the vast majority of doctors take in progressing from medical student to fully qualified consultant or general practitioner (GP), including an overview of postgraduate training and membership exams.

Chapter 2 Career routes—the 'alternative' routes. This includes descriptions of other career options such as specialty and associate specialist (SAS) roles, academia, the armed forces, working overseas, and jobs outside the NHS, as well as switching career paths.

Chapter 3 Specialty overviews. This includes a group of sections describing career progression in the major specialties—each option available at the end of the foundation programme is discussed separately. For example, if a doctor wanted to train in psychiatry, the relevant section would show them how to apply for specialty training, the necessary exams, and the options available as a final career (e.g. forensic psychiatry).

Chapter 4 Choosing careers and getting jobs. This outlines some of the considerations made in choosing a career. It also outlines the recruitment processes for the foundation programme and specialist training, and tips on how to be successful. Competition in different career routes is outlined, as is how to develop a competitive curriculum vitae (CV) and portfolio.

Chapter 5 Training and working in medical careers. These sections summarize the major changes in postgraduate medical training over recent years, particularly under *Modernising Medical Careers* (MMC) and following the *Shape of Training* review. They also describe the people and institutions providing and overseeing training (useful for interview preparation). Aspects important to working as a junior doctor, including pay, less-than-full-time training, and discrimination in medicine, particularly with regard to women are discussed, and the chapter concludes with debunking some common myths about medical careers.

Chapter 6 Career chapters. These two-page chapters cover 105 different careers in which doctors work, each one written by specialists in that career to give a unique insight into what their life and job are like. The first page describes the patients, the work, and the job in that specialty. The second page summarizes the specialty, giving an example of 'a day in the life' of specialists, the route to the career, and scales to compare the job to other jobs. The key to these scales is shown opposite. The chapters are arranged alphabetically to make them easier to look up.

Key to the summaries

A day in the life ...

These boxes give an example of a typical day in each specialty.

Myth	The popular myths about each job ...
Reality	... and the reality
Personality	Personality traits found in each specialty; these are not absolutes, just a guide
Best aspects	Why being a doctor in this specialty is the bee's knees
Worst aspects	The bits of the job that can make a doctor's blood boil
Route	The route to get into the specialty, and the necessary membership exams
Numbers	The number of trained doctors in the UK and the percentage of these posts filled by women where known
Locations	Where the job is based, e.g. in the community, all hospitals, larger hospitals, teaching hospitals, or specialist centres

Life	Graded according to the overall impact of the job on life outside medicine	Work
Boredom	Graded according to the risk of boredom or burnout	Burnout
Quiet on-call	Graded according to the 'severity' of on-calls, including number of calls, intensity of work, and the need to come into hospital	Busy on-call
Low salary	Most doctors earn a similar amount (p. 99); this scale shows potential earnings. This is just a guide, but doctors will need to work very hard in any specialty to get to the upper levels	High salary
Uncompetitive	Ranked according to competition ratios (pp.78–82) where available, otherwise the specialist's experience	Competitive

Medical careers terminology

Consultant The boss in each specialty (p. 12)

General practitioner (GP) Equivalent to a consultant, but in primary care (p. 13)

Specialty and associate specialist (SAS) doctors Experienced doctors in specialty doctor or associate specialist posts; the term also covers other non-training posts at a similar level (p. 19)

Specialty registrar (StR) A doctor in a specialty training programme. Levels are referred to as ST1, ST2, etc.

Core trainee (CT1–3) A doctor in core training in an uncoupled specialty training programme; equivalent to ST1–3

F2 Foundation programme training year 2

F1 Foundation programme training year 1

Outdated terms

Specialist registrar (SpR) Equivalent to ST3/4 and above

Senior house officer (SHO) Equivalent to F2, ST1–3, and CT1–3 (doctors in training and non-training jobs at this level are still often referred to as SHOs)

Pre-registration house officer (PRHO) Equivalent to F1

Other terms

Academic clinical fellowship Academic equivalent to ST1–3 (p. 23)

Annual review of competency progression (ARCP) Yearly review of the evidence collected by each trainee in their ePortfolio to decide if they meet the required standards for the trainee to progress in, or complete, training (p. 95)

Certificate of Completion of Training (CCT) Awarded at the end of specialty training which allows the doctor to work as a general practitioner (GP) or consultant (p. 36)

Certificate of Eligibility for General Practice Registration (CEGPR) and **Certificate of Eligibility for Specialist Registration (CESR)** Alternative awards for doctors who aren't eligible to apply for CCT, allowing them to work as a GP or consultant (p. 21)

Clinical supervisor (CS) A senior clinician supervising a trainee's clinical practice (p. 95)

Continuing professional development (CPD) Learning undertaken outside formal training, e.g. after CCT or in SAS roles

Educational supervisor (ES) A senior clinician with responsibility for the overall supervision of a trainee's educational progress (p. 95)

ePortfolio Online platform for documenting and recording achievements, feedback, and progress through training (p. 86)

Foundation programme Generic 2-year training programme after medical school (p. 4)

General Medical Council (GMC) The independent regulator of doctors in the UK; also regulates undergraduate and postgraduate education and training (p. 96)

Gold Guide A reference guide setting out arrangements for specialty registrars-available in the publications section of https://www.copmed.org.uk/

Modernising Medical Careers (MMC) Series of changes aimed at reforming junior doctor training (p. 92)

Less-than-full-time training (LTFTT) Foundation or specialist training in a part-time job (p. 97)

Run-through training Specialty training that starts at ST1 and continues through to CCT without further competitive application (p. 7)

Shape of Training review (2013) Independent review of postgraduate medical education chaired by Professor Sir David Greenaway (p. 93)

Specialty training GMC-approved training which leads to the award of a CCT (p. 7)

Training number All trainees in core or specialty training are allocated either a National Training Number (NTN) or Dean's/Deanery Reference Number (DRN) (p. 8)

Uncoupled training Training programme with a break and reapplication between core and specialist training (p. 7)

▌ Contributors

Less-than-full-time training

Dr Anna Moore
Registrar in Respiratory
Medicine and
Education Fellow
Barts Health NHS
Trust, London

Dr Ruth-Anna Macqueen
Co-Chair, BMA LTFT Forum
Registrar in Obstetrics and
Gynaecology
Barking, Havering and
Redbridge NHS Trust,
Romford

Academic medicine

Dr Ross Paterson
Senior Clinical
Research Fellow
Dementia Research Centre
and Dementia Research
Institute
UCL Queen Square Institute
of Neurology, London
Honorary Consultant
Neurologist
National Hospital
for Neurology and
Neurosurgery, Queen
Square, London

Dr Nikhil Sharma
Honorary Consultant
Neurologist
Department of Clinical and
Movement Neurosciences
UCL Queen Square Institute
of Neurology, London

Academic surgery

Ms Grainne Bourke
Honorary Clinical Associate
Professor Plastic and Hand
Surgery
Department of Plastic Surgery
Leeds Teaching Hospitals
NHS Trust, Leeds

Mr Ryckie Wade
NIHR Clinical Fellow in
Plastic Surgery
Department of Plastic
Surgery
Leeds Teaching Hospitals
Trust, Leeds

Acute internal medicine

Dr Luke Smith
Consultant in Acute and
General Internal Medicine
Guy's and St Thomas' NHS
Trust, London

Dr Ashkan Sadighi
Consultant in Acute
Medicine
West Middlesex Hospital,
Chelsea and Westminster
NHS Trust, London

Allergy

Dr Guy Scadding
Consultant in Allergy
Royal Brompton
Hospital, London

Anaesthetics

Dr James Dawson
Consultant Anaesthetist
Nottingham City Hospital,
Nottingham

Dr Will Tomlinson
Consultant Anaesthetist
Sheffield Teaching Hospitals
NHS Foundation Trust,
Sheffield

Armedforces: Army

Lt Col Paul Hunt
Defence Consultant in
Emergency Medicine
JHG (North)
James Cook University
Hospital, Middlesbrough

Armed forces: Royal Air Force Medical Officer

Gp Capt Ed Nicol
Consultant Cardiologist
Royal Brompton
Hospital, London

Sqn Ldr Robert Gifford
SpR in Endocrinology,
Diabetes, and General
Medicine
Edinburgh Centre for
Endocrinology and
Diabetes, Edinburgh

Armed forces: Royal Navy Medical Officer

Surg Cdr Michael Russell RN
Principal Medical Officer
Medical Centre, HMS Neptune
HM Naval Base Clyde, Faslane

Surg Lt Cdr Ela Stachow RN
Principal Medical Officer
HMS Prince of Wales

Audio vestibular medicine

Dr Rohani Omar
Specialist Registrar in
Audiovestibular Medicine
Great Ormond Street
Hospital, London

Dr Reeya Motha
Consultant Audiovestibular
Physician
Barts Health NHS
Trust, London

Aviation and space medicine

Sqn Ldr Bonnie Posselt
Specialty Registrar in Aviation
and Space Medicine
RAF Centre of Aviation
Medicine
RAF Henlow, Bedfordshire

Bariatric and metabolic surgery

Miss Roxanna Zakeri
Clinical Research Fellow in Bariatric Surgery
Centre for Obesity Research
University College
London, London

Mr Chetan Parmar
Consultant Upper Gastrointestinal and Bariatric Surgeon
Whittington
Hospital, London

Cardiology

Dr Joanna Lim
Consultant in Adult Congenital Heart Disease
John Radcliffe
Hospital, Oxford

Cardiothoracic surgery

Mr Jonathan Anderson
Consultant Cardiothoracic Surgeon
Hammersmith
Hospital, London

Chemical pathology

Dr Adrian Park
Consultant in Chemical Pathology
Department of Clinical Biochemistry
Addenbrooke's Hospital, Cambridge

Clinical genetics

Dr Jane Hurst
Consultant in Clinical Genetics
Great Ormond Street
Hospital, London

Dr Lara Menzies
Registrar in Clinical Genetics
Great Ormond Street
Hospital, London

Clinical neurophysiology

Prof Michael Koutroumanidis
Consultant Neurophysiologist
Guy's and St Thomas' NHS
Foundation Trust, London

Dr Lara Delaj
Consultant Neurologist
East Kent Hospitals
University NHS Foundation
Trust, Kent

Clinical oncology

Dr Yakhub Khan
Consultant Clinical Oncologist
Arden Cancer Centre
University Hospitals
Coventry and Warwickshire, Coventry

Clinical pharmacology and therapeutics

Dr Jeff Aronson
Consultant Physician and Clinical Pharmacologist
Nuffield Department of Primary Care Health Sciences, Oxford

Dermatology

Dr David de Berker
Consultant Dermatologist
University Hospitals Bristol
and Weston Foundation
Trust, Bristol

Diving and hyperbaric medicine

Dr Oliver Firth
Diving and Hyperbaric Physician
Director, Hyperdive Ltd

Ear, nose, and throat (ENT or otolaryngology)

Mr James Ramsden
Consultant ENT Surgeon
John Radcliffe
Hospital, Oxford

Ms Sonia Kumar
Consultant ENT Surgeon
John Radcliffe
Hospital, Oxford

Elderly medicine

Dr Emma Drydon
Registrar in Elderly and General Internal Medicine
Leeds Teaching Hospitals
NHS Trust, Leeds

Dr Sean Ninan
Consultant Geriatrician
Leeds Teaching Hospitals
NHS Trust, Leeds

Emergency medicine

Dr Jon Bailey
Registrar in Emergency and Intensive Care Medicine
Milton Keynes University
Hospital NHS Foundation
Trust, Milton Keynes

Emergency medicine: paediatric

Dr Jon Bailey
Registrar in Emergency and Intensive Care Medicine
Milton Keynes
University Hospital
NHS Foundation Trust, Milton Keynes

Dr Rebekah Caseley
Registrar in Paediatric Emergency Medicine
John Radcliffe
Hospital, Oxford

Emergency medicine: pre-hospital emergency medicine

Dr Emma Rowland
Clinical Lead in Emergency Medicine
Homerton University
Hospital, London

Endocrinology and diabetes

Dr Francesca Swords
Consultant Physician and Endocrinologist
Norfolk and Norwich
University NHS
Foundation Trust, Norwich

Expedition medicine

Dr Shona Main
Emergency Medicine Trainee and
Expedition Doctor
Adventure Medic, Edinburgh

Fertility medicine

Mr Matthew Prior
Consultant in Reproductive Medicine and Surgery
Newcastle Fertility Centre Biomedicine West Wing
International Centre for Life, Newcastle upon Tyne

Forensic medicine

Dr Meng Aw-Yong
Medical Director and Forensic Medical Examiner
Metropolitan Police Service, London
Associate Specialist in Emergency and Forensic Medicine
Hillingdon Hospital, Middlesex

Forensic pathology

Dr Sallyanne Collis
Consultant Forensic Pathologist
Forensic Pathology
Nine Edinburgh Bioquarter, Edinburgh

Gastroenterology

Dr Mark A Samaan
Consultant Gastroenterologist
Guy's and St Thomas' NHS Foundation Trust, London

General practice

Dr Hilary Audsley
General Practitioner
The Chestnuts Surgery, Sittingbourne

General practice: academic

Dr Kamal Mahtani
General Practitioner
Centre for Evidence-Based Medicine
Nuffield Department of Primary Care Health Sciences
University of Oxford, Oxford

General practice in rural settings

Dr Anna Roberts
General Practitioner
Charlotte Medical Practice
Lochfield Road Primary Care Centre, Dumfries

General practice in secure environments

Dr Jake Hard
General Practitioner
Royal College of General Practitioners, London

General practice: private practice

Dr Lawrence Gerlis
General Practitioner
Samedaydoctor
Marylebone, London

GP with extended roles

Dr Noel Baxter
General Practitioner
Primary Care Respiratory Society, Solihull

General surgery

Mr Oliver Warren
Consultant Colorectal and General Surgeon
Chelsea and Westminster Hospital, London

Mr Shengyang Qiu
Registrar in Colorectal and General Surgery
Chelsea and Westminster Hospital, London

Genitourinary medicine

Dr Anna Hartley
Consultant in Genitourinary Medicine
Leeds Sexual Health, Leeds

Dr Emily Clarke
Consultant in Genitourinary Medicine
Royal Liverpool University Hospital, Liverpool

Gynaecological oncology

Mr Phil Rolland
Gynaecological Oncologist
Gloucestershire Hospitals NHS Foundation Trust, Cheltenham

Haematology

Dr Alesia Khan
Consultant Haematologist
St James' University Hospital, Leeds

Hand surgery

Miss Lucy Cutler
Consultant Trauma and Orthopaedic Surgeon
University Hospitals of Leicester
Leicester Royal Infirmary, Leicester

Histopathology

Dr Matthew Clarke
Registrar in Histopathology
Institute of Cancer Research, London

Immunology

Dr Philip Bright
Consultant in Clinical Immunology
North Bristol NHS Trust
Southmead Hospital, Bristol

Dr Joe Unsworth
Consultant in Clinical Immunology
North Bristol NHS Trust
Southmead Hospital, Bristol

Infectious diseases

Dr Stephen Aston
Consultant in Infectious Diseases and General Internal Medicine
Liverpool University Hospitals NHS Foundation Trust, Liverpool

Dr Paul Hine
Consultant in Infectious Diseases and General Internal Medicine
Royal Liverpool University Hospital, Liverpool

Intensive care medicine

Dr Rob Ferguson
Consultant in Intensive Care and Emergency Medicine
York Teaching Hospital NHS Foundation Trust, York

Locuming full-time

Dr David McAlpine
Registrar Emergency Medicine
University of Cape Town, Cape Town, South Africa

Media medicine

Dr Ranj Singh
Locum Consultant In
Paediatric Emergency
Medicine
Evelina London Children's
Hospital, London

Medical education

Dr Kerry Calvo
Senior Clinical Teaching Fellow
UCL Medical School, Royal
Free Hospital, London

Medical entrepreneur

Dr Christopher N Floyd
CEO and Co-Founder,
Cranworth Medical Ltd
NIHR Clinical Lecturer in
Clinical Pharmacology
Kings College, London

Medical ethics

Dr Anna Smajdor
Associate Professor of
Practical Philosophy
University of Oslo,
Oslo, Norway

Medical management consultancy

Dr Sally Getgood
Director
Getgood Health Inc,
Ontario, Canada

Medical management

Dr Vin Diwakar
Regional Medical Director
NHS England and NHS
Improvement, London

Medical microbiology

Dr Philippa Matthews
Honorary Consultant in
Infectious Diseases and
Microbiology
Oxford University Hospitals
NHS Foundation Trust, Oxford

Medical oncology

Dr Adam Dangoor
Consultant Medical Oncologist
Bristol Haematology and
Oncology Centre
University of Bristol, Bristol

Medical politics

Dr Tom Dolphin
Consultant Anaesthetist
Imperial College Healthcare
NHS Trust, London

Médecins Sans Frontières

Dr Emily Shaw
Wellcome UCL
Clinical Fellow
Division of Infection and
Immunity
University College
London, London

Medico-legal adviser

Dr Caroline Osborne-White
Medical Telephone
Adviser
Medical and Dental
Defence Union of Scotland
(MDDUS), Glasgow

Metabolic medicine

Dr Rob Cramb
Consultant Chemical
Pathologist
Queen Elizabeth Hospital,
Birmingham

Dr Kate Shipman
Consultant Chemical
Pathologist
St Richard's Hospital,
Chichester

National healthcare policy and leadership

Prof Erika Denton
Honorary Professor of
Radiology
Norfolk and Norwich
University Hospital,
Norwich
National Advisor for Imaging
NHS Improvement and NHS
England

Dr Deborah Kirkham
Consultant in Genitourinary
and HIV Medicine
Croydon University Hospital,
Thornton Heath
Previous National Medical
Director's Clinical Fellow
NHS England and the *BMJ*

Neonatal medicine

Dr Richard Thwaites
Consultant Neonatologist
Queen Alexandra Hospital,
Portsmouth

Neurology

Dr Angelika Zarkali
Registrar in Neurology
Dementia Research Centre
UCL Queen Square Institute
of Neurology, London

Neurosurgery

Ms Eleni Maratos
Consultant Neurosurgeon
King's College
Hospital, London

Nuclear medicine

Dr Deborah Pencharz
Consultant in Nuclear
Medicine
Royal Free London NHS
Foundation Trust, London

Dr Thomas Wagner
Consultant in Nuclear
Medicine
Royal Free London
NHS Foundation Trust,
London

Obstetric medicine

Dr Paarul Prinja
Consultant Acute and
Obstetric Physician
New Cross Hospital,
Wolverhampton

Obstetrics and gynaecology

Mr Myles Taylor
Consultant Obstetrician
and Gynaecologist
Centre for Women's Health
Royal Devon and
Exeter NHS Foundation
Trust, Devon

Occupational medicine

Dr Paul Grime
Consultant Occupational
Physician
Cambridge University
Hospitals NHS Foundation
Trust, Cambridge

Oncoplastic breast surgery

Miss Laura Arthur
TIG Fellow in Oncoplastic
Breast Surgery
Royal Victoria Infirmary,
Newcastle upon Tyne

Mr Russell Bramhall
Consultant Plastic Surgeon
Canniesburn Plastic
Surgery Unit
Glasgow Royal Infirmary,
Glasgow

Ophthalmology

Mr David Lunt
Consultant Ophthalmologist
South Tees Hospitals
NHS Foundation Trust,
Middlesbrough

Prof Scott Fraser
Consultant Ophthalmologist
Sunderland Eye Infirmary,
Sunderland

Oral and maxillofacial surgery

Lt Col Johno Breeze
Consultant Oral and
Maxillofacial Surgeon
University Hospitals
Birmingham, Birmingham

Orthopaedic surgery

Mr Ian McDermott
Consultant Orthopaedic
Surgeon
London Sports
Orthopaedics, London

Paediatric cardiology

Dr Thomas Day
Registrar in Paediatric
Cardiology
Department of Paediatric
Cardiology
Evelina London Children's
Healthcare, London

Dr Sadia Quyam
Consultant Paediatric
Cardiologist
Department of Paediatric
Cardiology
Evelina London Children's
Healthcare, London

Paediatric surgery

Miss Joanna Stanwell
Consultant Neonatal
and Paediatric
Surgeon
Great Ormond Street
Hospital, London

Paediatrics

Dr Susie Minson
Consultant Paediatrician
Royal London Hospital
Barts Health NHS
Trust, London

Dr Miriam Fine-Goulden
Consultant in Paediatric
Intensive Care
Evelina London Children's
Hospital and South Thames
Retrieval Service for
Children
Guy's and St Thomas'
NHS Foundation Trust,
London

Paediatrics: community

Dr Rachel D'Souza
Consultant in Community
Paediatrics
Community Paediatric
Service
Children's Community
Health Services,
Manchester

Dr Juliet Court
Consultant Community
Paediatrician
Formerly at Manchester
Local Care Organisation,
Manchester

Pain management

Dr James Taylor
Consultant in Anaesthesia,
Critical Care, and Pain
Management
Bradford Teaching
Hospitals NHS Foundation
Trust, Bradford

Dr Karen Simpson
Consultant in Anaesthesia
and Pain Management
Leeds Teaching Hospitals
NHS Trust, Leeds

Palliative medicine

Dr Natasha Wiggins
Consultant in Palliative
Medicine
Great Western Hospitals
NHS Foundation Trust,
Swindon

Pharmaceutical medicine

Stevan R Emmett
Acting Chief Medical
Officer and Consultant
Pharmaceutical
Physician
Defence Science and
Technology Laboratory,
Salisbury

Plastic and reconstructive surgery

Mr Simon Eccles
Consultant Plastic
Surgeon
Chelsea and
Westminster Hospital,
London

Psychiatry: child and adolescent

Dr Rory Conn
Consultant Child and
Adolescent Psychiatrist
Devon Partnership Trust
Exeter

Dr Peter Hindley
Consultant Child
and Adolescent
Psychiatrist
Royal College
of Psychiatrists,
London

Psychiatry: forensic

Dr Daniel Whiting
NIHR Doctoral
Research Fellow
Department of
Psychiatry, University
of Oxford
Warneford Hospital,
Oxford

Psychiatry: general adult

Dr Jessica Harris
Consultant
Psychiatrist
John Radcliffe
Hospital, Oxford

Psychiatry: intellectual disability

Dr Kuljit Bhogal
Consultant Psychiatrist
Southern Health NHS
Foundation Trust

Psychiatry: medical psychotherapy

Dr Victoria Barker
Consultant Psychiatrist and
Medical Psychotherapist
Camden and Islington
Personality Disorder Service
Dartmouth Park Unit
Camden and Islington NHS
Foundation Trust, London

Dr Jon Patrick
Consultant Forensic
Psychiatrist and
Psychotherapist
The State Hospital, Carstairs

Psychiatry: old age

Dr Megan Theodoulou
Consultant Old Age
Psychiatrist
North Oxfordshire
Community Mental Health
Team for Older Adults
Nuffield Health Centre, Witney

Public health medicine

Dr Justin Varney
Director of Public Health
Birmingham City Council,
Birmingham

Radiology: diagnostic

Dr Alex Wilson
Registrar in Radiology
Royal London
Hospital, London

Radiology: interventional

Dr Farrukh Arfeen
Interventional
Radiology Fellow
Royal London
Hospital, London

Dr William Pleming
Interventional
Radiology Fellow
Royal London
Hospital, London

Rehabilitation medicine

Dr Manoj Sivan
Associate Clinical Professor
in Rehabilitation Medicine
University of Leeds and
Leeds Teaching Hospitals
NHS Trust, Leeds

Renal medicine

Dr Will White
Consultant in Renal
Medicine
Royal London
Hospital, London

Respiratory medicine

Dr Laura-Jane Smith
Consultant in Respiratory
Medicine
King's College
Hospital, London

Rheumatology

Dr James Galloway
Honorary Consultant in
Rheumatology
King's College
Hospital, London

Dr Neil Snowden
Consultant Rheumatologist
Pennine MSK Partnership
Integrated Care
Centre, Oldham

Sexual and reproductive healthcare

Dr Tracey Masters
Consultant in Sexual and
Reproductive Healthcare
Homerton University
Hospital NHS Foundation
Trust, London

Dr Kate Yarrow
Consultant in Sexual
and Reproductive
Healthcare
Maidstone and Tunbridge
Wells NHS Trust, Maidstone
and Tunbridge Wells

Spine surgery

Mr Paul Thorpe
Consultant Orthopaedic
Surgeon
Musgrove Park Hospital,
Taunton

Sports and exercise medicine

Dr Eleanor Tillett
Honorary Consultant
in Sport and Exercise
Medicine
University College
Hospital, London

Dr Farrah Jawad
Consultant in Sport,
Exercise, and
Musculoskeletal
Medicine
Homerton University
Hospital NHS Trust,
London

Stroke medicine

Dr Nicholas Evans
Clinical Lecturer in
Geriatric and Stroke
Medicine
Department of Clinical
Neurosciences
University of Cambridge,
Cambridge

Dr Iain McGurgan
Clinical Research Fellow
Centre for Prevention of
Stroke and Dementia
Nuffield Department of
Clinical Neurosciences
University of Oxford, Oxford

Transfusion medicine

Dr Heidi Doughty
Consultant in Transfusion
Medicine
NHS Blood and Transplant,
Birmingham

Dr Fateha Chowdhury
Consultant in Transfusion
Medicine
NHS Blood and
Transplant and St Mary's
Hospital, London

Transplant medicine

Dr Vicky Gerovasili
Consultant in Respiratory
and Transplant Medicine
Harefield Hospital,
Harefield, Uxbridge

Dr Kavita Dave
Specialty Registrar in
Respiratory and General
Internal Medicine
Royal Brompton and
Harefield NHS Trust, London

Transplant surgery

Mr Nikolaos Karydis
Consultant Transplant
Surgeon
Guy's Hospital, London

Trauma surgery

Mr Will Eardley
Consultant Orthopaedic
Trauma Surgeon
James Cook University
Hospital, Middlesbrough

Urogynaecology

Dr Rufus Cartwright
Consultant Urogynaecologist
Oxford University Hospitals
NHS Trust, Oxford

Urology

Mr John Beatty
Consultant Urological Surgeon
Leicester General Hospital
University Hospitals of
Leicester NHS Trust, Leicester

Vascular surgery

Mr Andrew Choong
Consultant Vascular and
Endovascular Surgeon
National University Heart
Centre, Singapore

Mr Eugene Ng
Vascular Surgeon
Westmead Hospital,
Sydney, Australia

Virology

Dr Mark Zuckerman
Consultant Virologist
King's College
Hospital, London

**Voluntary Service
Overseas (VSO)**

Prof Phil Heywood
Emeritus Professor of
Primary Care
University of Leeds,
Woodhouse, Leeds

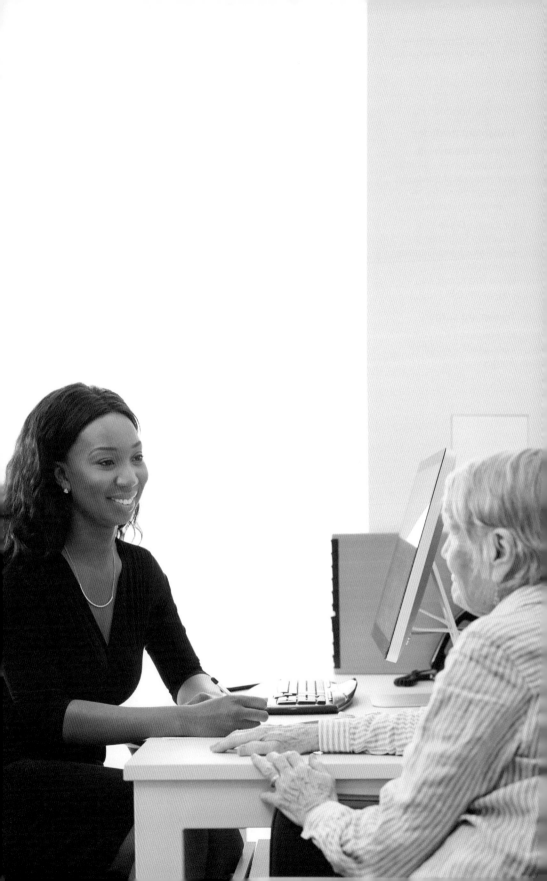

1

Career routes—the 'usual' route

Career overview

Most medical careers follow a similar basic pattern, as shown in Fig. 1.1. This chapter describes the main stages of a 'standard', or at least the most straightforward, medical career.

Medical school

It is essential for all doctors to have a medical degree (e.g. MB BS, MB ChB). There are 33 medical schools in the UK (a further six are accepting students but are yet to be approved by the General Medical Council (GMC))—each belongs to a parent university and is partly government-funded. Additionally, the UK's first independent medical school opened in 2015. Applications for courses are made online through the Universities and Colleges Admissions Service (https://www.ucas.com). Some students may need to complete a preliminary or gateway year due to their personal or academic circumstances.

- **Undergraduate medicine** Nearly all medical schools offer 5- to 6-year courses. Graduates may also undertake these courses as a second degree.
- **Graduate medicine** Two universities (Swansea and Warwick) have 'graduate-only' medical schools, but many others offer graduate entry programmes for those with a degree (usually 2:1 minimum). Courses take 4 years and competition for places is intense.

Intercalated degrees

In a year additional to the standard course, medical students can complete an additional Bachelor's or Master's degree. Students explore an area of interest in greater depth whilst developing research skills. Some universities allow selected students to undertake PhDs during their medical degree.

Foundation programme

(See p. 4.) New doctors must register with the GMC (p. 96) to start 2 years of generic training called the foundation programme (FP). This consists of salaried 3- to 6-month rotations in a variety of specialties. UK graduates are essentially guaranteed a place in FP training, but allocation to specific posts is competitive.

Early/core training

(See p. 7.) Successful completion of the FP enables doctors to enter a specialty training programme. For most, this starts with a period of early or core training where doctors learn generic and basic skills relevant to one or more specialties or subspecialties. Application is competitive for all programmes and there is no guarantee of getting a job.

Membership exams

(See p. 9.) Exams set by Royal Colleges and Faculties (p. 96) are specific to specialty in their content and format, and to the stage of training by which they must be completed. They are required in virtually all medical careers but can be difficult to pass and are often expensive. Not completing them in the specified time or number of attempts can mean completion of training is delayed or even prevented.

Further specialty training

(See p. 7.) Ultimately, training leads to the award of a Certificate of Completion of Training (CCT) (p. 36) which allows the doctor to work as a consultant or general practitioner (GP). Depending on the specialty, this may involve further competitive application to higher specialty training (HST) or **subspecialty training** (p. 12) programmes.

Consultant

(See p. 12.) This is the final career stage for hospital-based and some community-based specialties. In addition to taking ultimate responsibility for patients, the role involves training and supervising team members, and often management of the department itself.

General practitioner

(See p. 13.) In primary care, this is the final career stage equivalent to a consultant. GPs work with numerous services to promote health and provide medical care. Increasingly, secondary care services are moving into the community, with some GPs encouraged to develop specialist skills. There are also opportunities to develop business, management, academic, and teaching skills.

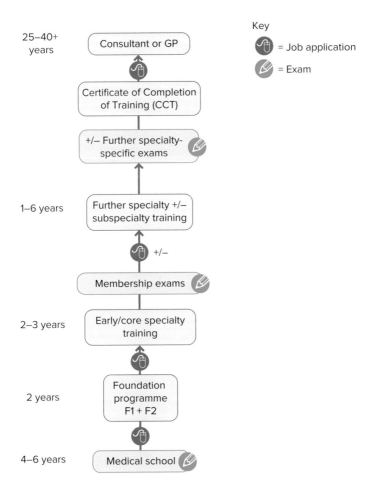

Figure 1.1 Overview of the 'standard' medical career.

Foundation programme

New doctors start the foundation programme (FP) after completing medical school. This is vocational training for 2 years, foundation year 1 (F1) and year 2 (F2), where doctors learn core skills and begin taking responsibility for patients. The FP is the only training pathway common to all clinical specialties. Full details of the FP and its requirements are outlined in the FP curriculum (available at https://foundationprogramme.nhs.uk).

F1 A 12-month internship typically comprising three 4-month placements—at least one in hospital medicine and usually one in surgery. F1s take supervised responsibility for patients and consolidate knowledge and skills acquired at medical school. The General Medical Council (GMC) grants new F1s **provisional registration** with a licence to practise. On completion of F1, the trainee is awarded a **Foundation Year 1 Certificate of Completion (F1CC)** after which the GMC issues a **Certificate of Experience**. The doctor then applies for **full registration** with a licence to practise, which is required to progress to F2.

F2 Twelve months comprising 2–4 placements, each lasting 3–6 months. Placements may be in any specialty, including at least one in community or primary care. Doctors further develop their skills and take on more clinical and management responsibilities. Successful completion of F2 leads to the award of a **Foundation Programme Certificate of Completion (FPCC)**, which is required to progress to core/specialty training (p. 7).

Each doctor completes F1 and F2 in the same geographical region (see foundation schools on p. 96 for more details). Most are allocated to FP jobs where all placements are known in advance. For others, allocation of F2 placements occurs at some point during F1. There are also 'stand-alone' F2 programmes available to doctors who have previously completed F1 or an equivalent internship, e.g. outside the UK.

Taster weeks

Usually taken as study leave in F2 to experience a specialty being considered as a career, often when not included as a formal FP placement. If approved by the educational supervisor (ES) (p. 95), tasters may be taken in any specialty and even outside their Trust or region.

Applying for the FP

The UK Foundation Programme Office (UKFPO) organizes the FP and allocates placements. UK graduates apply online during the final autumn of medical school, via the Oriel portal (https://www.oriel.nhs.uk). Applicants complete the situational judgement test (SJT) and Educational Performance Measure (EPM), with scores used to rank students. From 2025 all new UK doctors, home-grown and from overseas, also need to pass the Medical Licensing Assessment (MLA), which aims to set a minimum standard of required knowledge and skills.

SJT A 70-question assessment taken in the winter before F1 to test aptitude and attributes. Applicants rank or select the most appropriate responses to hypothetical scenarios likely to be encountered in F1. *(50 points)*
EPM Points are awarded for medical school performance, reported as deciles, from assessments chosen by each medical school. Currently, there are also points for additional degrees and academic achievements, but this may be scrapped from 2023. *(50 points)*

In theory, all UK graduates are guaranteed F1 jobs starting in August after completing their medical degree. However, in recent years, the FP has been oversubscribed. Lowest-ranking students form a reserve list; due to dropouts (e.g. exam failure), UK graduates, in practice, always get a job. The competitive element of applications means higher-scoring students are likely to be allocated their preferred posts and regions. Students with special circumstances (e.g. parental responsibilities) can request to be pre-allocated to a specific location. There may also be incentives to work in regions and specialties which traditionally have low recruitment and retention rates.

Does the specific foundation programme matter for a career?

The FP aims to provide generic training and focuses on developing core skills, e.g. communication, decision-making, etc. Not rotating through a specialty does not preclude applying for core/specialty training in it—FP jobs often provide useful career insights, but other ways to show commitment to a specialty include audits, taster weeks, and medical school electives.

Progression through the FP

The FP curriculum lists the outcomes doctors are expected to achieve during the programme. Over 96% of F1s and F2s successfully complete these by the end of their year. At the start of each placement, the FP doctor meets their supervisors (p. 95) to discuss their learning objectives. Supervisors provide reports to demonstrate completion of the required duration and assessments at the end of each placement. To be 'signed off' by their educational supervisor (ES) at the end of each year, doctors must complete all curriculum requirements. This includes completing formal assessments, as outlined in the next section below, and attaining 20 'foundation professional capabilities' (FPCs) describing key aspects of clinical and professional performance.

Supervised learning events (SLEs)

SLEs are assessments used to provide the trainee with constructive feedback to support continuing education and confirm attainment of skills and capabilities:

1) **Direct observation of procedural skills (DOPS)** The doctor is observed performing practical procedures and receives structured feedback.
2) **Case-based discussion (CBD)** The doctor presents and discusses a case in which they have been involved, and the assessor, usually a senior doctor, gives feedback on their clinical reasoning.
3) **Mini-clinical evaluation exercise (mini-CEX)** The doctor receives feedback on a directly observed patient interaction.
4) **Developing the clinical teacher** The doctor receives formal feedback on their teaching and presentation skills.

Additionally, each year, doctors must complete a self-assessment of performance and obtain a summary of **Team Assessment of Behaviour (TAB)** compiled anonymously from a selection of colleagues.

In England, the Horus ePortfolio (https://horus.hee.nhs.uk) is currently the online record for foundation SLEs, competences, and meetings. Scotland, Wales and NI currently use Turas (https://turasdashboard.nes.nhs.scot/). Keeping the ePortfolio up-to-date is a challenge, but it is essential to get the minimum requirements signed off. It is also a useful place to store reflections, certificates, and record achievements, particularly as it may be used in selection processes for core/specialty training.

Registering with the GMC

GMC registration is a legal requirement to practise medicine in the UK. For graduating UK students, the process is outlined in Fig. 1.2. Their personal details and identity are confirmed by the GMC, online and in person, before they complete an online application (http://www.gmc-uk.org). They are then given a unique GMC reference number, which remains the same throughout their career. Universities confirm which students pass their exams, and a 'GMC Online' account is set up for each of these students. Subject to a fitness-to-practise declaration (including details of health, convictions, and disciplinary actions) and payment of fees, students are provisionally registered with a licence to practise. Full registration is granted after successful completion of F1.

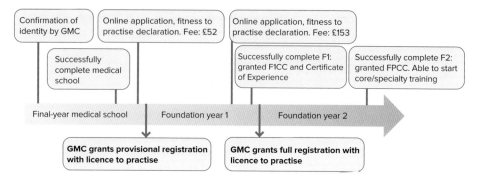

Figure 1.2 Process of General Medical Council (GMC) registration for UK medical graduates.

Specialty training

After the foundation programme (FP), the next stage is specialty training, as outlined in Fig. 1.3. Depending on the specialty, training takes 3–9 years, at the end of which doctors attain a Certificate of Completion of Training (CCT). There are over 60 CCT specialties, but no training pathway leads to a guaranteed consultant or general practitioner (GP) job. During training, doctors gain competences specified in the specialty's curriculum, and complete supervised learning events (SLEs), assessments, and exams. These and other training aspects are recorded in their ePortfolio (p. 86) which is reviewed each year at the annual review of competency progression (ARCP) (p. 95).

There are two types of training programme:

- **Run-through training** The doctor is guaranteed training in a single region from the first year of training (ST1) until they have finished training, provided they complete all necessary assessments and exams. There is no further competitive application to higher specialty training (HST), but trainees may have to compete for certain optional posts (e.g. subspecialty training). The most commonly undertaken run-through programme is **GP specialty training** (GPST) (p. 42). This lasts for 3–4 years and, after competitive application, is relatively straightforward: posts usually consist of 18 months in various hospital specialties and 18 months in general practice (GP).
- **Uncoupled training** The doctor applies for 'core' or basic training, which lasts for 2–3 years (e.g. core training year 1 (CT1), CT2 ± CT3), covering a range of related specialties. Following core training, there is further competitive application to an HST programme. Not everyone is successful on their first application, but once on a programme, training is guaranteed until attainment of a CCT, providing the required assessments and exams are completed.

Stand-alone training posts

There are a small number of short-term posts approved as equivalent to training at a given level, but which are not within a training programme. Such posts include Fixed Term Specialty Training Appointments (FTSTAs) and Locum Appointments for Training (LATs). It is not currently possible to attain a CCT by only doing these posts, but they may count towards training if the doctor is later accepted into a training programme. Numbers of these posts are dwindling in many places.

Do different routes matter?

For those committed to a particular specialty, there may be only one route to reach it (Table 1.1). For those interested in a few options, it is worth considering the advantages and disadvantages of different types of specialty training when making career decisions.

Run-through training

- **Advantages** Good job security; stay in the same region of the UK throughout; usually shorter training than the uncoupled route
- **Disadvantages** Not available for all career paths; difficult to change location during programme; final career decision immediately after the FP.

Uncoupled training

- **Advantages** More choice over eventual career specialty; longer time to decide before choosing a final career; easier to change location midway through training; clearer opportunities for career breaks (p. 101)
- **Disadvantages** Less job security; few options for those who fail to get an HST post; may be forced to change deanery between core training and HST; usually longer.

The *Gold Guide* (8th ed, 2020) states every trainee appointed to a specialty training pro-gramme will get a National Training Number (NTN) or Dean's/Deanery Reference Number (DRN). This is unique to the trainee and used for identification and workforce planning.

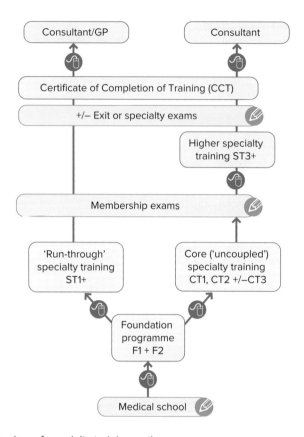

Figure 1.3 Overview of specialty training pathways.

Table 1.1 Specialties available through run-through and uncoupled training routes

Run-through training		Uncoupled training	
Child and adolescent psychiatry	p. 55	Anaesthetics	p. 39
Community sexual and reproductive health	p. 294	Emergency medicine	p. 37
Emergency medicine	p. 37	Intensive care medicine	p. 39
General practice	p. 42	Medical specialties	p. 44
Obstetrics and gynaecology	p. 47	Surgical specialties	p. 61
Ophthalmology	p. 64	Psychiatry specialties	p. 55
Some surgical specialties, e.g. neurosurgery	p. 61		
Paediatrics	p. 49		
Pathology	p. 52		
Public health	p. 57		
Radiology	p. 59		

▌Membership exams

The dreaded membership exams are essential to progress through specialty training. Many doctors find these the hardest exams they ever take. Several aspects make these exams unpleasant:

- Multiple parts to each exam, often using different formats, e.g. written, procedural, clinical
- Low pass rates, typically 35–45% for each part—many candidates fail at least one
- Expensive, plus costly revision courses (p. 10)
- Months of intense revision alongside a full-time job.

On the plus side, exams are more relevant to the job than ever and they undoubtably improve knowledge and clinical skills. Increasingly, there are exit exams at the end of specialty training to ensure trainees have reached the expected level of ability.

Available exams

Exams are administered by the Royal College or Faculty which governs specialty training. The acronyms of exams follow a formula: They start with 'M' (Membership) or 'F' (Fellowship), followed by whether the governing body is a Faculty (F) or Royal College (RC) and end with an abbreviation of the governing body:

- Anaesthetics (FRCA)
- Emergency medicine (FRCEM)
- Forensic and legal medicine (MFFLM)
- General practice (MRCGP)
- Intensive care medicine (FFICM)
- Medical specialties, i.e. physicians (MRCP; Specialty Certificate Exam)
- Obstetrics and gynaecology (MRCOG)
- Occupational medicine (MFOM)
- Ophthalmology (FRCOphth)
- Paediatrics and child health (MRCPCH)
- Pathology (FRCPath)
- Psychiatry (MRCPsych)
- Public health (MFPH)
- Sexual and reproductive healthcare (MFSRH)
- Sports and exercise medicine (FSEM)
- Surgical specialties (MRCS; FRCS)
- Radiology (FRCR)

Several other exams, e.g. Certificates or Diplomas, are also conducted by Royal Colleges and Faculties; these are (usually) not mandatory during training but may be helpful or required for special interest or subspecialty fields.

Exam format

Each membership exam is unique in structure and format. Some involve dissertations, laboratory skills, videoed consultations, or vivas. However, the majority of exams involve two formats:

- **Written exams** Usually multiple choice (MCQ), extended matching (EMQ), and best-of-five (BOF) questions, or a situational judgement test (SJT). Short answer questions (SAQ) are rare. Exams are time-pressured and test specialty-specific science and clinical knowledge.
- **Clinical exams** Multiple 'stations' with real patients, actors, or videos to test the candidate's history taking, clinical examination, professionalism, and procedural and communication skills. Each station tests specific skills, and most are time-pressured. Passing the exam is about looking like a doctor and demonstrating core abilities—candidates need excellent clinical skills, along with confidence.

Colleges mandate how many times candidates can sit each part of an exam. Nearly all have a maximum time period (in years), during which all parts need to be passed.

Costs

Costs vary between specialty and the type of exam. The following illustrates approximate costs. Bear in mind that there are often three or more parts to each exam, not including retakes.

- Exam: £170–1400+ for each part (compulsory exams are tax-deductible). Clinical parts cost the most.
- Written and online revision: variable, but around £30–200+.
- Courses: free to £1500+, depending on course duration and the type of exam.
- Travel and accommodation costs are often not refundable.

Most workplaces allow payment for courses to be taken from study leave budgets but rarely cover the cost of the actual exams.

When to take exams

Each specialty has eligibility criteria for sitting exams. Some can be taken immediately after medical school. Others require more experience as a doctor or in the specialty (see specialty overviews on pp. 35–66).

Important points for planning exams

1) Don't 'try out' a membership exam without really revising; this often starts an expensive and demoralizing pattern of repeated failure. Make each exam a top priority and aim to pass first time.
2) Avoid taking exams alongside other life events (e.g. weddings).
3) Take exams at the earliest opportunity, having acquired sufficient clinical experience to pass.
4) Think about the career path, e.g. Membership of the Royal College of Surgeons (MRCS) Part A can be sat during foundation years for those set on surgery—it's not a requirement to apply for CT1/ST1 training, but it shows commitment to specialty.

Revision

The exams are hard and will stretch even the best candidates. As a minimum, they require 4 weeks of intense revision (15–20 hours per week). Many doctors need more and often take study (or annual) leave before critical exams. Written exams often require revision using question banks, alongside additional reading. Clinical exams necessitate practising skills and getting feedback from peers and seniors, though a reasonable degree of reading is also required.

Exam resources

There is a competitive market for revision books, courses, and websites, so it's worth shopping around and requesting recommendations from colleagues or online. Courses can be expensive, but study budgets may cover fees. They give a good idea of what might come up and offer tips and tricks on how to answer questions. There are many websites with question banks for multiple membership exams such as https://www.onexamination.com and https://www.pastest.com.

Failing exams

Doctors are generally unaccustomed to failing at anything, but membership exams are difficult and failing is common. Failing does not make someone a bad doctor or not clever enough—often it means that other aspects of professional or social life took precedence over revision. Once the initial shock of failing has passed, it's important to be objective about the reasons for failure:

- **Poor exam technique** Questions can appear ambiguous and impossible to answer. Remember, exam boards have passed every written question, so there must be a logical reason to pick one answer over another. Confident practical performance requires lots of practice and an understanding of the expected standard.
- **Poor revision** Use focused revision; while it is important to have good background knowledge, this can develop throughout a career. Focus on subjects, and in formats, that regularly come up.
- **Insufficient revision** Maintaining a social life may indicate a need to hit the books harder, but it can also be difficult fitting revision around busy jobs. Plan ahead and start revising in plenty of time. Consider if there are future, less intensive jobs where life will be easier.
- **Exceptional circumstances** Some life events, e.g. illness, bereavement, etc., are unexpected and unavoidable despite the need to revise. Exam boards will take truly exceptional circumstances into account.
- **Bad luck** Keep trying—eventually most doctors pass!

Feedback from the exam board often gives a breakdown of marks which can suggest areas for improvement. Talk to colleagues who have taken the exams and discuss revision techniques.

Recurrent failure

If you cannot pass an exam, e.g. after three attempts, it is important you take a step back and think about your career. Are you doing a specialty that you enjoy and are good at? Do you need a break? Without passing exams, it may not be possible to progress to be a consultant or general practitioner (GP). In this event, specialty and associate specialist (SAS) posts (p. 19) in a supportive department may be a good career option.

▌ Consultant

This page describes the process of becoming a fully registered consultant. For the consultant career pathway, see p. 8. For the pathways of individual specialties, see specialty overviews (pp. 35–66).

Certificates and registration

To work as a consultant in the UK, it is a legal requirement for doctors to be admitted to the specialist register held by the General Medical Council (GMC). Full details are on the GMC website (https://www.gmc-uk.org) for each route to do this.

The most common route is to gain a **Certificate of Completion of Training (CCT)** by completing a GMC-approved specialty training programme:

1) Three to 6 months before completing training, the relevant Royal College or Faculty reviews evidence that the doctor has satisfied training requirements. They then make a recommendation to the GMC.
2) The GMC invites the trainee to complete an online application and pay fees (~£430). Application **must** be made within 12 months of the training completion date.
3) The application is processed and if successful, the doctor is awarded a CCT and automatically admitted to the specialist register.

Doctors may not be eligible to apply for a CCT if some or all of their training was in non-GMC-approved posts, including those who trained overseas. These doctors can apply for admittance to the specialist register through an alternative route, e.g. a **Certificate of Eligibility for Specialist Registration (CESR)** (p. 21). A CESR permits work under the same terms as a CCT.

Subspecialties

There are over 30 GMC-approved CCT subspecialties which are accessed through a main or 'parent' specialty (e.g. paediatric neurology is a CCT subspecialty of paediatrics). Subspecialty training completed by the time of application for a CCT in the parent specialty can be recognized on the specialist register at no extra cost. Subspecialties may be added to the register later, for a fee (~£300).

Consultant jobs

Trainees can apply for consultant posts up to 6 months prior to their training completion date. Competition is variable and may be fierce! There are two main methods for finding a post: first, by applying for an advertised job, e.g. on NHS Jobs (https://www.jobs.nhs.uk); and second, by being informed about a post by talking to incumbent consultants and/or clinical directors. This is not the 'old-boy network', but the result of preparation by the trainee, which also allows them to perfect their curriculum vitae (CV) and perform at their best at interview.

Applications for jobs usually involve interviews and presentations to a panel (often including a lay chair, senior hospital management, e.g. the chief executive, consultant(s) from the department, and others). If a post may be available soon, but not immediately, doctors may take a locum consultant post or a short-term 'post-CCT' job. If no post is likely in the foreseeable future, the trainee may need to rethink their particular field or location.

Acting up as a consultant (AUC)

During the last training year, doctors can work at consultant level whilst still being under a degree of supervision. It aids the transition from trainee to consultant—the roles are very different clinically and managerially. Many trainees find the experience a positive one.

Pay is dependent on seniority and additional activities undertaken. The starting salary is determined nationally and for full-time consultants is around £79 800 (p. 99).

General practitioner

This page describes the process of becoming a fully registered general practitioner (GP). For details of the GP career pathway, see p. 8. For GP jobs and lifestyle, see the following pages:

- GP (p. 172)
- Academic GP (p. 174)
- Private GP (p. 180)
- GP in a rural setting (p. 176)
- GP in secure environments (p. 178)
- GP with extended roles (p. 182).

Certificates and registration

To work as a GP in the UK, it is a legal requirement to be accepted onto the GP register held by the GMC. Full details are on the General Medical Council (GMC) website (https://www.gmc-uk.org) for each route to do this:

The most common route is to gain a **Certificate of Completion of Training (CCT)** by completing a GMC-approved GP specialty training (GPST) (p. 42) programme:

1) On starting GPST, trainees register with the Royal College of General Practitioners (RCGP). During training, they complete an ePortfolio (p. 86), evidencing their education and progress.
2) In the final 4 months, trainees are invited to apply for a CCT from the GMC and pay fees (~£430).
3) Once the final annual review of competency progression (ARCP) (p. 95) is complete, an application is automatically sent to the RCGP. The RCGP reviews evidence that training has been satisfactorily completed, then recommends to the GMC that the doctor should be awarded a CCT.
4) The GMC assesses the RCGP recommendation against the application made by the doctor. If successful, a CCT is awarded and the doctor is automatically entered onto the GP register.

Doctors may not be eligible to apply for a CCT if some or all of their training was in non-GMC-approved posts, including those who trained overseas. These doctors can apply for admittance to the GP register through an alternative route, e.g. a **Certificate of Eligibility for GP Registration (CEGPR)** (p. 21). A CEGPR permits work as a GP under the same terms as a CCT.

The GP register

All doctors working as fully qualified GPs in the UK, including those in temporary and locum posts, must be on the GP register. The complete list of everyone on this (and the specialist register) is not openly available, but you can check on the GMC website if a specific doctor is registered. Both trainee and fully qualified GPs also need to be accepted onto a **primary medical performer's list**—the process of this varies among the devolved nations.

GP jobs

The following are the main types of GP jobs:

- **Independent contractors (partners)** 'own' their practice, alone or in a consortium, which have contracts to provide services. Alongside clinical work, they manage their practice and staff, and have a say in how the business is run. Salary is partly determined by surgery performance and is usually between £70 000 and £120 000.

- **Salaried GPs** are employed by independent contractors (or by primary care organizations). Salary, usually between £50 000 and £100 000, is determined by experience and working pattern, and is not affected by the practice's income. Jobs are less likely to include management roles.
- **Locum GPs** are employed to cover specific sessions or a fixed period, e.g. due to absence of a permanent member of staff. Salaries vary.
- **Private GPs** Patients pay directly for consultations and treatment. They may work independently or as part of a consortium, or be employed by a private organization.

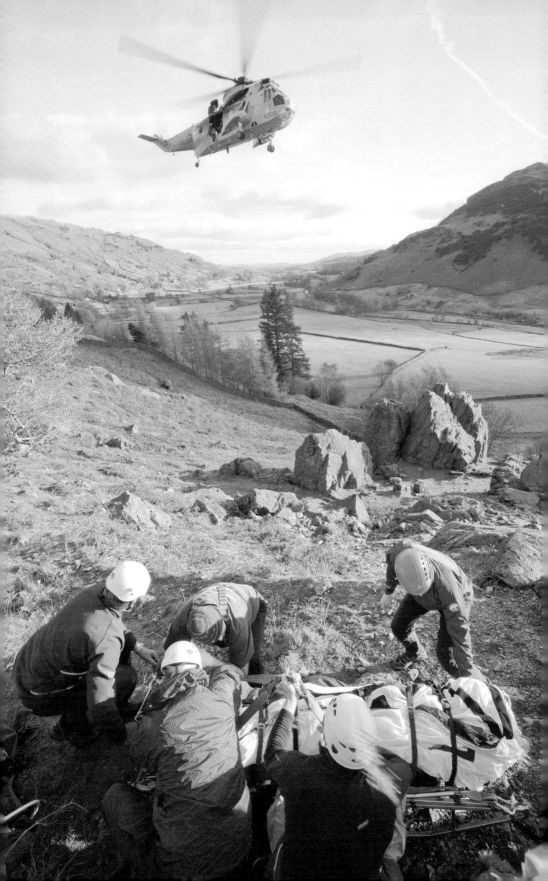

2

Career routes—the 'alternative' routes

▌Alternative routes

Although many medical careers follow a similar trajectory as that outlined in Chapter 1 (p. 1), there are many other ways to work and train. This chapter outlines some of the more common alternatives to the 'typical' career.

Specialty and associate specialist doctors

Not every doctor becomes a general practitioner (GP) or a consultant and a proportion will stay in non-training service positions. Roles are variable—broadly, specialty and associate specialist (SAS) doctors perform similar clinical activities to other doctors. However, they are not in a training path towards becoming a consultant or a GP and, at senior levels, they have less responsibility and accountability. SAS roles may offer the ideal career structure, combining the excitement of clinical practice with greater flexibility. For some, they may be the best option after being unable to secure a training post or pass membership exams (p. 9).

As shown in Fig. 2.1, SAS doctors can competitively apply for training posts if they meet eligibility criteria: they often need to obtain a certificate or document confirming they have the same competences as trainees applying at that level. Some move to consultant posts through routes alternative to standard training pathways, e.g. by obtaining a Certificate of Eligibility for Specialist Registration (CESR) or the GP equivalent (see p. 21 for details). These routes can be lengthy, complex, and expensive processes with no guarantee of success.

- **Good points** Establishment in a department; not moving every few months; no time pressure for exams; excellent experience and full range of clinical activities; reduced administration; opportunities for additional roles, e.g. lecturing.
- **Bad points** Can be difficult to transfer to training/consultant jobs; limited career progression and training opportunities; often perceived as lower status; service provision work and wide variation in job plans; variable pay (p. 99); less independence.

SAS roles and terms

As a minimum, SAS doctors must complete the foundation programme (FP) (p. 4) or demonstrate they have achieved FP competences in other posts or overseas. Responsibilities depend on the needs of the specialty or department, and job planning is negotiable. Formal access to training in SAS jobs is desirable, but not guaranteed. SAS roles depend on previous training and experience:

- **Associate specialist** Senior doctor with >10 years' postgraduate experience. They work in a permanent role in a defined specialty and are responsible to a named consultant. Officially, this grade is closed to new entrants.
- **Specialty doctor** Doctor with >4 years' postgraduate training, including at least 2 years in a relevant specialty. Pay progression is linked to meeting competence 'thresholds', demonstrating participation in job planning, professional development, and appraisal.
- **Trust/staff grade** Doctor at trainee level working in a permanent, non-training service provision job. They are not automatically covered by national contracts (p. 99); terms and conditions are set by the employing Trust.

Locum Appointment for Training (LAT) Temporary post approved for training, which counts towards a Certificate of Completion of Training (CCT) if the doctor subsequently joins a specialty training programme.
Locum Appointment for Service (LAS) Temporary post not approved for training; these posts do not count towards a CCT but can be used for alternative certifications (p. 21).

- **Clinical fellow** Doctor undertaking a job to gain specialty or subspecialty experience, usually for a fixed term. Service provision may be combined with research/teaching/ leadership roles and higher degrees or qualifications. Doctors often take these roles between training stages or after CCT (p. 36)—not to be confused with academic clinical fellows (ACFs) (p. 23).

Exams

Unlike in training posts, membership exams are not always required. Benefit remains in taking exams, diplomas, or certificates to develop specialty or subspecialty interests, or to demonstrate competences for future applications, e.g. to training programmes.

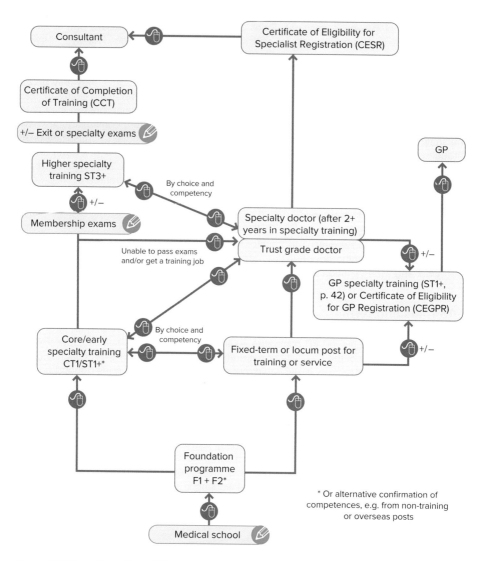

Figure 2.1 Overview of specialty and associate specialist (SAS) roles.

For further information

NHS Employers SAS doctors website. https://www.nhsemployers.org/pay-pensions-and-reward/medical-staff/sas-doctors

Alternatives to a Certificate of Completion of Training (CCT)

The aim of medical training is for doctors to attain the skills, knowledge, capabilities, and experience to fulfil their role as a consultant or general practitioner (GP)—doctors meeting these requirements can be entered onto the specialist or GP register held by the General Medical Council (GMC). Doctors who successfully complete a GMC-approved training programme and are awarded a CCT (p. 36) are automatically entered onto the relevant register. However, this is not the only route, and for doctors who have completed some or all of training outside approved programmes, the GMC will accept evidence that they have trained to an equivalent standard.

Certificate of Eligibility for Specialist Registration (CESR) or GP Registration (CEGPR)

Doctors who can demonstrate that they do not require additional specialty training because they have gained equivalent competencies in non-approved posts, e.g. in specialty and associate specialist (SAS) roles (p. 19) or overseas, can apply to the GMC for a CESR or CEGPR. Each specialty (including general practice) has clear guidance available on the GMC website (https://www.gmc-uk.org) detailing the required documents and evidence (e.g. qualifications, employment records, appraisals, assessments, etc.). Application costs around £1640 (compared to £430 for CCT). Completing the process can take over six months and requires the doctor to provide around 1000 pages of evidence. There is no guarantee of success, although the GMC will provide feedback for those who are unsuccessful; the doctor can also appeal the decision (for an additional fee).

> Unlike a CCT, a CESR or CEGPR is not automatically recognized in other European countries. Currently, specialists and GPs who trained on the continent usually have their qualification mutually recognized in the UK. It is unclear if this will change as a result of the UK leaving the European Union (EU).

CESR or CEGPR via the Combined Programme (CESR CP or CEGPR CP)

Doctors who complete only part of a GMC-approved training programme have previously applied for a CESR or CEGPR via the Combined Programme. Such doctors have gained experience before starting their training programme, e.g. in a different specialty or in non-training posts in the UK or overseas. These include doctors starting a specialty training programme at a higher level (e.g. ST5 instead of ST3) and those who enter at the normal level but gain approval to complete an accelerated programme of training. Recent changes mean that such trainees are now able to apply for a CCT, which can also be retrospectively applied for.

CEGPR via the Approved Programme (CEGPR AP)

Doctors in a GP specialty training programme who have not passed one part of MRCGP (p. 43) by the time they complete training may be able to apply for a CEGPR AP. The final part must be passed within 12 months of finishing training or they will need to apply for a CEGPR. The GMC invites eligible doctors to apply shortly after exam results are published. Application fees are the same as applying for a CEGPR (~£1640).

▌Switching career paths

Inevitably, some doctors will want to change career paths during their working life. Some realize they have made the wrong career choice or develop other interests. As priorities change over time, doctors may turn to careers which offer more opportunities for progression or a better work–life balance.

The perennial lack of flexibility in training is a contributing factor to junior doctor dissatisfaction and issues with workforce retention. It is therefore understandable that improving flexibility has been an underlying principle of several reforms and evaluations of postgraduate medical training. These include *Modernising Medical Careers* (MMC) (p. 92), the *Shape of Training* review (p. 93), and the 2017 General Medical Council (GMC) report *Adapting for the Future*.

Transferring to a different specialty

Doctors already in a training programme who hope to switch to a different specialty need to apply through the normal process of competitive application; if unsuccessful, they can continue in their existing programme. Trainees must meet eligibility criteria for the new specialty. However, they may find it tricky to demonstrate 'commitment' to the new specialty, particularly as their portfolio (p. 86) and curriculum vitae (CV) (p. 85) are likely to be tailored to the original career. They may need a break between programmes to build experience, e.g. in non-training jobs or to undertake additional qualifications. For other jobs, e.g. radiology, experience in other fields can be valuable and may permit application to a higher training level than for applicants straight from the foundation programme (FP).

> It often takes a lot of courage to leave a training programme, particularly when a great deal of time and effort have been invested into getting there. It is important to carefully consider your reasons for leaving and think about your ambitions for the future. It is vital to speak to your programme director or postgraduate dean (p. 95) in advance, and it can be helpful to discuss with peers, seniors, friends, and family.

Transferrable skills

Doctors transferring to a different specialty training programme may be able to reduce their training duration by up to 2 years (but nearly always less). Relevant skills gained in the previous training programme may be recognized through a process known as the Accreditation of Transferable Competences Framework (ATCF). Previously, this has only been possible when transferring between a limited number of pre-defined specialties; where the ATCF was not applicable, training could be protracted, with doctors having to repeat or demonstrate previously-acquired competences.

However, as specialty curriculums in future will have to include generic competences, there will be greater opportunity to map cross-specialty skills acquired in any training programme (and potentially in non-training posts): 'gap analysis' may be used to identify outcomes yet to be achieved and adjust the likely duration of training accordingly. Time will tell how well this process works in practice, and trainees will still need to complete the minimum training duration in the new specialty.

Pay

Pay under the 2016 contract (p. 99) is related to stage or grade of training, rather than years of service as under the 2002 contract. Therefore, there may be a significant reduction in pay for those who transfer to a different specialty, which is often started at a lower training grade. This may be particularly noticeable for doctors who have completed training in one specialty and wish to retrain in a different specialty (e.g. it's not uncommon for hospital doctors to retrain in general practice), unless pay protection or other incentives are introduced.

Academic career

All doctors are encouraged to participate in teaching and research during their careers, but some have formal roles in academia. Academics are found in every specialty, from general practice (p. 42) to medicine (p. 44) and surgery (p. 61). They are involved in a range of scholarly activities, aiming to push the boundaries of medicine by pioneering new treatments, investigations, and practices.

The career route described is not the only way into academia, but it is the most direct. Doctors with sufficient research and clinical experience can transfer between clinical and academic pathways. However, academic jobs are highly competitive and require academic excellence (e.g. distinction in medical degree, publications, first class Bachelor's degree) and references from academic supervisors.

The National Institute for Health Research (NIHR)

Government body that is the largest funder of NHS research, including for individuals undertaking clinical research.

Training

The following training pathway, as summarized in Fig. 2.2, applies to most specialties, with the exception of general practice: academic general practice training differs in each UK country but essentially lasts for 4 years. Around 25% of time is spent in academia and the rest in clinical practice. Research degrees (PhD/MD) and further academic training can be undertaken after completing GP training.

- **Undergraduate** Medical students can take time out of their medical degree to undertake an intercalated or additional degree (Bachelor's, Master's, and in a handful of cases, PhDs). This typically involves a period of research. Scholarships and bursaries are available to fund outstanding students or projects.
- **Foundation programme (FP)** Around 7% of FP posts are in the Academic Foundation Programme (AFP). AFP placements include four months in academic posts, usually during F2. Other posts are in clinical rotations identical to those in the standard FP, but with additional opportunities for research or teaching.
- **Specialty training** Following the FP or AFP, trainees apply for academic clinical fellowships (ACFs). ACFs are equivalent to core training, lasting up to three years—75% of time is in clinical practice; the other 25% is in academia, providing opportunities to prepare applications for research fellowships. Clinical specialty may be allocated before or during the ACF.

The processes, terminology, and funding of academic jobs differ greatly. Details are beyond the scope of this book—check information from administrative bodies before applying.

- **Research fellowship** During ACFs, trainees develop plans for a period of research (usually 3–4 years), typically used as the basis of a PhD/MD. Research is completed during a fixed-term research fellowship. Those who already have a PhD/MD undertake postdoctoral work. After their research fellowship, ACFs return to complete clinical specialty training without further competitive application, or apply for a clinical lectureship (CL).
- **CL** For senior trainees with a higher degree (PhD/MD). CLs last 4 years, or until CCT, and doctors spend half of their time in teaching and/or research. There may be some full-time clinical work to allow completion of specialty training and preparation for consultant jobs or senior lectureships.

'Honorary consultants' are employed by higher education institutions as academics of at least senior lecturer level and also work clinically in the NHS at consultant level.

Academic trainees have protected time for research but, despite having less time working clinically, they must still attain or complete the same competences, assessments, and exams as non-academic trainees.

Funding

It really is all about the money—academics have to apply for funding to support their research, e.g. from charities or national bodies such as the NIHR. One advantage of formal academic programmes is that trainees have supervisors and mentors throughout the process.

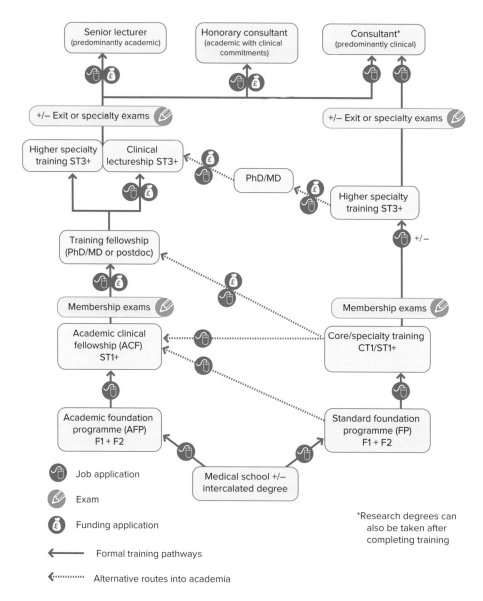

Figure 2.2 Overview of academic training pathways (except general practice).

For further information

UK Foundation Programme, Academic Foundation Programme. https://foundationpro-gramme.nhs.uk/programmes/2-year-foundation-programme/academic-training/

NIHR Integrated Academic Training information. https://www.nihr.ac.uk/explore-nihr/academy-programmes/integrated-academic-training.htm

▌ Armed forces career

Doctors in the armed forces are trained as officers alongside their medical training, as outlined in Fig. 2.3. Defence medicine can be very diverse since doctors often follow their patients to wherever they are stationed, including war zones. There are three services within the armed forces (known collectively as the Defence Medical Services) and training follows a similar pattern in each:

- Army (p. 120)
- Royal Air Force (p. 122)
- Royal Navy (p. 124).

Training

Medical school Students can apply for bursaries/cadetships whilst at university. Each of the forces has its own selection process—successful applicants usually receive funding for a set duration during medical school. This is around £3000–17000 per year, often with an additional lump sum on completing basic training and payment of university tuition fees. In return, the doctor must work for the armed forces for a fixed time (at least 6 years) once they are fully registered with the General Medical Council (GMC) (p. 96). While the money is attractive, the commitment is binding and expensive to buy out of.

Foundation programme (FP) Medical cadets must complete the FP (p. 4) after medical school. They apply through the standard FP process but are usually allocated to programmes aligned to Ministry of Defence Hospital Units (MDHUs). These are within NHS hospitals but treat both military and civilian personnel.

> In addition to basic training, all military doctors have a period of comprehensive medical military training. Competition for posts is often tough, and successful application also depends on fitting medical eligibility criteria and having a reasonable fitness level.

Specialty training The structure is similar to standard training pathways, but military doctors also develop skills to manage in environments not typically encountered in the NHS (e.g. war zones, submarines). After foundation year 2 (F2), doctors have further military training, followed by 1–3 years as a general duties medical officer (GDMO), a role similar to a GP specialist registrar, which may mean deployment overseas. They then choose a clinical specialty; the options are restricted to those required by the armed forces (e.g. it is not possible to train in paediatrics, geriatrics, or obstetrics and gynaecology (O&G) in the Navy).

Military specialty training posts are set aside for military doctors. Despite applying through national recruitment processes, they are only in competition with other military doctors. If they leave the armed forces during specialty training, they will lose their training post, so hospital doctors often need to sign up for at least a further 2 years of service to complete training.

Post-CCT After completing training, doctors can continue to work in the armed forces, e.g.:

- As a GP, usually working as the registered medical officer (RMO) of a regiment. They follow their regiment on all its activities, including training and deployment.
- As a consultant working in an MDHU; they may still be required to go on deployment.

Doctors can also join the armed forces after having completed training through the 'standard' route. They need to commit to at least 3 years of service (but may be welcomed by a generous bonus).

Exams

It is essential to pass membership exams required in specialty training. There is no difference in the specific exams between the armed forces and other medical careers.

Pay

In addition to bursaries and other incentives, military doctors are usually paid more (by up to 25%) than the basic salary of their non-military colleagues (p. 99).

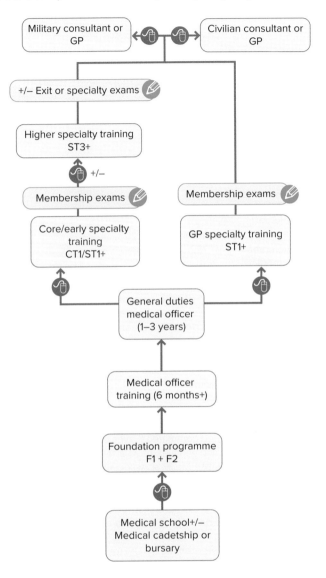

Figure 2.3 Overview of medical careers in the Armed Forces.

For further information

Government information on Defence Medical Services. https://www.gov.uk/govern-ment/groups/defence-medical-services

'Off the beaten path' and portfolio careers

There are many careers where medical training provides unique and highly valued insights, and jobs that require doctors' skills in different environments. The possibilities are endless, but such roles are diverse and uncommon—as such, there's no standard career path. Some examples are described in more detail on the following pages:

- Diving and hyperbaric medicine (p. 148)
- Entrepreneur (p. 208)
- Expedition doctor (p. 162)
- General practitioner (GP) in secure environments (p. 178)
- Forensic medicine (p. 166)
- Media medicine (p. 204)
- Medical education (p. 206)
- Medical management (p. 214)
- Medical politics (p. 220)
- Medico-legal adviser (p.224)
- National healthcare policy and leadership (p. 228)
- Overseas aid; volunteering (p. 222 and p. 318)
- Pharmaceutical medicine (p. 264).

When considering these types of jobs:

1) Most doctors undertake them part-time or as portfolio careers alongside 'standard' medical jobs. This may be financially and personally rewarding. However, they can have significant time pressures and come with great risk, whether financial, e.g. investing personal capital, or personal—some doctors simply take on too much!
2) Often, the more experience a doctor has, the more capable they are for these jobs. Completing the foundation programme (FP) and fully registering with the General Medical Council (GMC) are usually essential, and a Certificate of Completion of Training (CCT) (or equivalent) is advantageous.

Training

Medical school Joining societies and committees gives experience in areas of interest, plus organization and leadership skills. Universities have a range of such activities, e.g. student councils. Organizations, e.g. the British Medical Association (BMA), have student branches, and others have internships (e.g. the World Health Organization (WHO)).

FP Specific placements are unlikely to have a great bearing on non-standard careers. However, consider taster weeks (p. 4) to explore outside the box. Natural breaks in training, e.g. after FP or core training, provide opportunities to explore and gain skills, insights, or qualifications.

Specialty training Time 'out of programme' (OOP) (p. 101) provides protected time to explore other paths and develop skills or research in specific fields. Formal schemes facilitating non-clinical experience are available, e.g. fellowships through the Faculty of Medical Leadership and Management (https://www.fmlm.ac.uk/).

Experience Many jobs require doctors to develop experience and additional skills (e.g. writing or presentation skills, problem-solving, ethical analysis, coding, etc.) alongside training, as shown in Fig. 2.4. It is often necessary to have developed such skills to a high level before someone will pay for them.

Textbooks, patient information, clinical trial reports, medical 'problem pages', and blogs all have more depth when written by those with a medical background. Even Casualty (other medical dramas are available) has medical advisers, ensuring its story lines don't stray too far from the realms of possibility (at least clinically). Writing is time-consuming and comes with little financial reward initially—this improves with increasing clinical and writing experience.

Exams and qualifications

Completion of membership exams (p. 9) is an important marker of clinical ability and experience. Exams ensure the doctor has key knowledge in their specialty, and medical opinion is often given more weight if backed by membership-level experience and qualifications. Also consider what courses and qualifications will help in a future career; the following examples (often as certificates, diplomas, or degrees) can be taken as part-time or even online courses:

- **Non-clinical** For example, law, management, education, Masters of Business Administration (MBA), app development
- **Clinical** For example, mountain medicine, tropical medicine and hygiene, remote medicine, forensic medicine.

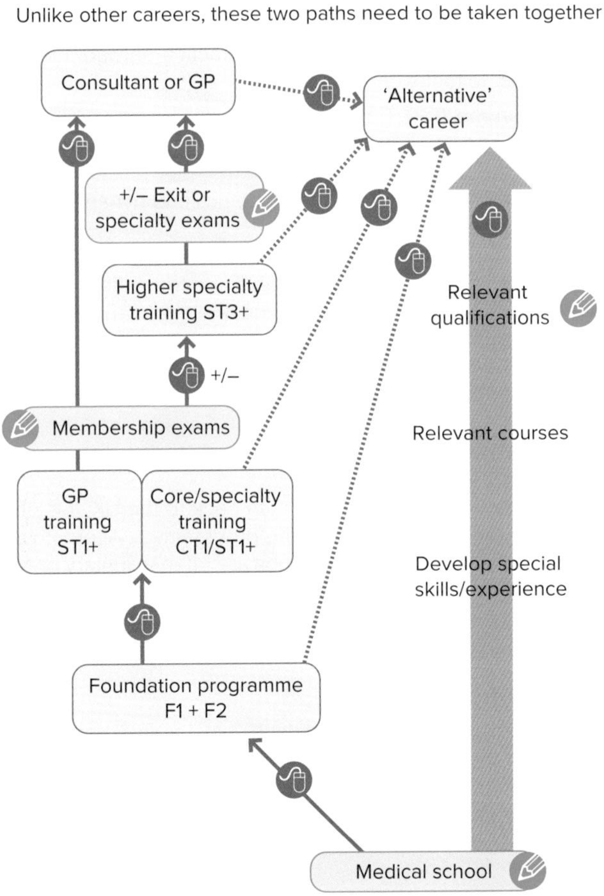

Figure 2.4 Training in 'alternative' careers related to medicine.

▌Overseas career

Medicine offers fantastic opportunities to travel. As outlined in Fig. 2.5, there are three broad categories of career that take doctors overseas:

1) **Voluntary/aid work** In countries with under-resourced medical services or recent disasters, doctors can have a huge impact on people's lives and health. Alongside making a difference, living and working in different cultures can be life changing. Two examples of this type of work include:
   - Médecins Sans Frontières (MSF) (p. 222)
   - Voluntary Service Overseas (VSO) (p. 318).

2) **Training/practising in a foreign country** (also see p. 103) A UK medical degree is acceptable proof of medical training for most countries. However, doctors may also need to speak the local language and pass additional exams. Training pathways differ between countries and describing each is beyond the scope of this book. UK doctors often undertake a period of service in Australia or New Zealand since no further exams are currently required.

3) **Travelling as an expert** Specialists (particularly academics) may be invited to share their expertise at conferences or in hospitals and universities overseas.

Training

Medical school Some universities take part in student exchange programmes which provide UK trainees with opportunities to experience practice abroad. Electives are typically taken overseas (with variable focus on medical practices).

- **Foundation programme (FP)** Completing the FP is usually required to work abroad and enables the trainee to re-enter the UK training system afterwards. If planning to work abroad after the FP, choose a programme with placements that cover broad areas, e.g. GP, emergency medicine, and obstetrics and gynaecology (O&G), or a specialty likely to be entered as a career.
- **The 'F3'** More than 50% of doctors take a break between foundation and specialty training (p. 101). Many continue clinical work in some form either in the UK or overseas. Although this rarely counts towards UK training, the experience is useful and may help in specialty training applications.
- **Specialty training** Overseas research or fellowship programmes, and bursaries and scholarships are available to support trainees in out-of-programme (OOP) placements (p. 101); 1-year 'post-CCT' fellowships (typically in Canada, the USA, Australia, etc.) are sometimes taken between completing training and starting a consultant post, often for subspecialty training.
- **Long term** For those who aren't keen to rush back to the UK, it is often possible, but usually competitive, to join overseas training programmes. Alternatively, some doctors devote an entire career to overseas aid—jobs are often voluntary or offer a minimal stipend, but increasing experience makes it possible to earn a salary. Examples include the World Health Organization (WHO) and the United Nations (UN). Armed forces doctors (p. 26) are likely to travel throughout their career on deployment.

Exams and qualifications

Completing membership exams before undertaking voluntary/aid work helps develop knowledge necessary to deal with difficult situations and makes it easier to obtain jobs upon return. Consider other qualifications which may help—the most common of these is the Diploma in Tropical Medicine and Hygiene, which is usually taken as a short (approximately 3 months) intensive course costing £6000+. Part-time courses and funding support (e.g. scholarships, bursaries) are available.

Other considerations

Financial considerations are essential to ensure an overseas job is a viable option, e.g. salary, cost of living, tax, pensions, etc. Medical indemnity is required and maintaining General Medical Council (GMC) registration is advisable as there may be problems re-registering if you wish to return to UK practice. Safety can't be guaranteed, so get travel and health advice in advance.

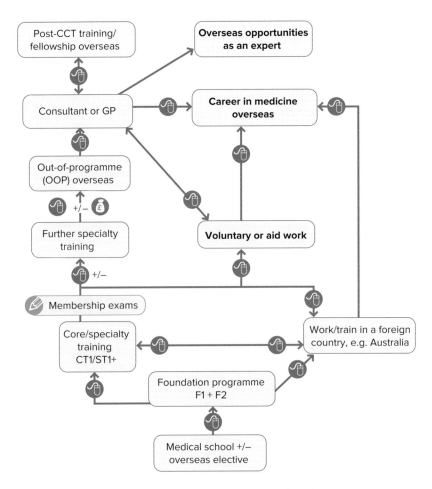

Figure 2.5 Overview of opportunities and pathways to work and train overseas.

▌Leaving clinical medicine

Careers in medicine don't have to last a lifetime. Whether doctors find they do not enjoy clinical work, feel they've had enough, or just want to explore something different, there are many options available. Whilst a medical degree is a vocational qualification, it also counts as a normal degree and is highly regarded as such. Additionally, working as a doctor develops and demonstrates a range of skills transferrable to other sectors, whether that is clinical knowledge or related skills, e.g. teamwork, leadership, and organization.

Before leaving, doctors should consider the following:

- Is the problem clinical practice or just the current job/hospital/city/country?
- Would changing to a different specialty help?
- Would a break be sufficient? See the section on taking time out (p. 101).
- Is there a chance of wanting to return to clinical medicine? Try not to burn bridges.
- What are the financial implications of leaving medicine?
- Are additional qualifications or courses required before starting a different career?
- Will a different career lead to greater happiness?

When considering a career change, try to establish what aspects of a job matter and how the new career matches these. Starting a new career or expanding an existing side-line is likely to take time, planning, and motivation—it may be worth taking part-time or locum clinical work to cover life expenses whilst working things out. Talk to people already doing your intended job about the good and bad aspects and ensure that it meets your needs and ambitions better than a medical career. The grass is greener where it's watered, not just because it's on the other side of the fence. Consider Table 2.1.

Careers related to medicine

There are many non-clinical jobs where medical experience will be a huge asset, or even an essential requirement. Doctors have worked (or found themselves) in roles from advising the government to founding med tech start-ups and advising investment firms, and have even had successful careers on the comedy circuit. Jobs are likely to be advertised outside of the usual clinical websites, e.g. NHS Jobs, Oriel, etc., and it is essential to find out where the adverts will be. This book presents some of the more common options; however, the list is by no means exhaustive:

- Entrepreneur (p. 208)
- Medico-legal advisor (p. 224)
- Medical consultancy (p. 212)
- Media medicine (p. 204)
- Medical education (p. 206)
- Medical ethics (p. 210)
- Medical management (p. 214)
- Medical politics (p. 220)
- National healthcare policy and leadership (p. 228)
- Pharmaceutical medicine (p. 264).

Careers unrelated to medicine

Alongside diagnostic skills and the ability to cannulate whilst half asleep, doctors also develop many transferrable skills. It is important to highlight these in a CV (p. 85) whilst removing the medical jargon. Key skills include: time management, prioritization, communication (written and oral), presentations, management, teamwork, decision-making, coping with stress, and teaching.

Try to network with people in the new career to help guide the changeover process and suggest ways to find employment. Few organizations function like the NHS, so be careful not to assume things will be done in the same way.

Table 2.1 Aspects to consider when leaving clinical medicine

Where?	When?	Who?	How?	(For) What?
Location	Full-time	Your skills and attributes	Qualifications	Income
e.g. home, office	Part-time		Competitive application and interview processes	Career progression
e.g. home, abroad	Flexible working	Potential clients and colleagues		Perks, e.g. cars, bonuses
e.g. rural, town, city	Shifts		Starting a business	Flexibility
				Work–life balance
				Achieve a goal
				Autonomy

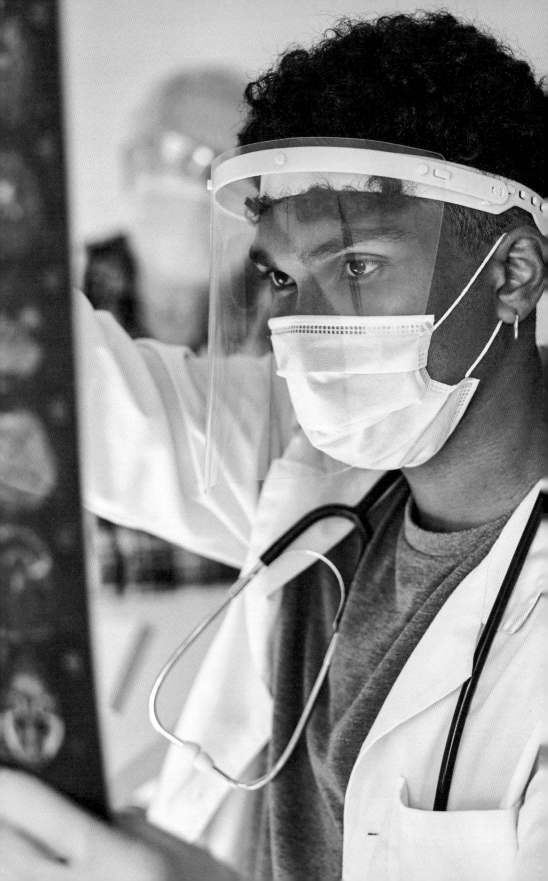

3
Specialty overviews

Introduction

This chapter contains an overview of the training pathways in the most common clinical specialties. It outlines the training structures, application processes, and exams needed to complete specialty training (which always starts after the foundation programme (FP) (p. 4)). However, the specifics are frequently updated, so it's also important to check with the relevant Royal Colleges, Faculties, and deaneries.

Training pathway glossary—see Table 3.1 for common abbreviations

Specialty A branch of practice in a specified area, e.g. cardiology, general practice (GP), neurosurgery, paediatrics, histopathology, etc. In the UK, all main specialties have a GMC-approved training pathway.

Subspecialty Practice in a specific part of a broader field which is reached via a main (or 'parent') specialty. Many also have GMC-approved training pathways.

Special interest An area of expertise within a specialty, but which is not a recognized subspecialty.

Basic or core training Trainees learn the fundamentals of clinical practice central to a specialty through experience in a broad range of associated fields. It leads to one or more specialties, depending on the training structure (p. 7).

Membership exams Exams set by Royal Colleges and Faculties which need to be passed during training (p. 9).

Higher specialty training (HST) Later stages of specialty training which leads to the award of a Certificate of Completion of Training (CCT).

CCT Awarded on completing a GMC-approved specialty training programme, which allows the doctor to work as a consultant or general practitioner (GP).

Dual CCTs (previously joint CCTs) Some training pathways allow (or mandate) simultaneous training in two related specialties, ultimately leading to a CCT in both. Trainees need to get into both pathways via open competition, and duration of training increases by up to 24 months compared to single CCT training (if available).

Table 3.1 Common abbreviations

ACCS	Acute care common stem	**GMC**	General Medical Council
AM	Acute medicine	**GP**	General practice/practitioner
ARCP	Annual Review of Competence Progression	**GPwERs**	GP with extended roles
BBT	Broad-based training	**HST**	Higher specialty trainee/training
CCT	Certificate of Completion of Training	**ICM**	Intensive care medicine
CIT	Combined infection training	**IMT**	Internal medicine trainee/training
CMT	Core medical trainee/training	**MSRA**	Multi-Specialty Recruitment Assessment
CST	Core surgical trainee/training	**NTN**	National Training Number
CT	Core trainee/training	**OSCE**	Objective structured clinical exam
ED	Emergency department	**SCE**	Specialty Certificate Examination
EM	Emergency medicine	**SJT**	Situational judgement test
FP	Foundation programme	**ST**	Specialty trainee/training

▋ Acute care common stem (ACCS)

This is a 3-year core training pathway (CT1–3) in the hospital specialties most involved in acute and critical care (Fig. 3.1).

Training

Year 1 and Year 2 Six months in emergency medicine (EM), 6 months in acute medicine (AM), and 3 months minimum in each of anaesthetics and intensive care medicine (ICM).

Year 3 is in the exit specialty applied to for ACCS training, which is one of:

- **AM** (p. 114) Treating adult patients referred from the emergency department (ED) or GP in the critical first 24–72 hours of a medical admission
- **Anaesthetics** (p. 39 and p. 118) Provides general and regional anaesthetic and analgesia for procedures, surgery, and obstetric cases, etc.
- **EM** (p. 154) Front line of acute adult and paediatric hospital care. Involves the assessment and management of all patients, from the critically ill to the walking wounded.

> Despite some overlap in competences and assessments required by different ACCS streams, switching between paths is difficult and almost always requires further competitive application.

HST Following ACCS, trainees competitively apply for HST posts (ST3/4) in their exit specialty and/or ICM (p. 200). During HST, trainees can also apply for subspecialty training in pre-hospital emergency medicine (PHEM) (p. 158). ACCS-AM is equivalent to internal medicine training (IMT) (p. 44); trainees completing either programme can apply for HST in any medical specialty (p. 44).

There are other routes into anaesthetics (p. 39) and AM (p. 44). The following are alternative routes into EM:

- Run-through training from ST1
- Defined route of entry into EM (DRE-EM): ST3 posts available for doctors with 2 years of relevant experience, e.g. in core surgical training (CST) (p. 61), ACCS-AM or anaesthetics, or non-training jobs. There is no further competitive application for HST (ST4+).

Preparation

Most FP jobs have rotations in one or more of the above specialties due to the current emphasis on increasing acute care provision. 'Taster weeks' are also helpful.

Applications

All applications are competitive and made online via the national recruitment portal Oriel (p. 73). Applications for ACCS-anaesthetics and ACCS-AM are made to core anaesthetics training (CAT) (p. 39) and IMT (p. 44), respectively; preference for ACCS is made later in the selection process. Candidates are shortlisted using scores from application forms; the highest-ranking candidates are invited to interview.

Exams

No exams are necessary to apply for ACCS but are required for HST:

- **Anaesthetics** Primary Fellowship of the Royal College of Anaesthetists (FRCA) (p. 40) required for ST3; Final FRCA required for CCT
- **AM** Membership of the Royal College of Physicians (MRCP) (p. 45) required for HST; Specialty Certificate Exam (SCE) required for CCT
- **EM** Membership of the Royal College of Emergency Medicine (MRCEM) Primary (a single best answer (SBA)) paper), MRCEM Intermediate SBA paper, and MRCEM

objective structured clinical exam (OSCE) required to apply for ST4. Fellowship (FRCEM) required for CCT. This involves an SBA paper and an OSCE exam.

ACCS vs core training

Although longer than traditional core training programmes, ACCS trainees gain additional experience and competences in acute care, particularly in procedural skills, e.g. airway management, which may not otherwise be encountered. Going into HST, ACCS trainees may have less experience in the specialty applied for than core trainees, due to time spent in other ACCS specialties. Completing ACCS in one exit specialty doesn't necessarily provide eligibility to apply for HST in another.

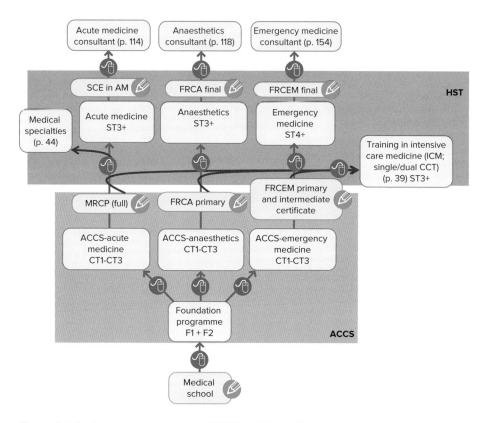

Figure 3.1 Acute care common stem (ACCS) training pathways.

For further information

The Intercollegiate Committee for Acute Care Common Stem Training (ICACCST). Web: https://www.accs.ac.uk/accs Email: accs@rcoa.ac.uk

The Royal College of Emergency Medicine (RCEM). Tel: 020 7404 1999. Web: https://www.rcem.ac.uk Twitter: @RCollEM

▍Anaesthetics

Anaesthetics is the largest single hospital-based specialty, with over 7000 consultants practising in the UK. Traditionally, anaesthetists provide perioperative care and analgesia, sedation, or anaesthesia for surgical procedures. They are increasingly involved in critical care and are (thankfully) found at the head-end in most crash calls. Anaesthetists can develop special interests and expertise in a range of areas, including cardiothoracic, neurosurgical, or paediatric anaesthesia, and pain medicine (p. 260). They can also competitively apply for additional training in one of:

- **Pre-hospital emergency medicine (PHEM)** (p. 158) A subspecialty of acute care common stem (ACCS) specialties (p. 37) and intensive care medicine (ICM) involving the assessment and management of emergencies outside the hospital
- **ICM** (p. 200) Care exclusively of critically ill patients requiring high levels of observation and organ support. Simultaneous training (i.e. dual CCT) is currently possible with several specialties involving overlapping skills, e.g. anaesthetics, emergency medicine (EM), acute/renal/respiratory medicine.

Training
Anaesthetics training (Fig. 3.2) starts in one of two ways:

- **Core anaesthetics training (CAT)** (CT1–2) A 2-year programme with rotations in anaesthetics and ICM
- **ACCS–anaesthetics** (p. 37) A 3-year programme with rotations in associated acute specialties for year 1 and 2, followed by a year in anaesthetics at the same level as CT2 in CAT.

HST Following core training in either pathway, trainees competitively apply to HST in anaesthetics (ST3+); a 5-year training programme leading to a CCT in anaesthetics. HST is divided into:

- **Intermediate training** (ST3–4) Introduces trainees to specialist anaesthetics, e.g. cardiothoracic and neuroanaesthesia
- **Higher training** (ST5+) 1 year in general anaesthetics and 1 year in an optional unit of training, e.g. pain medicine, military anaesthesia, anaesthesia in developing countries
- **Advanced training** (usually ST7) Trainees build expertise in chosen area(s) of anaesthesia and develop professional skills, e.g. management.

Paediatric ICM
Anaesthetics trainees can apply for subspecialty training in paediatric ICM via the paediatric NTN Grid (p. 50).

Preparation
Some FP jobs include ICM or anaesthetics. Experience can be gained in other acute specialties such as EM and surgery. It's a competitive specialty; look at the person specifications (p. 83) well in advance. Keeping a logbook of procedural skills and showing an interest through tasters, research, and audits will support applications.

Applications
All applications are competitive and made online via the national recruitment portal Oriel (p. 73). Application to CAT or ACCS–anaesthetics is a single process, with candidates choosing later whether to be considered for one or both. Candidates are shortlisted using scores from application forms; the highest ranking candidates are invited to interview.

Exams

No exams are required to start CAT or ACCS-anaesthetics. Fellowship of the Royal College of Anaesthetists (FRCA) must be completed during training. It has two components (Primary and Final):

- **Primary FRCA** An exam in three parts—a multiple-choice question (MCQ)-based exam, a practical objective structured clinical exam (OSCE), and a structured oral exam (SOE). Each section must be passed before sitting Final FRCA.
- **Final FRCA** An MCQ-based exam, then an SOE. Both parts need to be passed within 7 years of passing Primary FRCA.

Fellowship of the Faculty of Intensive Care Medicine (FFICM) is needed for a CCT in ICM. There is no Primary FFICM at present, so trainees must hold one of Membership of the Royal College of Physicians (MRCP) (p. 45), Primary FRCA, or Primary Fellowship of the Royal College of Emergency Medicine (FRCEM) (p. 37) before sitting the FFICM Final. This consists of an MCQ-based exam, then a practical OSCE/SOE.

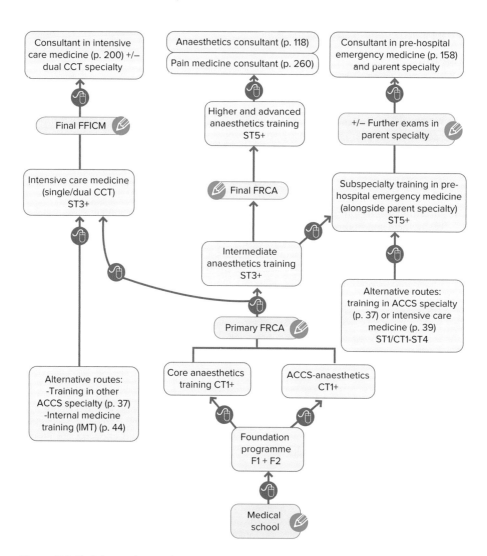

Figure 3.2 Training pathways in anaesthetics.

█ General practice

General practitioners (GPs) (p. 172) work in the community, treating patients of any age or complaint. They also have vital roles in health promotion and are the gateway to most hospital services. It is a diverse specialty, with opportunities for management, business, and academia. There are over 40 000 GPs in the UK and some have specific roles, including:

- **Academic GP** (p. 174) GP with formal roles in research or education
- **GP with extended roles** (GPwERs) (p. 182) GP with expertise beyond that developed through standard training
- **Performing minor surgical procedures** For example, removing skin tags, varicose veins.

Patient demographics, budgets, and workloads are determined by the area covered; the life of a rural GP (p. 176) can be miles away from life in a big city.

Training

As shown in Fig. 3.3, training is in a 3-year run-through programme (ST1–3) known as **GP specialty training (GPST)**. The first 18–24 months is in hospital specialties, e.g. emergency medicine (EM), paediatrics, obstetrics and gynaecology (O&G), etc. Trainees work as supervised GP registrars for the remainder. Increasingly, 4-year training schemes are available, including academic clinical fellowships (ACFs) (p. 23) and educational scholarships.

Broad-based training

A 2-year core training pathway currently only available in Scotland and Northern Ireland. Trainees spend 6 months in each of GP, internal medicine, paediatrics, and psychiatry. They then automatically enter one of these specialties at ST2 (paediatrics and GP) or CT2 (internal medicine and psychiatry).

It is relatively common to switch from hospital specialties to GPST; some doctors may be supported to complete a shortened GPST programme, depending on previous training and experience (p. 22). Switching from GP to hospital specialties can be more difficult.

GPwER Qualified GPs undertake further training, research, or qualifications to gain knowledge and skills in a specific area. This can be determined by personal interests, prior experience, or the needs of the practice or local area.

Preparation

The majority of FP posts include a rotation in community-based medicine, typically GP. All FP experience is relevant, but deliberately reflecting on psychosocial aspects of care and public health issues is beneficial.

Applications

Applications are via a national 3-stage process managed by the GP National Recruitment Office (GPNRO):

1) **Application form** for factual information only (i.e. work history) submitted online via Oriel (p. 73). Applicants also preference training regions. Note: some regions are historically undersubscribed and attract a one-off bonus (currently £20 000) for new GPSTs.
2) **Multi-Specialty Recruitment Assessment (MSRA):** computer-based exam used to rank and allocate applicants to deaneries. Candidates scoring over 550 (approximately the top 10%) are automatically given posts and do not attend the selection centre.
3) **Selection centre** at the allocated deanery involving observed simulated tasks and written assessments. Scores are used to rank applicants and allocate posts.

Exams

No exams are required for application. Trainees need Membership of the Royal College of General Practitioners (MRCGP) for CCT. MRCGP comprises three integrated sections:

- **Applied Knowledge Test (AKT)** A 3-hour computer-based test of clinical medicine, with sections of critical appraisal and health informatics. Taken during or after ST2
- **Clinical Skills Assessment (CSA)** A 13-station objective structured clinical exam (OSCE) on clinical assessment and management, professionalism, and communication skills. Taken during ST3
- **Workplace-Based Assessment (WPBA)** Trainees complete a set number of WPBAs which provide opportunities to gain feedback from supervisors and colleagues, and to reflect on their day-to-day practice.

Diplomas Many GPs take diplomas during training. Common examples include the Diploma of Child Health (DCH) and the Diploma of the Royal College of Obstetricians and Gynaecologists (DRCOG). Exams are similar to membership exams (p. 9), with GP-specific content.

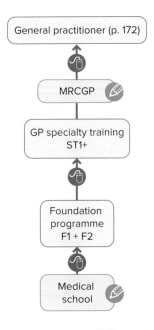

Figure 3.3 Training pathway in general practice (GP).

For further information

The Royal College of General Practitioners (RCGP). Tel: 020 3188 7400 Web: https://www.rcgp.org.uk Email: info@rcgp.org.uk Twitter: @rcgp

GP National Recruitment Office (GPNRO). Web: https://gprecruitment.hee.nhs.uk/ Email: gpnro@hee.nhs.uk Twitter: @GPNRO

Medical specialties

The medical specialties are a large group of hospital-based non-surgical jobs managing adult patients. Medics (or physicians) range from generalists dealing with the breadth of medical conditions to subspecialty experts. Many jobs mix ward- and clinic-based medicine, with some also performing practical or laboratory procedures. Table 3.2 lists the medical specialties divided into two groups (see the section on training below for further details).

In some paths, additional subspecialty training is available, e.g. metabolic medicine (p. 226) and stroke medicine (p. 300)—a subspecialty of several specialties, including cardiology, AM, and neurology.

Training

As shown in Fig. 3.4, training is in uncoupled programmes (p. 7), starting with core training. 2-year core medical training (CMT) was replaced by internal medicine training (IMT) in 2019. IMT takes 3 years and includes rotations in several medical specialties, with mandated time in intensive care medicine (ICM), geriatrics, and outpatients. Alternatively, doctors can complete acute care common stem–acute medicine (ACCS-AM) (p. 37).

HST Core training is followed by competitive application for HST (ST3+). Training lasts 4–6 years, and each specialty has its own curriculum and required competences. From 2022, 'Group 1' specialties will start HST at ST4 and simultaneously train in internal medicine (the feared and revered 'Med Reg' role). Confusingly, 'Group 2' specialties, occupational medicine (p. 242), and ICM (p. 200) will continue to recruit to ST3 after 2 years of IMT (or 3 years of ACCS-AM)—dual CCT in internal medicine will not be mandatory.

HST in several medical specialties is also accessible from other training programmes, e.g. GP, paediatrics, etc., so check person specifications in advance (p. 83). More details are also available in the career chapters (p. 109).

Table 3.2 Two groups of medical specialties

Group 1 specialties	Group 2 specialties
Acute medicine (AM) (p. 114)	Allergy (p. 116)
Cardiology (p. 132)	Audiovestibular medicine (p. 126)
Clinical pharmacology and therapeutics (p. 144)	Aviation and space medicine (p. 128)
Endocrinology and diabetes (p. 160)	Clinical genetics (p. 138)
Gastroenterology (p. 170)	Clinical neurophysiology (p. 140)
Genitourinary medicine (p. 186)	Dermatology (p. 146)
Geriatric medicine (p. 152)	Haematology (p. 190)
Infectious diseases (p. 198) without dual CCT in pathology specialty (p. 52)	Immunology (p. 196)
Neurology (p. 232)	Infectious diseases (p. 198) with dual CCT in pathology specialty (p. 52)
Palliative medicine (p. 262)	Medical oncology (p. 218)
Renal medicine (p. 288)	Medical ophthalmology
Respiratory medicine (p. 290)	Nuclear medicine (p. 236)
Rheumatology (p. 292)	Paediatric cardiology (p. 252)
	Pharmaceutical medicine (p. 264)
	Rehabilitation medicine (p. 286)
	Sport and exercise medicine (SEM) (p. 298)

Preparation

All FP jobs include a placement in hospital medicine. Experience in relevant specialties, e.g. emergency medicine (EM), ICM, etc., is useful. Consider tasters, audits, research, and courses for particularly competitive specialties (p. 80).

Applications

Applications are competitive and made online via the national recruitment portal Oriel (except for pharmaceutical medicine—for details, see the Faculty of Pharmaceutical Medicine website at https://www.fpm.org.uk). Recruitment to IMT and ACCS-AM is in a single process, with preference for one or both given later. Eligible applicants are shortlisted using application forms, with the highest-scoring applicants invited for interview.

Exams

Trainees from IMT or ACCS-AM need Membership of the Royal College of Physicians (MRCP) to start HST. The exam is in two parts:

- **Part 1:** multiple-choice question (MCQ)-based exam in two papers, testing understanding of common and important disorders and clinical science
- **Part 2:** Two parts, sat in any order after passing Part 1:
  - **Written:** MCQ-based exam testing application of clinical knowledge and decision-making
  - **Practical Assessment of Clinical Examination Skills (PACES):** objective structured clinical exam (OSCE)-based exam assessing examination, diagnostic, communication, and management skills.

Some specialties also require completion of a Specialty Certificate Examination (SCE), diploma, or knowledge-based assessment to attain CCT.

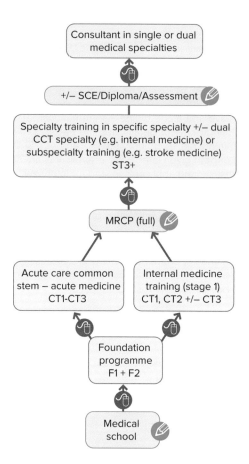

Figure 3.4 Training pathway in medical specialties.

For further information

The Joint Royal Colleges of Physicians Training Board (JRCPTB). Tel: 020 3075 1249. Web: https://www.jrcptb.org.uk Twitter: @JRCPTB

Physician Specialty Recruitment Office (PSRO). IMT website: https://www. IMTrecruitment.org.uk Twitter: @ct1recruitment

Specialty training website: https://www.st3recruitment.org.uk Twitter: @st3recruitment

Obstetrics and gynaecology

Training in obstetrics and gynaecology (O&G) (p. 240) is the starting point for specialties and subspecialties relating to women's healthcare, the female reproductive system, and reproduction. Most involve surgical management combined with medical care.

- **Gynaecology** Medical and surgical care for disorders of the female reproductive system. Usually also includes management of early, uncomplicated pregnancy
- **Obstetrics** Management of later-stage or complicated pregnancy, and of surgical or complicated childbirth.

Training

As shown in Fig. 3.5, training is in a 7-year run-through programme from ST1. This is based on a core curriculum, which also incorporates ultrasound training:

- **Basic level** (ST1–2) General experience in managing acute obstetric and gynaecological presentations
- **Intermediate level** (ST3–5) Development particularly of technical skills, with the aim of performing procedures under indirect supervision (i.e. with a consultant nearby) by ST5
- **Advanced level** (ST6–7) Progress to independent practice. Opportunity to develop subspecialty interests either by completing subspecialty training (see below) or by taking at least two of the 20+ available Advanced Training Skills Modules (ATSMs), e.g. menopause, colposcopy, medical education, etc.

Subspecialty training Two clinical years + 1 year in research. At any point after ST5 and passing Membership of the Royal College of Obstetricians and Gynaecologists (MRCOG) Part 2 (see below), trainees can competitively apply to one of four subspecialties:

- **Gynaecological oncology** (p. 188) Deals with the management of gynaecological cancers
- **Maternal and fetal medicine** Focuses on the medical and surgical management of high-risk pregnancies due to maternal or fetal disorders or disease
- **Subfertility and reproductive medicine** (p. 164) Prevention, diagnosis, and management of reproductive problems, including assistance or maintenance of reproductive capacity
- **Urogynaecology** (p. 310) Diagnosis and treatment of incontinence and pelvic floor disorders in women.

Obstetric medicine (p. 238) deals with medical problems in pregnancy. It is available as an ATSM in O&G specialty training. Trainees in a medical specialty (p. 44) can also develop it as a specialist interest (or 'credential') by gaining experience out of programme (p. 101) or after CCT.

Preparation

Four-month placements in O&G are relatively common in the FP, but experience can also be gained in emergency medicine (EM), GP, and genitourinary medicine (GUM). Evidence of some experience in O&G is important for successful application to specialty training, and any research, tasters, audits, electives, etc. are very useful.

Applications

ST1 applications are made through a national process. Longlisting is based on an online application form completed on the national recruitment portal Oriel (p. 73). All eligible applicants are invited to sit the Multi-Specialty Recruitment Assessment (MSRA) (p. 74). Candidates scoring highly enough are invited to interview. Candidates with relevant experience outside the FP, e.g. in non-training posts, can apply directly at ST3, but competition is high.

Exams

No exams are necessary to apply for O&G training, but passing MRCOG is required for CCT. Each part needs to be passed sequentially:

- **Part 1** Written exam (single best answer (SBA)) in two papers on basic and clinical sciences relevant to O&G. It can be taken at any time after medical school and is required to progress to ST3.
- **Part 2** Written exam (extended matching questions and SBA) assessing application of knowledge in clinical scenarios.
- **Part 3** Clinical assessment in a circuit of 14 tasks, assessing core knowledge, skills, and competences. Completion of Part 3 is needed to progress to ST6.

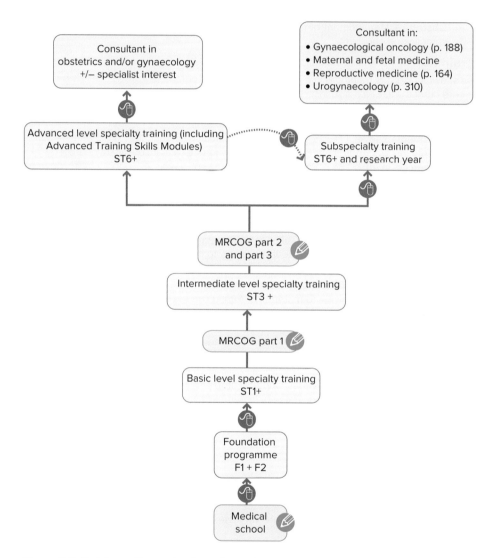

Figure 3.5 Training pathways in obstetrics and gynaecology (O&G).

For further information

The Royal College of Obstetricians and Gynaecologists (RCOG). Tel: 020 7772 6200.
Web: https://www.rcog.org.uk Twitter: @RCObsGyn

Paediatrics

Paediatrics is the basis for a range of hospital- and community-based specialties and subspecialties related to the management and prevention of disease in babies, children, and adolescents. It is broadly divided into:

- **General paediatrics** (p. 256) The largest group; a hospital-based job providing acute and long-term medical management. Many develop special interests, e.g. perinatal medicine.
- **Community paediatrics** (p. 258) Subspecialty involving work outside the hospital environment, assessing and managing patients with developmental, social, or behavioural problems and physical disabilities. Specialists are frequently involved in safeguarding issues, e.g. child abuse and neglect.
- **Neonatal medicine** (p. 230) Subspecialty involved in the care of newborn babies, including those born prematurely or with problems at birth.
- **Subspecialty paediatrics** Paediatricians trained in one of 15 other subspecialties:
  - Child mental health
  - Allergy, immunology, and infectious diseases
  - Clinical pharmacology
  - Diabetes and endocrinology
  - Emergency medicine (p. 156)
  - Gastroenterology, hepatology, and nutrition
  - Inherited metabolic medicine
  - Intensive care medicine
  - Nephrology
  - Neurodisability
  - Neurology
  - Oncology
  - Palliative medicine
  - Respiratory medicine
  - Rheumatology.

Training
As shown in Fig. 3.6, training is in an 8-year run-through programme from ST1:

- **Level 1** (ST1–3) Basic principles of paediatrics, with rotations in general paediatrics and neonatology
- **Level 2** (ST4–5) 12 months in general paediatrics and 6 months in each of neonatology and community paediatrics
- **Level 3** (ST6–8+) Advanced training in either general paediatrics, with up to 12 months in subspecialty training, or solely subspecialty training.

Other specialties have paediatric branches, including pathology, psychiatry, radiology, and surgery. Recruitment is to the named specialty rather than to paediatrics. **Paediatric cardiology** (p. 252) can be entered after either core training in adult medicine (p. 44) (requires additional paediatric training) or Level 1 paediatric training.

Preparation
Little time is spent in paediatrics during medical school, so gaining further insight is advisable. Some FP jobs include paediatric rotations, and experience can be gained in related specialties, e.g. GP and emergency medicine (EM). Tasters, research, and audits are helpful, particularly for subspecialties.

Applications

ST1 applications are made via the national recruitment portal Oriel (p. 73). Eligible applicants are ranked based on interview score. Candidates with relevant experience outside the FP, e.g. in non-training posts, can apply directly at ST2, ST3, or ST4 level, but competition may be high.

Subspecialties Application for subspecialties is through **National Training Number (NTN) Grid recruitment**. Each year, available training posts in each region are submitted to the Grid. Following competitive application via Oriel, candidates are matched to posts.

Level 3 trainees and post-CCT paediatricians not completing Grid subspecialty training can undertake a Special Interest (SPIN) module in one of the subspecialty areas. SPIN modules are not recognized by the GMC as formal subspecialty training but allow the doctor to be involved in providing specialist care.

Exams

No exams are required to apply for ST1/2 posts. Membership of the Royal College of Paediatrics and Child Health (MRCPCH) is required to enter Level 2 training. MRCPCH is in four parts: three written papers and one clinical exam. The written papers combine extended matching questions (EMQs), best-of-five (BOF), and true/false questions and can be taken in any order:

- **MRCPCH Foundation of Practice** Core elements of assessment and clinical decision-making in paediatrics
- **MRCPCH Theory and Science** Fundamentals of pharmacology and physiology, and principles of evidence-based practice
- **MRCPCH Applied Knowledge in Practice** Two papers testing clinical knowledge and decision-making, using data interpretation and case histories.

MRCPCH clinical Ten objective structured clinical exam (OSCE)-style stations assessing paediatric assessment and management, taken after passing all written exams.

Additionally, trainees in their penultimate year complete the Specialty Trainee Assessment of Readiness for Tenure (RCPCHStart). This helps to identify areas on which to focus in their last year and practice scenarios with which they may be faced as a new consultant.

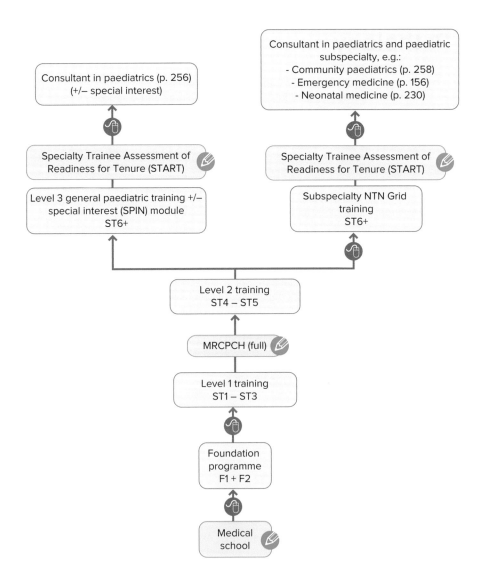

Figure 3.6 Training pathways in paediatrics.

For further information

The Royal College of Paediatrics and Child Health (RCPCH). Tel: 020 7092 6000.
Web: https://www.rcpch.ac.uk Email: enquiries@rcpch.ac.uk Twitter: @RCPCHtweets

Pathology

Many people think all pathology is 'histopathology', but the term encompasses several specialties and subspecialties using various techniques to study and diagnose disease. Most work occurs in the laboratory, but many jobs involve some patient contact. The following are the most common areas of specialization, but there are other fields determined by patient group (e.g. paediatric and perinatal) or disease site (e.g. neuropathology):

- **Chemical pathology** (p. 136) Interpreting biochemical tests and using them to advise or manage patient care
- **Histopathology** (p. 194) Diagnosing disease from tissue samples, encompassing surgical pathology, autopsy, and cytopathology. Subspecialties related to histopathology include forensic pathology (p. 168) and neuropathology.

Training

As shown in Fig. 3.7, training in each specialty is in 5- to 6-year run-through programmes (ST1+). Training in related (sub)specialties begins after a minimum time in basic training and may involve further competitive selection. Some subspecialties are also accessible from other training programmes, so check person specifications in advance.

Preparation

There are a handful of FP jobs with rotations in pathology. Chemical pathology and biochemistry are involved in all specialties on some level, e.g. interpretation of lab results. Tasters, electives, observerships, and relevant higher degrees provide insight and knowledge, and are valuable in showing commitment to specialty.

Applications

Applications are made on the national recruitment portal Oriel (p. 73). Most recruitment is via national processes involving shortlisting, followed by face-to-face assessment at interview or a selection centre. A handful of specialties still require separate applications if applying to more than one region.

Exams

No exams are required to apply, but specialty-specific Fellowship of the Royal College of Pathologists (FRCPath) exams are needed for CCT. FRCPath is in two parts:

- **Part 1** Always includes a written exam (e.g. extended matching questions (EMQs)/multiple-choice questions (MCQs)/short answer questions (SAQs)); some specialties also include a practical exam
- **Part 2** Taken after Part 1 and 2+ years of specialty training. They are a combination of practical laboratory assessments, written essays or exam questions, and viva-style exams.

Early-stage trainees also need to pass 'Stage A exams' which require the interpretation of data, microscopy, and photos in a circuit of tasks. This forms a major part of determining whether trainees can progress.

Medical specialties involving pathology

- **Haematology** (p. 190) and **immunology** (p. 196) are medical specialties (see p. 44 for further details) specializing in blood cells, but with a large laboratory component.
- **Medical microbiology** (p. 216), **infectious diseases and tropical medicine** (p. 198), and **virology** (p. 316) are specialties involving identification of disease-causing microbes from fluid or tissue samples, and providing or advising management.
- **Metabolic medicine** (p. 226) is a subspecialty of internal medicine and chemical pathology (see above). Specialists manage patients with metabolic disorders (e.g. dyslipidaemias, artificial nutrition, etc.).

Training

As shown in Fig. 3.7, following completion of core training in medicine (p. 44), trainees competitively apply for specialty training (ST3+) in one of:

- **Metabolic medicine** As a subspecialty of internal medicine or chemical pathology
- **Combined infection training (CIT)** A 2-year common training pathway for medical microbiology, medical virology, infectious diseases, and tropical medicine; posts are linked to one of these specialties for HST. Trainees can dual CCT with internal medicine or another CIT specialty.

Preparation

Several FP jobs have rotations in one or more medical specialties involving pathology. Interpretation of tests relevant to these specialties is involved in almost all specialties on some level. Tasters, electives, observerships, and relevant higher degrees provide insight and knowledge, and are valuable in showing commitment to specialty.

Applications

Applications are made on the national recruitment portal Oriel (p. 73) and are usually via national processes, with preferences for available posts made after interviews.

Exams

Application for specialty and subspecialty training requires full Membership of the Royal College of Physicians (MRCP) (p. 45). Additionally:

- Metabolic medicine: trainees in internal medicine submit a research dissertation; chemical pathology trainees need FRCPath as above.
- Trainees in CIT specialties take the written (MCQ) FRCPath Part 1/Combined Infection Certificate Exam (CICE); microbiology and virology trainees also need to pass FRCPath Part 2 before completing training.

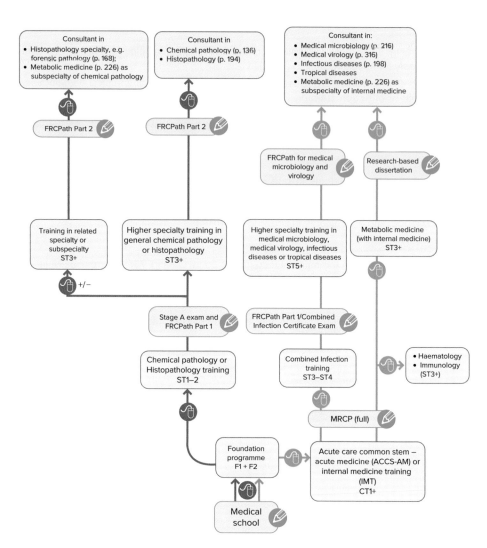

Figure 3.7 Training pathways in pathology specialties (blue arrows) and medical specialties (p. 44) which include pathology (green arrows).

For further information

The Royal College of Pathologists (RCPath). Tel: 020 7451 6700 Web: https://www.rcpath.org Email info@rcpath.org Twitter: @RCPath

▌ Psychiatry

Psychiatry is a diverse specialty encompassing several hospital- and community-based roles relating to mental health. Psychiatrists almost never work alone and are normally part of a large multidisciplinary team (MDT).

Training

As shown in Fig. 3.8, training starts with a 3-year core training programme (CT1–3) involving rotations in a range of psychiatric specialties, with a minimum of 12 months in general adult psychiatry. On completion of CT3 and obtaining Membership of the Royal College of Psychiatrists (MRCPsych) (see below), trainees competitively apply to HST in one of:

- **Child and adolescent psychiatry** (p. 268) Specialists in managing patients under 18 years with neurodevelopmental disorders (e.g. autism) and disorders found in adults (e.g. schizophrenia). There is an emphasis on working with families and community agencies. At the time of writing, run-through training (ST1+) is being piloted. Note: child mental health is a separate paediatric subspecialty (p. 49).
- **Forensic psychiatry** (p. 270) Management of psychiatric and psychosocial disorders in those in prisons or secure units. Specialists require in-depth knowledge of legal systems and often act as expert witnesses in court.
- **General adult psychiatry** (p. 272) The largest group of psychiatrists, managing psychiatric disorders in patients aged 18–65 years in inpatient and outpatient settings.
- **Psychiatry of intellectual disability** (p. 274) Psychiatric disorders are more common in people with intellectual disabilities. These specialists provide community-based treatment. They also manage related neurodevelopmental disorders or other illness (e.g. cerebral palsy, epilepsy).
- **Medical psychotherapy** (p. 276) Specialists who use talking and activity-based therapies to manage (mainly) psychological disorders (e.g. adjustment disorders, anxiety states).
- **Old age psychiatry** (p. 278) A workforce increasing with the ageing population which manages mental health problems in patients (typically) over 65 years, including degenerative disorders (e.g. dementia).

Attainment of CCT normally takes 3 years from starting HST (ST4–6) but may be extended in those training in dual CCT specialties, e.g. forensic psychotherapy. During/post-HST, general adult psychiatrists can develop special interests in several fields:

- **Liaison psychiatry** Specializes in providing psychiatric care for general hospital patients
- **Addictions psychiatry** Management of patients with drug and alcohol addiction
- **Rehabilitation** Restoration of community function to people with mental illness
- **Other** Including eating disorders, neuropsychiatry, and perinatal psychiatry.

Preparation

Psychiatry jobs are common in the FP. Experience can also be gained in related specialties, e.g. GP, emergency medicine (EM), paediatrics. Tasters in psychiatric specialties and relevant audits or research are useful.

Applications

Applications for CT1/ST1 and ST4 are made via the national recruitment portal Oriel (p. 73). Applicants are shortlisted using an online application form. Selection and allocation to posts are based on ranking of scores after interview.

Exams

No exams are required to apply for core training, but MRCPsych is needed to apply for HST (i.e. ST4). MRCPsych is in three parts: two written, and the Clinical Assessment of Skills and Competencies (CASC).

The written papers can be sat in any order:

- **Paper A** Can be sat by any fully registered doctor, i.e. post-F1; 200 questions (multiple-choice questions (MCQs) and extended matching questions (EMQs)) covering core elements of theory and basic science in psychiatry.
- **Paper B** Recommended to be sat after 12 months of psychiatry experience/training. A third of the paper is on 'Critical Review', i.e. of research, and statistics; the rest is on clinical topics in psychiatry.

The **CASC** is an OSCE-based exam of assessment, examination, clinical management, and communication skills. It can only be taken after passing both written exams and at least 24 months in psychiatry training. An Assessment Portfolio must also be successfully completed.

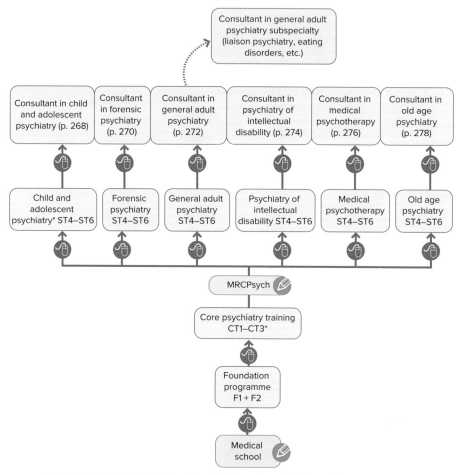

*Run-through training available for child and adolescent psychiatry from ST1

Also, some dual training posts, e.g. general adult and old age psychiatry

Figure 3.8 Training pathways in psychiatry.

For further information

The Royal College of Psychiatrists (RCPsych). Tel: 020 7235 2351. Web: www.rcpsych.ac.uk Twitter: @rcpsych

Public health

Public health is a unique specialty as it deals with the health of populations rather than of individuals. It is competitive, with applications accepted from non-medical graduates with relevant experience, as well as from doctors. The roles available are numerous and varied; they can involve anything from public relations to research but broadly involve projects aiming to protect and improve health and services.

Training
As shown in Fig. 3.9, training is in a 5-year run-through programme (p. 7) from ST1. Provided required targets and assessments are met, training is guaranteed until CCT.
   Training is in three stages:
- **Phase 1** Gaining basic knowledge, including formally through a higher degree (e.g. Masters or Diploma in Public Health)
- **Phase 2** Development of skills and competences, taking on defined service work
- **Phase 3** Consolidation of skills and knowledge; performing advanced skills in public health; development of special interests, e.g. health protection or health and social service quality.

Time out of training can be taken, e.g. for research or a higher degree (PhD/MD), between Phases 2 and 3.

Preparation
Some time at medical school is devoted to public health principles and several universities offer an intercalated degree in public health. FP posts in public health are rare, but experience can be gained in related posts, e.g. GP. Tasters can help gain more insight into the career, and related audits and research can make an application stand out.

Applications
Applications are made via the national online recruitment portal Oriel (p. 73). Eligible applicants are invited to sit written tests assessing numerical and critical reasoning, and a situational judgement test (SJT). Scores are used to rank applicants, with the top candidates invited for face-to-face assessment at a selection centre. Trainees switching from other fields may be eligible for shortened training time if they have previously gained relevant competences.

Exams
No exams are required to apply for ST1. Membership of the Faculty of Public Health (MFPH) is required to attain CCT. This is a 2-part examination which can be taken at any time, including by doctors who are not in public health training:

Diplomate exam Written exam in two parts (Paper I and II), each in two parts sat over 2 days. The exam assesses understanding of the scientific basis of public health, e.g. applied statistics, health economics. Passing leads to Diplomate Membership (DFPH).

Final membership exam The Objective Structured Public Health Exam (OSPHE) comprises six practical stations assessing applied knowledge, skills, and attitudes of everyday public health issues. Stations can include mock presentations or meetings with the press or members of the public. Passing leads to full MFPH.

   Members and non-members of the Faculty of Public Health (FPH) are automatically elected to Fellowship after admittance to the GMC specialist register, e.g. after completing a training programme. Fellows can nominate other professionals working at consultant level in public health or related fields for Fellowship by distinction.

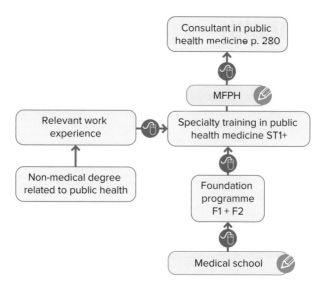

Figure 3.9 Training pathways in public health medicine.

For further information

The Faculty of Public Health (FPH). Web: https://www.fph.org.uk Twitter: @FPH

▌Radiology

Radiologists use a variety of modalities to diagnose, monitor, and treat pathologies that can be visualized on screen. There are two main areas:

- **Clinical radiology** (p. 282) Often thought of as 'diagnostic' radiology. Work mostly involves interpreting images (e.g. magnetic resonance imaging (MRI), computed tomography (CT), X-ray, ultrasound) to answer specific questions about cases. They also perform minor procedures which are more successful or safer under imaging guidance.
- **Interventional radiology** (IR) (p. 284) Performs minimally invasive procedures for diagnosis and treatment under direct imaging. There are three main areas of specialization within IR: vascular, non-vascular, and neuroradiology.

Training

As shown in Fig. 3.10, training in clinical radiology is in a 5-year run-though programme (p. 7):

- ST1–3 trainees learn clinical radiological techniques for imaging of any anatomical area.
- From ST4, trainees develop special interests in at least one field defined by anatomical area (e.g. breast, cardiac), patient demographic (e.g. paediatric, emergency), or imaging modality (e.g. MRI). Alternatively, trainees enter IR training (ST4–6)—although a recognized subspecialty of clinical radiology this does not lead to a separate CCT.

Growing demand for imaging studies has effectively led to a shortage of radiologists. Training has been facilitated by one of the world's largest e-learning platforms The Radiology Integrated Training Initiative (R-ITI). Additionally, dedicated radiology academies (in Plymouth, Norwich, and Leeds and West Yorkshire) have been established to increase the number of trainees.

There are two other radiological specialties which do not train through this pathway:

- **Clinical oncology** (p. 142) Non-surgical management of cancer patients, administering radiotherapy and systemic therapies. Specialty training (ST3–7) is co-ordinated by the Royal College of Radiologists (RCR).
- **Nuclear medicine** (p. 236) Applied use of free radioactive materials for clinical and research purposes (but not radiotherapy). An expanding field due to increasing use of radiolabelled material, positron emission tomography (PET), and gamma cameras. HST (ST3–6) is co-ordinated by the Royal College of Physicians (RCP).

Preparation

There are no specific radiology posts during the FP. Requesting and interpreting radiological studies features in hospital-based jobs, particularly acute medicine (AM), surgery, and emergency medicine (EM). Radiology is competitive; tasters, relevant research, and audits are valuable at application. Radiology courses heighten knowledge and demonstrate commitment to specialty.

Applications

Applications are made online via the national recruitment portal Oriel (p. 73). Eligible applicants sit the Specialty Recruitment Assessment (SRA), which is used to score and rank applicants. Those scoring highly are invited to face-to-face assessment at a selection centre. There is no standardized application process for IR and posts are usually recruited to locally (often via Oriel).

Exams

Clinical radiology No exams are required for application to ST1. Fellowship of the Royal College of Radiologists (FRCR) is required for CCT. It has two parts: First FRCR Exam (sat during the first training year), then the Final FRCR Exam:

- **First FRCR Exam** Two modules taken together or separately:
  - Physics—multiple-choice questions (MCQs) of UK radiation legislation and scientific principles
  - Anatomy—image viewing of the whole body.
- **Final FRCR Exam** Two parts taken at separate sittings:
  - Part A—six written papers (single best answer (SBA)) over 3 days covering modules related to the core curriculum.
  - Part B—practical assessments in a single week of two image reporting sessions and an oral exam.

Clinical oncology Membership of the Royal College of Physicians (MRCP) (p. 45) needed to apply; FRCR in Clinical Oncology required for CCT.

Nuclear medicine MRCP (p. 45) needed to apply; Diploma in Nuclear Medicine required for CCT.

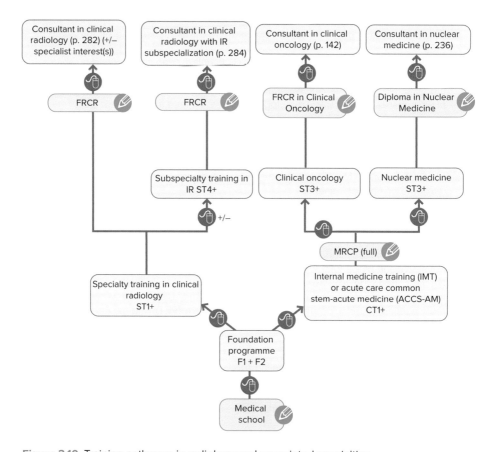

Figure 3.10 Training pathways in radiology and associated specialties.

For further information

The Royal College of Radiologists (RCR). Tel: 020 7405 1282. Web: https://www.rcr.ac.uk
Twitter: @RCRadiologists

▌Surgical specialties

The surgical specialties involve invasive procedures to remove, repair, or remodel a patient's pathology or anatomy. Details on each specialty can be found on the following pages:

- Cardiothoracic surgery (p. 134); subspecialty in congenital cardiac surgery
- Ear, nose, and throat (ENT) (otolaryngology) (p. 150)
- General surgery (p. 184)
- Neurosurgery (p. 234)
- Ophthalmology (p. 246)
- Oral and maxillofacial surgery (OMFS) (p. 248)
- Paediatric surgery (p. 254)
- Plastic surgery (p. 266)
- Trauma and orthopaedic surgery (T&O) (p. 308 and p. 250)
- Urology (p. 312)
- Vascular surgery (p. 314).

Entry and progress through training are not uniform across surgical specialties. Standardized curricula in each specialty have now been adopted by all relevant Royal Colleges, even if training pathways differ. The pathway for most surgical careers is outlined below, except OMFS, ENT, and ophthalmology which are discussed on p. 64.

Training

Training generally starts in 2-year core surgical training (CST (CT1-2)), as shown in Fig. 3.11. Trainees gain basic surgical experience and specialty-specific competences. CST can be:

- **Themed** 12–20 months in a pre-defined surgical specialty, with the remainder in allied specialties. This gives trainees more exposure to the designated specialty, but it can be difficult to change tack during training and core surgical competences still need to be obtained.
- **Generic** Training with rotations in a variety of specialties. Trainees are exposed to a wider range of fields and skills but, on applying for higher specialty training (HST), may have less experience in any one specialty. It can therefore be difficult to build a competitive CV.

The number and type of available CST posts differ greatly between years and regions. Check websites of individual specialties before applying.

After CST, trainees competitively apply for HST (ST3+). Due to limited numbers of posts and fierce competition, many trainees are not successful on their first application. There are numerous clinical fellow, staff grade (p. 77), or locum jobs available to gain further experience before reapplying. HST programmes vary, depending on specialty, but broadly last 5–8 years, with opportunities to develop special interests in later stages.

> Run-through training (p. 7) is currently available (but not compulsory) for neurosurgery and cardiothoracic surgery and, in Scotland, T&O. The *Improving Surgical Training* (IST) report, published in 2015, has also led to pilots of run-through training in specialties, including general surgery, urology, T&O, and vascular surgery.

Preparation

Many FP jobs include 3–4 months in general surgery and many have rotations in other specialties, typically T&O or ENT. Experience in associated specialties, particularly emergency medicine (EM) and intensive care medicine (ICM), is useful. Tasters and attending basic surgical courses give important insight into skills and requirements.

Applications

Applications for CST and run-through training posts are made via the national recruitment portal Oriel (p. 73). Shortlisted applicants are interviewed at a national selection centre. HST jobs also have competitive entry through national processes.

Exams

No exams are required to apply for CST. Intercollegiate Membership of the Royal College of Surgeons (MRCS) is required for HST. The exam is in two parts and can be sat by any medical graduate; passing Part A is required to sit Part B:

- **Part A** Two multiple-choice question (MCQ) papers sat on the same day: (1) applied basic science and (2) principles of surgery in general
- **Part B** An 18-station objective structured clinical exam (OSCE) exam covering applied surgical knowledge and clinical, procedural, and communication skills.

The Joint Surgical Colleges' Fellowship Examination (JSCFE – although Fellowship of the Royal College of Surgeons (FRCS) is actually awarded) is a specialty-specific summative assessment in two parts (one written, one OSCE). It is required to complete training in all surgical specialties (except ophthalmology).

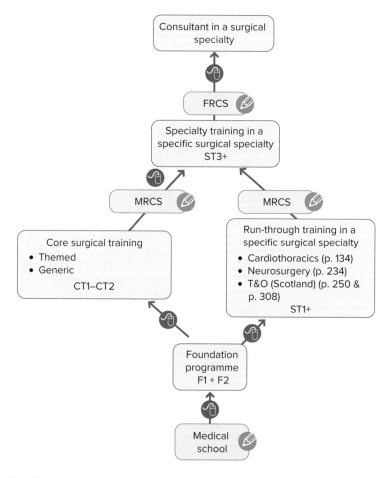

Figure 3.11 Training pathways in most surgical specialties.

For further information

The Joint Committee on Surgical Training (JCST). Tel: 020 7869 6299. Web: https://www.jcst.org Email: jcst@jcst.org Twitter: @JCST_Surgery

The Association of Surgeons in Training (ASiT). Tel: 020 7869 6681. Web: https://www.asit.org Email: info@asit.org Twitter: @ASiTofficial

▌ Further surgical specialties

Oral and maxillofacial surgery

Training

As shown in Fig. 3.12, training uniquely requires both a medical degree (e.g. MB BS) and a dental degree (e.g. BDS); some universities offer shortened 3- or 4-year programmes for the second degree. Medical graduates complete the FP before starting a dental degree but do not need to then complete dental foundation training. Alternatively, a dental degree can be undertaken after core surgical training (CST) (p. 61).

Trainees who have both degrees and have completed at least 12 months in CST (p. 61) can competitively apply to 5-year oral and maxillofacial surgery (OMFS) specialty training (ST3–7). Run-through training (ST1+) is also available. There may be further competitive selection for advanced training, e.g. head and neck oncology; specialist fields may also be entered via associated specialties, e.g. plastic surgery.

Applications

CST application is described on p. 62. ST3 OMFS applications are made via the national recruitment portal Oriel, and includes assessment at interview.

Exams

Membership of the Royal College of Surgeons (MRCS) (p. 62) required for HST (ST3+) in OMFS; trainees must pass the specialty-specific FRCS (OMFS) exam (see p. 62) for CCT. Trainees who did dentistry as the first degree sit exams for Membership of the Joint Dental Faculties (MJDF) or Membership of the Faculty of Dental Surgeons (MFDS). These exams are desirable but aren't essential in OMFS training.

ENT (otolaryngology)

Training

Training (Fig. 3.12) is in a similar format to that described on p. 61, with trainees completing CST, then applying for HST (ST3–8). There is an ongoing pilot for run-through training from ST1.

Applications

Applications for CST is described on p. 62. ST1 and ST3 ENT applications are co-ordinated through similar national processes, including an online application form on Oriel (p. 73) and interview.

Exams

- MRCS (ENT) is required for HST. This involves passing Part A MRCS (p. 62) and Part 2 of the Diploma of Otolaryngology–Head and Neck Surgery (DO-HNS), a 28-station objective structured clinical exam (OSCE). Alternatively, trainees can sit both parts of MRCS (p. 62) and both parts of the DOHNS (Part 1 is a written exam) which also allows them to apply for other specialties, e.g. plastic surgery.
- FRCS (Otolaryngology) needed for CCT.

Ophthalmology

Training

Training (Fig. 3.12) is usually in a 7-year run-through programme (ST1–7). However, candidates with 24 months' experience in ophthalmology, e.g. in non-training posts and the necessary competences, can apply at ST3 level.

Applications

Applicants to run-through training are shortlisted using an application form (via Oriel) (p. 73), then are invited to sit the Multi-Specialty Recruitment Assessment (MSRA); those scoring highly enough are invited for interview. ST3 application involves an interview but does not require sitting the MSRA.

Exams

No exams are required to start ST1 training. Fellowship of the Royal College of Ophthalmologists (FRCOphth) and attainment of the refraction certificate is required for CCT:

- **Part 1 FRCOphth** Written exam on basic science and theoretical optics. To be passed before ST3
- **Refraction certificate** A 12-station OSCE on retinoscopy and refraction. To be passed before ST4
- **Part 2 FRCOphth** Written exam covering the entire ophthalmology curriculum. Successful candidates then take a practical exam (viva and OSCE) 8–10 weeks later. Both to be passed by the end of ST7.

Preparation

A handful of FP posts have rotations in these specialties. Experience can be gained in associated specialties, e.g. general surgery and emergency medicine (EM). Tasters, audit, research (ideally presented at relevant conferences or published in journals), and related courses build a strong CV for application.

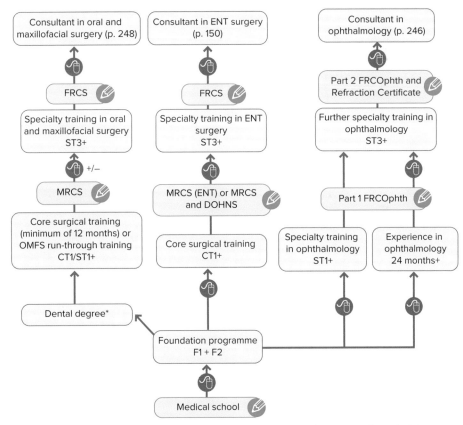

*Both medical and dental degrees needed for OMFS training. Dental degree may alternatively be obtained after core surgical training

Figure 3.12 Training pathways in oral and maxillofacial surgery (OMFS), ear, nose, and throat (ENT) surgery, and ophthalmology.

For further information

British Association of Oral and Maxillofacial Surgeons (BAOMS). Tel: 020 74058074. Web: https://www.baoms.org.uk Email: office@baoms.org.uk Twitter: @BAOMSOfficial

ENT UK. Tel: 020 7404 8373. Web: https://www.entuk.org Email: entuk@entuk.org Twitter: @ENT_UK

The Royal College of Ophthalmologists (RCOphth). Web: https://www.rcophth.ac.uk Twitter: @RCOphth

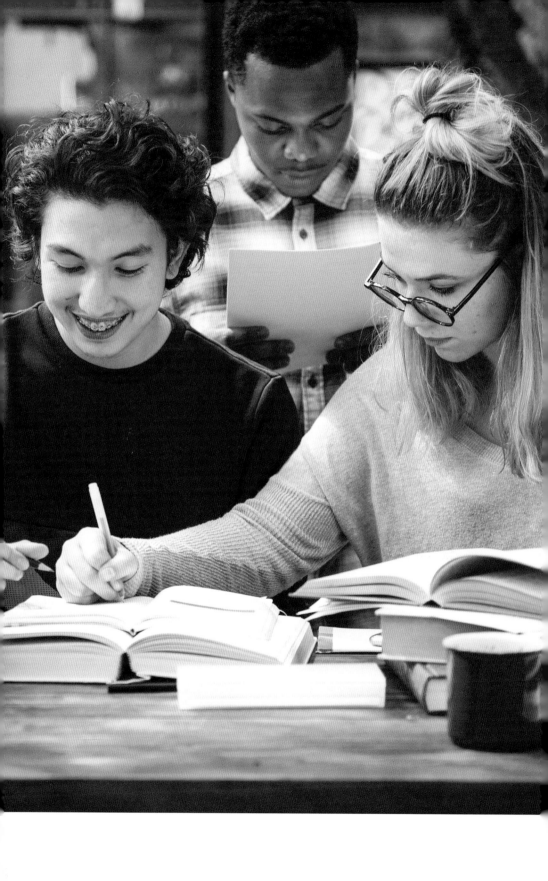

4

Choosing careers and getting jobs

Choosing a career

As this book demonstrates, there are a wealth of career options available to those with a medical degree. This can make deciding on a career path more difficult as there are numerous considerations to be taken into account. In addition, the current training structure has been criticized for making doctors choose a career without much opportunity to explore their options. It also lacks flexibility in allowing them to change paths later—some progress is, however, under way to try and address these issues (p. 93). Work has a huge impact on day-to-day life and happiness, so it is important to think carefully about what really matters when choosing a career.

Priorities

Every medical career offers a range of working patterns and lifestyles. The career chapters (pp. 110–318) give an impression of how each career compares. Key priorities to consider include:

- Frequency/intensity of on-calls
- Less-than-full-time/flexible working options
- Salary and private work
- Location, e.g. hospital or community
- Extracurricular interests, e.g. research
- Being part of a team
- Independence and autonomy
- Domestic and foreign travel.

Skills

Different doctors are good at different things. This can determine what type of job suits them, although nearly all jobs will require most of the below skills to varying degrees. See the career chapters (pp. 110–318) for a guide to the skills required in each career, e.g.:

- Communication skills
- Practical/technical ability
- Thinking/academic ability
- Attention to detail
- Managerial skills
- Teamwork/leadership skills
- Business/financial skills
- Dealing with a variety of patients/systems
- Dealing with a subset of patients/systems
- Ability to work under pressure
- Coping with responsibility
- Writing and presentation skills.

Type of work

Similarly, different aspects of medicine appeal to different people. Roles, responsibilities, and opportunities also vary between careers. See the sections entitled 'The work' and 'Extras' in the career chapters (pp. 110–318). Common types of work include:

- Clinics
- Ward rounds
- Procedures
- Operations
- Emergencies
- Laboratory work
- Research
- Teaching
- Management
- Imaging
- Advisory roles
- Leadership/organizational roles.

Competition

Despite recent (often negative) media attention and high-profile disputes between doctors and regulatory bodies such as the Department of Health, medicine remains a competitive field. A doctor's experience and achievements determine which careers they are able to pursue. Most doctors have sufficient ability to succeed in any specialty, but they may need to work extremely hard through their medical studies and early career to achieve the necessary qualifications and CV. See pp. 78–82 for competition ratios, and individual career chapters (pp. 110–318) for estimates of competitiveness by career.

Finding jobs

Foundation programme

Available programmes are advertised on the national recruitment portal Oriel (p. 73). Applicants to the 2-year foundation programme (FP) submit an online application and rank all 20 foundation schools (p. 96), also known as units of application (UoAs), in order of preference. They can also apply for specialized foundation programmes (SFPs), previously known as academic FPs, in up to two UoAs (see p. 87 for more details). After applications have been scored and candidates ranked, applicants are allocated to a UoA. The process of allocating candidates to individual programmes differs between foundation schools. For further details, see https://foundationprogramme.nhs.uk and websites of UoAs. Some students are pre-allocated to a UoA due to special circumstances, e.g. caring responsibilities. Pairs of students who feel unable to risk separation can link applications, ensuring allocation to the same UoA.

Core and specialty training

Nearly all vacancies are advertised on the national recruitment portal Oriel (p. 73). Details of application processes, including timetables (e.g. for applications and interviews) and eligibility criteria, can be found on Oriel, as well as on websites of relevant governing bodies and deaneries. Aside from a few exceptions (e.g. academic jobs), a single organization is usually responsible for recruitment to all jobs in a programme or specialty across England, Scotland, and Wales. Northern Ireland (typically) has separate recruitment processes. Applicants are usually ranked based on academic achievements, computer-based testing, and/or face-to-face assessments; highest scoring candidates are allocated to their preferred posts.

Consultant and GP jobs

Temporary and permanent consultant (p. 12) and GP (p. 13) jobs are advertised on the NHS jobs website (https://www.jobs.nhs.uk). Jobs are also often found through word of mouth and may additionally be listed on other websites, including BMJ Careers, Trust/Practice websites, and even LinkedIn.

Other routes

Clinical fellow (p. 77) Hospitals often recruit doctors for non-training or education/research-based roles. Although candidates often hear about these jobs by word of mouth, they are also advertised on the NHS jobs website and usually websites of the employing organization(s).

Word of mouth Whilst changes to recruitment pathways over recent decades have lessened the impact of the 'old boy network', medicine is a small world and people talk. For a competitive job at consultant level, it is important to be known and liked by the department. Showing interest and visiting departments remain an essential part of getting a job.

Locuming (p. 202) Be aware that the process of signing up to locum agencies can take months. Choosing the right agency is important, as coverage of regions and specialties differ. It may be more straightforward to join the internal locum 'bank' of a particular Trust. However, these are increasingly managed by private companies.

Contacting organizations Some jobs need to be created rather than found. For specific research interests, it is worth contacting leaders in the field to see if they can offer a suitable post. If pursuing careers outside the NHS, contacting organizations directly, even if it feels like a long shot, is a good way to begin.

Search engines Some vacancies are advertised outside of the NHS Jobs website or Oriel, particularly if non-clinical or in fields where doctors are typically employed by private organizations, e.g. pharmaceutical medicine (p. 264). It is essential to find out where these are advertised and an online search is usually helpful. Companies and agencies will have websites detailing application processes and contacts.

Surviving the recruitment system

Application processes for training programmes differ between specialties; specifics are beyond the scope of this book, so check online before applying. Helpfully, virtually all applications are now made online via the national recruitment portal Oriel (https://www.oriel.nhs.uk). Application windows, known as 'rounds', are set nationally—there are usually two rounds each year, but available specialties and regions often differ between them.

The required 'essential' and 'desirable' experience, achievements, e.g. membership exams, and attributes are detailed in specialty-specific '**person specifications**'. These are available on Oriel, websites of deaneries, Royal Colleges/Faculties, and Health Education England (HEE) (https://specialtytraining.hee.nhs.uk). It is **essential** to review these as early as possible before application to ensure requirements are met.

Choosing jobs

During the application process, candidates rank regions and/or posts in order of preference.

- If applying for competitive posts, consider including less competitive backup choices. Accepting a less preferred option is not mandatory but might provide a valuable opportunity to get into the field. Competition ratios are outlined on pp. 78–82.
- Consider whether the location or the specialty is more important. Switching career paths (p. 22) or regions during training can be difficult, and specialties may not re-accept applicants who have previously dropped out.

Application forms

It is essential to complete **all** sections and answer **honestly**. For some specialties, application forms only collect information used to longlist candidates; all eligible applicants are invited for further assessment (see the section 'Assessments', below). Others score forms to shortlist candidates; those ranked highest are invited for further assessment. There may be 'white-space' questions that are not scored but signpost areas to discuss at interview. Show completed forms to as many people as possible, including peers, supervisors, seniors, and friends and family (if only for spelling and grammar). It may be useful for applicants who don't have English as their first language to ask a native English speaker.

CV points Application forms used for shortlisting usually ask about publications, posters, presentations, audits, courses, and exams. Diversity scores more highly than excellence in a single area, i.e. one good example per category beats 20 publications and nothing else. **Do not lie** or exaggerate; being unable to provide proof will harm scores or even be considered a probity issue.

Experience It helps to spend time in the chosen specialty to demonstrate interest. Note: some posts specify a maximum or minimum duration that candidates may have spent working in that specialty before starting training.

Assessments

Increasingly, standardized computer-based assessments are used to test core knowledge and skills. This may be followed by interview or selection centre assessment to form an overall score. Sample questions, mock papers, and tutorials are available online. Preparation and a good working knowledge of relevant documents, e.g. the GMC's *Good Medical Practice*, are important. Tests usually involve ranking answers or single-best answer, extended matching, or multiple-choice questions:

- **Situational judgement test (SJT)** Challenging professional situations where applicants judge possible responses

- **Multi-Specialty Recruitment Assessment (MSRA)** A test in two parts—one on professional dilemmas (an SJT) and one involving clinical problem-solving.

Interviews/selection centres (p. 75) Format and how to book slots are communicated via email and/or Oriel. Note: there are no interviews for non-specialized FP jobs.

Portfolio A well-organized portfolio is essential. Guidance is provided on how the specialty wants the physical portfolio (p. 86) to be arranged.

Interviews and selection centres

Each specialty has its own format for face-to-face assessments but may include the following:

- **Portfolio station** Discussion of career to date, professional development and values, and career intentions
- **Presentation station** Short presentation on a specialty-specific topic followed by Q&A
- **Clinical station** Discussion of diagnosis and clinical management of a patient
- **Task-orientated station** Demonstrating skills relevant to the specialty, e.g. data interpretation, suturing
- **Ethics station** Discussion of the ethical considerations of a patient or professional scenario
- **Management and leadership station** Discussion of professional and safety considerations of a clinical or non-clinical scenario
- **Simulated tasks** Actors playing a part, e.g. as a colleague, patient, or relative, with the candidate interacting in a professional capacity
- **Group discussion** Groups of candidates discuss clinical or non-clinical situations, demonstrating qualities such as teamworking and leadership.

Interviews often use standardized questions and mark schemes, based around the qualities described in the person specification (p. 83). Global scores have several components, e.g.:

- Communication skills
- Preparedness and enthusiasm
- Portfolio structure and content
- Professionalism
- Suitability for post
- Knowledge and problem-solving.

Marks may be lost by displaying 'negative' attributes, e.g. requiring prompts to answers, missing or misinterpreting important information, or giving answers not in line with GMC standards or *Good Medical Practice*.

Preparation

Knowing what to expect makes it easier to be relaxed and make a favourable impression:

- Thoroughly read all guidance documents to ensure the format is fully understood.
- Talk to doctors who have previously been through the process. Ask them about the format and questions asked. Senior colleagues may be interviewers and give an insider's view.
- Consider what qualities are being assessed. These are stated in the person specification (p. 83) and GMC guidance, e.g. *Good Medical Practice*.
- Know your portfolio inside out. Find examples demonstrating attributes detailed in the person specification, e.g. teamworking, reflective practice, leadership, etc., and how your experiences helped you develop.
- Practise interview techniques with peers and senior colleagues to improve style and familiarity with common questions.

What to take The recruitment office will instruct which documents to bring to confirm eligibility, e.g. passport, GMC certificate, proof of visa/work permit status, proof of address, etc. An up-to-date portfolio (p. 86) is usually also required.

What to wear Appearance has a huge impact at interviews. Aim to appear as a safe, responsible, and professional doctor who deserves to be trained in the specialty of the interviewer(s). Candidates should dress smartly, e.g. a suit and tie, trousers/skirt suit, or a smart top and trousers/skirt, but be comfortable.

On the day

Interviewers are nearly all doctors and, on the whole, friendly and trying to help maximize interviewees' potential. Try to relax and be yourself. Take time to think about the answers, rather than say the first thought that occurs. If in doubt, ask the interviewer to repeat the question. Keep answers succinct and to the point. Interviewers are looking for doctors with whom they want to work, so appearing enthusiastic and approachable gives a good impression.

What happens next?

Overall assessment scores are used to rank candidates. Applicants are then matched to jobs, based on their previously stated preferences. The highest scoring candidate will get their first-choice post. The second highest will get their first-choice post unless this was the same as the highest-scoring candidate—in this case, they will get their second-choice job, and so on. Those not scoring highly enough to be allocated a job are placed on a reserve list. There is a set time period for accepting or rejecting posts. In this time, candidates can 'up-grade' to a post they ranked higher if someone who was originally offered that post rejects it.

And if you don't get a job ...

It's relatively common not to be offered a job after a round of applications. This may be a shock and can be distressing, but it is vital to reflect and consider why the application was unsuccessful, e.g.:

- Not meeting the eligibility criteria—check the person specification (p. 83) carefully
- Not preferencing sufficient jobs on the application form
- Applying to competitive specialties/regions
- Lack of experience or CV points
- Poor performance in assessments—review feedback carefully.

Improving the CV Not being invited to interviews suggests the need to gain additional points for shortlisting. Time between rounds can be used to follow the suggestions on p. 83.

Improving interview/selection centre performance Face-to-face assessments are a brief chance to make a good impression. Practice and an understanding of the format and re-quired standard are important. Reflect on feedback after an unsuccessful interview. A poorly or incorrectly presented portfolio is likely to irritate interviewers and lose marks.

> It's possible to be deemed 'unappointable' following an interview/selection centre. Unappointable candidates may have: (1) failed to gain a set minimum number of marks; and/or (2) demonstrated a serious lack of clinical or professional knowledge (including over-exaggerating or lying about achievements or putting confidential information in their portfolio).

Further application rounds Some, but not all, specialties run two rounds of applications each year. Core and run-through training applications run from November to March for jobs starting in August. Higher specialty training (HST) applications run from January to April for August to October starts. A second round of applications follows each window by a few months.
Not getting a training job the first time is rarely a disaster and can provide opportunities to gain additional experience:

- **Clinical fellow posts** Fixed-term, non-training posts, usually for 6–12 months, to pro-vide clinical cover for a service or department. They give clinical experience similar to trainees and some may be combined with protected time to develop teaching, lead-ership, or research skills. There is no shortage of these posts across the country, and some may be 'created' for the right applicant. Look on NHS Jobs (https://www.jobs.nhs.uk) and Trust websites, and speak to consultants in departments of interest.
- **Time out** Use the time to work in different countries or travel, making sure you gain relevant experience (even if not strictly clinical) to justify the career break.
- **Research jobs** These offer unique insights into a specialty and look good on the CV. Find roles at NHS Jobs, and speak to heads of departments in hospitals or research institutions.
- **Locuming** Pays the bills, but not always useful as training. Prolonged locuming rarely looks good on a CV, unless the time was also used to do something else 'worthwhile', e.g. audits, research, sitting exams, exploring other interests/careers.

Competition for CT1/ST1 applications

Health Education England (HEE) (https://www.hee.nhs.uk) publishes figures on UK-wide competition for training in each specialty at CT1/ST1 level[1]. Table 4.1 summarizes these figures for Round 1 applications in 2019, and competition ratios in 2018 for comparison.

Competition ratios change year-on-year; Table 4.1 acts only as a guide. It is also worth remembering that some applicants will be deemed ineligible for longlisting (p. 73), and some will apply for more than one specialty. In 2017, just over 46% of applicants applied for two or more specialties[2].

Competition varies not only between specialty, but also between regions; some are significantly more oversubscribed than others. Taking internal medicine training (IMT) and acute care common stem–acute medicine (ACCS-AM) as an example, in 2019, 97% of posts in London were filled in the first recruitment round, compared to 44% of posts in the Peninsula region (South West England).[3] However, practically all posts across the UK were filled following Round 2 applications.

Clearly there are vast differences in the number of posts available in each specialty, which is an important consideration when applying. Although the actual number of posts changes each year, fewer available jobs are likely to make a specialty more competitive. Also, not all specialties necessarily have posts in every region, meaning applicants may have to be flexible about where they train if they are set on a particular career path.

The key message from these figures is that medicine is competitive and in some specialties, only the 'best', or best prepared, will get their first choice of job. To achieve this, it is necessary to have above-average achievements (p. 83), a good CV (p. 85), a well-written application form (p. 73), and polished skills for face-to-face assessment (p. 75).

[1] Health Education England. Competition ratios 2018 and 2019. Available at: https://specialtytraining.hee.nhs.uk/Competition-Ratios

[2] Health Education England. (2017). 2017—CT1/ST1 competition ratios. Available at: https://specialtytraining.hee.nhs.uk/Competition-Ratios

[3] IMT Recruitment. Fill rate data 14–19: IMT 2019 fill-rates by region. NHS & Royal College of Physicians. Available at: https://www.imtrecruitment.org.uk/documents

Table 4.1 Competition ratios for CT1/ST1 specialty applications in 2018–19

CT1/ST1 specialty	Applications 2019	Available posts 2019	Competition ratio 2019	Competition ratio 2018
Community sexual and reproductive health	83	7	11.86	9.30
Public health medicine	804	86	9.35	9.67
Child and adolescent psychiatry	120	14	8.57	8.55
Cardiothoracic surgery	101	12	8.42	8.18
Neurosurgery	157	24	6.54	4.47
Oral and maxillofacial surgery	29	7	4.14	4.38
Clinical radiology	1095	302	3.63	3.75
Ophthalmology	356	110	3.24	3.74
Core surgical training	1896	648	2.93	2.94
Anaesthetics and acute care common stem (ACCS)–anaesthetics	1333	568	2.35	2.46
Emergency medicine and ACCS–emergency medicine	777	363	2.14	1.90
Histopathology	194	93	2.09	1.84
Obstetrics and gynaecology	529	262	2.02	1.86
Core psychiatry training	814	473	1.72	1.48
Internal medicine training and ACCS-acute medicine	2229	1563	1.43	1.50
General practice	5166	3861	1.34	1.33
Paediatrics	564	476	1.18	1.30
Total 2019	**16 247**	**8869**		

Note: no data available for broad-based training or run-through surgical training pilots.

Source: data from Health Education England, on behalf of Northern Ireland Medical and Dental Training Agency, NHS Education for Scotland, and Health Education and Training Wales. Available at: https://specialtytraining.hee.nhs.uk/Competition-Ratios

Competition for ST3/ST4 applications

Health Education England (HEE) (https://www.hee.nhs.uk) also publishes figures on UK-wide competition for specialty training at ST3/4 level[4]. Tables 4.2, 4.3, 4.4, and 4.5 summarize these figures for Round 1 applications in 2019, and competition ratios in 2018 for comparison.

Table 4.2 Competition ratios for ST1 specialty applications for medical specialties in 2018–19

Specialty*	Applications received 2019	Posts available 2019	Competition ratio 2019	Competition ratio 2018
Acute medicine	322	110	2.93	1.96
Allergy	10	2	5.00	11.00
Audiovestibular medicine	7	5	1.40	3.00
Cardiology	426	127	3.35	2.56
Clinical genetics	27	14	1.93	2.69
Clinical neurophysiology	23	7	3.29	1.54
Clinical pharmacology and therapeutics	14	12	1.17	1.00
Combined infection training	144	65	2.22	1.81
Dermatology	132	39	3.38	3.13
Endocrinology and diabetes	234	120	1.95	1.44
Gastroenterology	273	92	2.97	2.51
Genitourinary medicine	20	46	0.43	0.59
Geriatric medicine	248	211	1.18	1.26
Haematology	145	86	1.69	1.60
Immunology	19	6	3.17	2.11
Medical oncology	151	41	3.68	2.20
Medical ophthalmology	12	7	1.71	1.33
Metabolic medicine	12	17	0.71	0.82
Neurology	138	52	2.65	2.63
Nuclear medicine	7	2	3.50	2.67
Occupational medicine	25	9	2.78	2.36
Paediatric cardiology	40	10	4.00	2.77
Palliative medicine	91	24	3.79	2.79
Rehabilitation medicine	23	26	0.88	1.18
Renal medicine	150	66	2.27	1.51
Respiratory medicine	267	101	2.64	2.35
Rheumatology	102	29	3.52	2.40
Sport and exercise medicine	42	14	3.00	2.67
Overall	3104	1340		

* Data not available for aviation and space medicine.

Source: data from Health Education England, on behalf of Northern Ireland Medical and Dental Training Agency, NHS Education for Scotland, and Health Education and Training Wales. Available at: https://specialtytraining.hee.nhs.uk/Competition-Ratios

[4] Health Education England. Competition ratios 2018 and 2019. Available at: https://specialtytraining.hee.nhs.uk/Competition-Ratios

Table 4.3 Competition ratios for ST1 specialty applications for surgical specialties in 2018–19

Specialty	Applications received 2019	Posts available 2019	Competition ratio 2019	Competition ratio 2018
Cardiothoracic surgery	35	7	5.00	3.67
General and vascular surgery	428	198	2.16	1.54
Neurosurgery	21	3	7.00	6.00
Oral and maxillofacial surgery	23	24	0.96	1.40
Otolaryngology (ear, nose, and throat)	136	53	2.57	2.36
Paediatric surgery	41	16	2.56	4.20
Plastic surgery	149	38	3.92	4.19
Trauma and orthopaedics	519	167	3.11	2.88
Urology	141	68	2.07	2.66
Overall	1493	574		

Source: data from Health Education England, on behalf of Northern Ireland Medical and Dental Training Agency, NHS Education for Scotland, and Health Education and Training Wales. Available at: https://specialtytraining.hee.nhs.uk/Competition-Ratios

Table 4.4 Competition ratios for ST1 specialty applications for psychiatry specialties in 2018–19

Specialty	Applications received 2019	Posts available 2019	Competition ratio 2019	Competition ratio 2018
Child and adolescent psychiatry	70	73	0.96	0.77
Forensic psychiatry	35	31	1.13	1.29
General and old age psychiatry	80	72	1.11	1.11
General adult psychiatry	182	184	0.99	1.02
Medical psychotherapy	8	3	2.67	3.00
Old age psychiatry	62	57	1.09	0.79
Psychiatry of intellectual disability	26	58	0.45	0.35
Overall**	463	478		

** Not shown are other dual psychiatric specialties which contributed 14 posts in 2019.

Source: data from Health Education England, on behalf of Northern Ireland Medical and Dental Training Agency, NHS Education for Scotland, and Health Education and Training Wales. Available at: https://specialtytraining.hee.nhs.uk/Competition-Ratios

Table 4.5 Competition ratios for ST1 specialty applications for other specialties in 2018–19

Specialty	Applications received 2019	Posts available 2019	Competition ratio 2019	Competition ratio 2018
Anaesthetics	575	377	1.53	1.36
Clinical oncology	135	54	2.50	2.32
Diagnostic neuropathology	5	3	1.67	0.83
Emergency medicine ST3	88	60	1.47	1.10
Emergency medicine ST4	81	57	1.42	1.13
Intensive care medicine	305	171	1.78	1.73
Obstetrics and gynaecology	261	78	3.35	2.84
Paediatric and perinatal pathology	3	4	0.75	Unknown
Paediatrics ST3	123	39	3.15	1.50
Paediatrics ST4	126	57	2.21	1.27

Source: data from Health Education England, on behalf of Northern Ireland Medical and Dental Training Agency, NHS Education for Scotland, and Health Education and Training Wales. Available at: https://specialtytraining.hee. nhs.uk/Competition-Ratios

Many of the same issues affecting competition for jobs at CT1/ ST1 level (p. 78) also apply at ST3/4 level. Therefore, to have the best chance of securing a job in a desired location, it is important to continue maintaining an above-average CV, a logbook (where appropriate), and a portfolio (p. 86), and be active about getting involved in teaching, audits, and research.

▌Staying competitive

Medicine is competitive—getting into medical school is only the start. Doctors must be objective about their CV and experience to progress in their chosen career. All advertised training programmes have a **'person specification'** which specifies: (1) 'eligibility criteria', i.e. the basic requirements to apply; and (2) 'selection criteria' detailing achievements and attributes required and expected of applicants. The below are generic to most jobs, but it is vital to look at the relevant document before applying.

Achievements and qualifications

Medical school can seem arduous and comes with an array of distractions from studying. However, medical school performance and academic achievements comprise 50% of the score used to rank applicants for foundation programme (FP) posts (p. 4). These remain useful for subsequent applications, in some cases even at consultant/GP level.

Intercalated degrees Most undergraduate medical students take intercalated degrees (p. 3). The variety of subjects is vast, so an idea about future career is useful. Intercalated degrees score points in applications (equivalent to degrees completed before medical school), usually with more points if awarded first class honours.

Postgraduate qualifications From low to high status: certificates, diplomas, masters (MSc or equivalent), and doctorates (medical doctorates (MD) and PhDs). Time commitment varies; many diplomas/MSc courses can be completed alongside a full-time job (e.g. part time, distance learning). Doctorates are a commitment of at least 2 years full time.

Membership exams (p. 9) These are essential to progress through training. Taking the initial parts early on demonstrates commitment to specialty. Note: all exams have a maximum number of retakes and/or time to pass, so it is important to plan when to take them.

Prizes/awards Any prize looks good on a CV (and is often accompanied by financial reward). Prizes can be local, regional, national, or international. Opportunities include research presentations, prize exams, and essay writing. Some are surprisingly uncompetitive, so be proactive.

Publications Any publication will make an applicant stand out. The ideal is as 'first author' of original research in a peer-reviewed journal. Others include letters, reviews, and case reports. Early in training, a single publication makes a big difference; more are needed in higher-impact journals to maintain advantage as careers progress.

Presentations Research can be submitted to conferences as abstracts. The best are selected for oral presentations. More abstracts are accepted as poster presentations, which attract fewer points but are still worthwhile. The highest-status conferences are international, but there are many national and local ones.

Teaching The importance of doctors as effective teachers is increasingly recognized. Experience and training in teaching (e.g. PG Cert in Medical Education) may score points.

Quality improvement/audit Although a mandatory part of training, demonstration of active and effective participation in improving quality and safety is highly desirable. It is even more useful if it generates a prize, publication, or presentation.

What standard is the competition?

Applicants may be competing with doctors with significant academic experience gained in the UK or overseas, and doctors changing career direction who have accumulated achievements and qualifications. It is highly variable between specialties how much these are 'worth' for applications. For example, applicants to GP training are ranked only on performance in the Multi-Specialty Recruitment Assessment (MSRA) (p. 74) and selection centre (p. 75), not on prior achievements. Most specialties use achievements to longlist candidates and identify who to invite for interview, but once there, it's all still to play for (p. 75).

Demonstrating an interest

The phrase 'commitment to specialty' appears frequently in person specifications and is often discussed at interview. Essentially, this is proof that applicants really want to train in that specialty. This reduces the likelihood of trainees struggling or dropping out and, importantly, applicants demonstrate insight into their potential career. Any experience can influence career choice (for better or worse), so consider the following:

- **Medical student selected study modules** Students choose optional modules from a list of suitable specialties outside the core curriculum. If a specialty of interest is not on the list, then consider approaching a consultant or GP in that field to create a new one.
- **Medical student elective** A unique chance to experience a specialty, travel the world, and have fun! Experience in prestigious institutions can be useful for really competitive specialties. Although the likelihood of performing procedures is greater in developing countries, ensure that there is enough supervision to avoid being put in unsafe situations.
- **Keep a logbook/record** Be proactive in attending clinics, procedures, and operations. Recording anonymized details of interesting cases is an excellent way of developing interest and understanding.
- **Taster weeks** (p. 4) During the FP, usually in F2, trainees can spend a week working in, or observing, a specialty or job of their choice. Be imaginative and look for interesting options; they do not have to be in clinical practice or in the current place of work. It is also an opportunity to talk to people at varying career stages to gain further insight.
- **Research project** An excellent way to show dedication to a specialty whilst developing generic research skills, e.g. statistical analysis, and possibly getting published. Other than in academic posts (p. 23), research usually has to be undertaken alongside specialty training, or for students, during an intercalated degree or as a project in the holidays; financial support or scholarships may be available.
- **Postgraduate qualifications** For example, a diploma or masters in the specialty or a relevant subject. Some can be done alongside medical training, i.e. part time or distance learning.
- **Courses** Rarely contribute to shortlisting points but show commitment to specialty. An increasing variety are available, from teaching to simulation, including Advanced Life Support (ALS) and Advanced Trauma Life Support (ATLS).
- **Societies** Practically all specialties and subspecialties have a Society, Association, Faculty, or Royal College. Contact details for these can be found in relevant career chapters (pp. 110–318). Many have options for student/junior doctor membership, and this is an excellent way to hear about opportunities.
- **Conferences** Information about conferences can be found online, or through trainees or relevant organizations as mentioned earlier. Attending conferences shows commitment and provides an understanding of current and important issues in the specialty.
- **Extracurricular activities** Application forms or interviewers may ask about achievements outside work which demonstrate significant strengths, skills, and determination. Common examples include sporting achievements and charity work.

Getting the balance right

Some doctors spend every waking minute aiming to further their medical career, whilst others choose just to do their job. Neither extreme is wrong and there is a spectrum in between. It is important for trainees to think about where they fit on this spectrum and assess which careers are compatible. An incompatible choice is likely to lead to frustration with colleagues or job applications. Gauge the competitiveness of a specialty and what each 'expects' of its potential trainees; for example, GP applications don't formally ask about academic or altruistic achievements. Other specialties want irrefutable proof of commitment, seemingly since birth.

Curriculum vitae

A curriculum vitae (CV) is a document that summarizes a person from a professional point of view, including education, qualifications, employment, and achievements. They are primarily used during job applications, especially for non-clinical, non-training, and more senior clinical jobs (e.g. consultant/GP posts).

CVs should be kept up-to-date and relevant—employers won't be interested in A-level grades in consultant interviews! Adapt the CV for each post applied for, emphasizing experience relevant to the specialty, job, or location. The CV is an important part of the physical portfolio brought to interview—it is an opportunity to promote yourself to the recruitment panel, giving them better insight into what you can bring to the role. There are plenty of example formats online, but CVs should include:

Personal details Full name, date of birth (± age in brackets), contact details (address, telephone numbers, email), and GMC number. Consider post-nominals, career aspirations, and current post. Senior doctors may want to include a title page with just their name and qualifications.

Memberships List memberships of professional bodies, e.g. MRCP, FRCEM, MRCPsych.

Qualifications List significant qualifications, including doctorates, masters and bachelor's degrees, diplomas, and medical degree ± A-levels. Start with the most recent and include the awarding institution, grade, and date, e.g. 2019, BMedSci (Hons), First Class, University of Manchester.

Awards, prizes, and distinctions List, with the most recent first. Include the name of the award, the reason it was awarded, the awarding institution, and dates. If appropriate, consider categorizing, e.g. international, national, regional, local.

Employment Starting with the most recent, list all relevant jobs; early in medical careers, this may include non-medical jobs and education, e.g. university, secondary school. Include dates, institutions, educational supervisors, and important roles (e.g. managing acute admissions, leadership, teaching).

Publications List, with the most recent first. Provide information in this order: authors (include all authors, but highlight your own name), title, journal title (can be abbreviated to standard journal abbreviations), year, date, volume, and pages. A quick approach is to copy the reference from PubMed (https://pubmed.ncbi.nlm.nih.gov). Those with numerous publications should either display a selection (most impressive/relevant) or put them in categories in order of status: peer-reviewed original research, peer-reviewed reviews, reports, letters, abstracts, textbooks.

Presentations Include presentations at conferences, invited lectures, grand rounds, departmental presentations, and journal clubs. The more senior the applicant, the more selective this list will become.

Audit/quality improvement List these, with the most recent first, including a brief description of the aim, methods, results, conclusions, and impact.

Other sections A CV is a very personal document and it should reflect the applicant. Some people choose to include the following: personal statement, other interests, e.g. hobbies, extracurricular achievements, teaching experience, management experience, research interests, etc. A description of why they are suitable for the job can be included in the CV or a covering letter.

Referees It is usual practice to include two referees, who **must** be asked if they are willing to provide a reference prior to submitting the CV; each referee should be sent a copy of the updated CV. Include the referee's name, position, institution, and contact details. Referees may be different to the ones provided for online applications, which usually specify the most recent clinical and educational supervisors.

Portfolios and ePortfolios

A portfolio is an organized presentation of a doctor's educational, professional, and personal achievements. This includes:

- A copy of the CV
- Degree and exam certificates
- Prizes and awards
- Audits/quality improvement and research
- Publications and posters
- Academic experience, e.g. courses, teaching, logbooks, reflections
- Feedback
- Additional and non-academic achievements.

Hard-copy portfolios are kept in a normal ring-binder; some choose to push the boat out with a leather bound or monogramed version. Whilst first impressions count, it is the content that matters. Keeping an up-to-date and well-organized portfolio avoids the pre-interview panic of trying to work out into which box in your parents' garage you stuffed your BSc certificate. For training jobs, many specialties are prescriptive about how a portfolio must be presented at interview. Failure to do so frustrates interviewers and is likely to lose points.

ePortfolio

In addition to keeping a formal portfolio, all doctors are now expected to maintain an electronic portfolio (ePortfolio). The platform on which this is kept depends on the stage and specialty and there are a number available, e.g. Horus (https://horus.hee.nhs.uk) and the NHS Education for Scotland ePortfolio (https://www.nhseportfolios.org)—formal training programmes will mandate which of the platforms to use. Some may also be used when out of training, usually for a fee. The ePortfolio is intended to collate evidence of the knowledge, skills, and attributes a doctor has attained during a job or stage of training. They are almost universally used during annual appraisals or the annual review of competency progression (ARCP) (p. 95), and occasionally at interviews. Generally, ePortfolios include:

- Personal details
- Details of current and previous posts
- Workplace-based assessments or supervised learning events (p. 5)
- Logbooks, e.g. procedures, operations, clinics
- Teaching records
- Curricular items or competences to be signed off
- Personal reflection, e.g. cases, career goals
- Feedback
- Supervisor meetings and reports.

Sounds easy?

Unfortunately, the majority of trainees are not given protected time to complete their ePortfolio and it must therefore be squeezed between clinical duties or done in their own time. It is therefore very easy, but ill-advised, to abandon it until just before the ARCP which determines if a trainee can progress, e.g. to the next training year, or complete training. Due to the frequent redesign and redevelopment of both ePortfolio platforms and specialty curricula, it is not uncommon for supervisors (as well as trainees) to be unfamiliar with the layout and even the content of an ePortfolio.

If used well, the ePortfolio is invaluable for both learning, e.g. gaining feedback, reflecting, etc., and demonstrating skills and knowledge. Sadly, many trainees and supervisors miss the point, seeing it as a mainly (pointless) tick-box exercise. However, resistance is futile—the ePortfolio is here to stay. Furthermore, you will find yourself having to complete a somewhat similar ePortfolio as a consultant, to inform the appraisal and revalidation process, so it is something you can never escape. With a little effort (and often hindsight), it can be a truly useful resource.

Applying for academic training

The recruitment process for academic jobs (p. 23) runs in parallel to mainstream posts but has several important differences. One similarity is that jobs are advertised and applied for via the national recruitment portal Oriel (https://www.oriel.nhs.uk) (p. 73).

Specialized (formerly academic) Foundation Programme

After submitting a mainstream foundation programme (FP) application (p. 72), applicants apply for Specialized Foundation Programme (SFP) jobs in up to two foundation schools (or units of application (UoAs)). Candidates complete separate SFP application forms, unique to each UoA, which ask for further details, e.g. research experience, educational achievements, etc. Each UoA scores applications in its own way, meaning identical answers to 'white-space' questions may be scored differently. Applications are used to shortlist applicants; the highest-scoring candidates are invited to interview (face-to-face or video-call/telephone). The interview score is added to the candidate's academic decile score (p. 4). All candidates must also get a satisfactory situational judgement test (SJT) score. Candidates unsuccessful in getting an SFP post are allocated a standard FP job (p. 4).

Core and higher specialty training

Applications open earlier than non-academic applications. The academic application form has more white-space questions, focusing on research, teaching, prizes, presentations, and publications. In addition to clinical referees, candidates provide academic reference(s), e.g. by supervisors from previous research posts or degrees. The application form is used to shortlist candidates to invite for interview.

Candidates who do not already hold a National Training Number (NTN) (p. 8) in the specialty applied to for academic training must also complete a standard training application form—this asks if they wish to be considered only for academic posts or additionally for non-academic jobs.

Recruitment is organized locally by the relevant deanery/region, rather than nationally. There are set windows for job applications which can be found on Oriel, Health Education England (HEE), and National Institute for Health Research (NIHR) websites. Applications are made individually to available posts and candidates can apply for as many posts as they wish. Each post can be advertised in up to three specialties and across multiple training levels. For example, there may be a single post to which only one candidate will be recruited either in dermatology at ST1, ST2 or ST3 or in public health at ST1. Candidates are therefore potentially competing to be the best applicant across multiple specialties and against more experienced clinicians.

The interview lasts for at least 30 minutes and the format is variable between posts and regions. Some have stations similar to mainstream interviews (p. 75); others have a single interview by a panel. Interviewers will include clinicians, academics, and lay representatives who assess the candidate against the general academic person specification. Academic questions focus on career aspirations, research interests, and potential as a researcher. Candidates must bring a physical portfolio to demonstrate their qualifications and previous experience.

To be appointed, candidates must score highly in the academic interview and get through 'clinical benchmarking'. This means that at some point prior to starting academic training, they must have been through the mainstream interview process in that specialty and deemed 'appointable' (p. 77). Their score in the mainstream interview is not used to rank for academic jobs.

After the interview Successful applicants are given an academic NTN (NTN(A)). There is a second (or even third) round of academic applications later in the year, but each specialty is unlikely to be offered in every region.

▌ Applying from overseas

Requirements

For better or worse, Brexit has happened and as a result the UK immigration system will change. Find up-to-date information in the Visa and Immigration section on https://www.gov.uk, and information specifically for doctors on https://www.nhsemployers.org. This is a complex and evolving area, and the process depends on individual circumstances.

Visas International medical graduates (IMGs) from outside the European Economic Area (EEA) (and possibly in future from within it) need a Tier 2 (general) visa. To apply, a licensed employer provides a certificate of sponsorship and confirms the salary. These statements contribute to a points-based system which includes English language ability. There is a fee of over £400 per visa.

Immigration Post-Brexit immigration requirements for European Union (EU), EEA, and Swiss citizens and other nationals are currently unclear. Currently, doctors on Tier 2 visas who have lived and worked in the UK for over 5 years and earn >£35 800 can apply to work and live in the UK permanently.

General Medical Council (GMC) All doctors must register and obtain a licence from the GMC. Again, the application process depends on the nationality and where the doctor obtained their primary medical qualification (PMQ). It may change after Brexit, but currently:

- **Both a medical degree from and citizenship of an EEA country or Switzerland** Provided the PMQ is on the GMC's approved list (available on the GMC website at https://www.gmc-uk.org), the applicant applies online, then attends an identity check at GMC offices with original documentation, qualifications, evidence of English language capabilities, references, etc.
- **Either a medical degree from and/or a national of any other country** Applicants must demonstrate their medical ability via one of:
  - Professional and Linguistic Assessment Boards (PLAB): a two-part exam—a multiple-choice question (MCQ) exam and a clinical exam
  - Sponsorship by a medical college or pre-approved Trust, department, or fellowship scheme
  - Membership exams (p. 9)
  - Eligibility for admittance to the specialist or GP register (e.g. Certificate of Eligibility for Specialist Registration (CESR)) (p. 21).

From 2023, IMGs who would have sat the PLAB must pass the Medical Licensing Assessment (MLA) which UK graduates will also sit. This sets minimum standards of safe practice, transcending nationality and country of education.

Language Doctors must demonstrate English language proficiency by one of the following: PMQ undertaken in English; a recognized English language test (e.g. International English Language Testing System (IELTS)); or providing a reference from an employer in an English-speaking country.

Types of jobs

Foundation programme (FP) (p. 4) A 2-year internship following medical school. Posts are guaranteed to UK medical graduates, with unfilled places available for IMGs. Applicants need a PMQ accepted by the GMC and written approval from the Dean of the medical school. Those who have completed an internship overseas can apply to stand-alone F2 jobs (p. 4).

Specialty training (p. 7), **and specialty and associate specialists (SAS)** (p. 19) Currently, medical jobs (except in public health) are considered 'shortage occupations', meaning application and allocation for posts are not restricted to, or prioritized for, UK graduates. IMGs eligible to work in the UK can therefore competitively apply to any UK training programme. Applicants will need evidence they have attained FP competencies (not necessarily in the FP) and meet all other entry criteria as detailed in the person specification (p. 83). Further details

can be found in HEE application guidance (https://specialtytraining.hee.nhs.uk/Recruitment/
Application-guidance).

Consultant/GP (pp. 12–13) Doctors trained outside the UK can apply through the CESR
or Certificate of Eligibility for GP Registration (CEGPR) routes (p. 21) to be admitted to the
specialist/GP register. GPs new to the NHS complete an induction and returner scheme
managed by the GP National Recruitment Office (https://gprecruitment.hee.nhs.uk/), and also
need to be on a primary medical performers list.

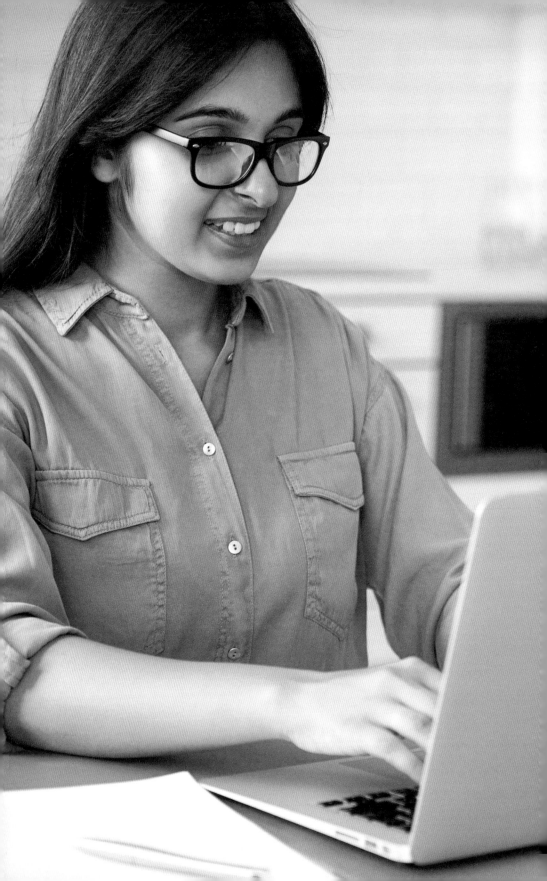

5

Training and working in medical careers

Postgraduate training: Modernising Medical Careers

The postgraduate training system in the UK has undergone three wholesale changes in living memory and numerous more subtle evolutions. Despite appearing in constant flux, many aspects of training remain the same and the overall route to consultant or general practitioner (GP) will remain recognizable in the future.

History

Prior to the Calman reforms of 1996, there was little structure to postgraduate medical training. There were four training grades (pre-registration house officer (PRHO), senior house officer (SHO), registrar, and senior registrar) and the onus was on junior doctors to arrange their next posts at 6-monthly or yearly intervals. Posts could be anywhere in the country, involving multiple applications. Training was based on gaining experience in apprenticeship-type models, with no defined end point. Senior registrars could stay in posts for years, even decades, waiting for the right consultant job.

Structuring training was instigated by the then Chief Medical Officer (CMO) Sir Kenneth Calman. Rotations were standardized and the registrar and senior registrar grades were replaced with a single, time-limited specialist registrar (SpR) grade. Training culminated in a Certificate of Completion of Specialist Training (CCST), with 6 months' grace to find a consultant post. Once accepted on an SpR rotation, training was secure in one region. Training jobs were limited, which unfortunately created a 'lost tribe' of SHO-level doctors waiting for posts. The next CMO Sir Liam Donaldson published 'Unfinished Business' in 2002, highlighting the plight of doctors marking time as SHOs. A scheme to address this by further structuring training was proposed, forming the basis of Modernising Medical Careers (MMC).

Modernising Medical Careers

MMC aimed to streamline training and ensure trainees achieved defined competences rather than just training for a set length of time. It was launched in 2005 with the arrival of the foundation programme (FP) (p. 4). The subsequent introduction of run-through training (p. 7) meant trainees often made decisions on their final specialty far earlier than many felt ready to. This was compounded by the apparent inflexibility of training routes. Competences and their assessments have also been criticized for settling for the minimum standard rather than encouraging doctors to excel.

However, the biggest problem for MMC was the immediate transition to the new recruitment process in August 2007. For potential SpRs, this led to a high number of doctors competing for a limited number of training posts. This perceived unfairness was exacerbated by difficulties with the national electronic application process: the Medical Training Application Service (MTAS). The scheme, used for both FP and specialty training applications, was deeply flawed in terms of selection and shortlisting criteria, professional involvement, and actual delivery. MTAS was consequently abandoned and, after a period of deaneries sorting out allocations locally, was replaced by the Foundation Programme Application System (FPAS). FPAS also had teething issues but formed the prototype for the Oriel portal which is now used (quite successfully) for practically all training programme applications.

In short, MMC was not welcomed by doctors, leading to actual protests, an apology from the Health Secretary at the time, Patricia Hewitt, and ultimately an independent inquiry chaired by Professor Sir John Tooke. The subsequent report published in 2008 encouraged postgraduate medical education to produce the best doctors possible, largely by overhauling governance of training and better defining the responsibilities and expectations of trainees and training organizations.

Postgraduate training: Shape of Training

Shape of Training (SoT) (2013) was an independent review of postgraduate medical education, chaired by Professor Sir David Greenaway. The review built on several recommendations from the *Tooke Report* (2008)—primarily those focused on developing a medical workforce adapted to the UK's ageing and increasingly comorbid population. Additionally, there is currently something of a retention crisis in many specialties, with doctors increasingly taking time out of training, switching pathways, or leaving clinical practice altogether. SoT proposed several recommendations on how to adapt medical training to address these issues, with the principle ones being:

1) To train more doctors able to provide general (rather than specialist) care in a variety of settings
2) To train specialists according to the local needs of the population
3) To better prepare doctors for working in multi-professional teams
4) To increase flexibility in work patterns, specialization, and development of non-clinical skills.

Training

In future, training after the foundation programme (FP) (p. 4) is likely to move into 'broad-based' training programmes involving rotations in groups of similar specialties, e.g. surgical specialties, medical specialties, those related to women's health, etc. Doctors can then develop transferrable skills that can be used in different settings, which also (theoretically) makes switching specialties easier.

Training is expected to take 6–8 years from graduation. For some specialties, this implies reducing the current length of training. Training would only produce generalists in that field; some consultants/general practitioners (GPs) could go on to gain 'credentials' demonstrating their knowledge and skills as specialists or subspecialists. Additionally, within training, doctors will be able to spend up to a year developing non-clinical skills, e.g. education, leadership, management, etc. There will also be greater flexibility for academics to step in and out of clinical training.

Assessment

The current competency-based assessment system means most curricula clearly define specific behaviours, skills, and knowledge trainees need to attain. The aim is for these specifics to be superseded by more overarching generic 'professional capabilities'. Colleges and educational bodies have already begun the process of overhauling curricula to bring them in line with recommendations.

Implementation

Trainees in some specialties, particularly those involving operations and procedures, already find it hard to attain the required experience. Concerns have been raised as to how to achieve this in even less time. SoT suggests training will only be provided in 'high-quality clinical placements' with increased protected training time. As is currently the case, it is difficult to see how these measures will overcome the demands of service provision and the fragmentation of training caused by rotas and limitations on working hours.

Having learnt hard lessons from the disastrous introduction of MMC, SoT also aims to minimize disruption of training adaptations on doctors. Largely this means changes will be phased in and nationally co-ordinated. Changes have started to be implemented, e.g. transition of 2-year core medical training (CMT) to 3-year internal medicine training (IMT)

(p. 44). However, even this is not straightforward, as over half of the current 'medical' specialties will continue to recruit after 2, and not 3, years of IMT.

Predicting how to train a workforce best able to thrive in the future is inevitably tricky; SoT attempts to address several competing interests, e.g. training vs service provision, need for generalists vs need for specialists, flexibility vs structure. Time will tell whether a balance can be struck that suits all parties.

Overseeing education

A vast and complex network of people and organizations oversee, deliver, support, assess, and evaluate training from graduation to Certificate of Completion of Training (CCT) (p. 36). Overviews of their main roles and functions are outlined in the following sections.

The people

Clinical supervisor (CS) A senior clinician (usually consultant or general practitioner (GP)) responsible for overseeing the clinical work of a trainee during a specific placement or rotation. They should provide appropriate training opportunities, supervised learning events (SLEs) (p. 5), constructive feedback, and support to ensure that time spent in the placement is productive and worthwhile. They usually need to complete a report about the trainee's progress at the end of the placement.

Educational supervisor (ES) A senior clinician (usually consultant or GP) responsible for the overall supervision of a trainee's education over one or more placements. The ES may or may not also be the trainee's CS, and the trainee may or may not work with their ES clinically. Either way, the ES should meet regularly with the trainee. The role is complex and requires additional training in supervision. Generally, it involves discussing trainees' learning needs and objectives, using the ePortfolio to assess learning and progression, discussing career decisions, and identifying and supporting trainees who are struggling. They also provide reports, usually towards the end of a training year.

Foundation or training programme director (FPD/TPD) The individual (usually senior consultant/GP) who has responsibility for managing and quality-assuring a training programme on behalf of the deanery (see below). They work with, and support, the head of school and/or the postgraduate dean and those locally responsible for training, e.g. ES, to make sure programmes deliver suitable and effective training. They are involved in reviewing each trainee's development at their annual review of competency progression (ARCP).

> The **ARCP** is the process by which trainees are reviewed on a yearly basis to ensure they are working safely and progressing according to the requirements set out in their curriculum. Most ARCPs are done without the trainee actually being present (called *in absentia*), but trainees should be provided with full details about what is required, e.g. number of SLEs, exams, logbooks, etc., well in advance. The trainee's entire ePortfolio and a self-declaration about their work, including involvement in any complaints or serious incidents, are reviewed. From this, the ARCP panel, which includes the programme director, decides if the trainee is progressing as expected or whether they need additional evidence or more time in training or haven't done enough to progress.

Director of medical education (DME) A senior individual appointed by Trusts or NHS Boards. They take responsibility for ensuring that local postgraduate education is of the high standard required regionally and nationally. They work closely with the postgraduate dean to develop and oversee the wider educational agenda and support supervisors and educators.

Postgraduate dean The individual with overall responsibility for overseeing and managing postgraduate training from foundation programme (FP) to completion of specialty training in a specified region (i.e. the deanery or an office of a public body, e.g. Health Education England (HEE)). They work with a large team, DMEs, and programme directors to ensure programmes are delivered according to General Medical Council (GMC)-approved curricula.

The places

Training occurs in workplaces appropriate for doctors to develop the knowledge and skills they need according to their curriculum. Some of the key organizations that oversee training are outlined below—there are some variations between regions and the devolved nations.

Deaneries Successful applicants to a training programme are allocated to a specified geographical region encompassing one or more Trusts/organizations. The name of the body responsible for managing and delivering postgraduate training across each region has been rebranded several times over the years. Usually it is referred to as 'the deanery', e.g. North Western deanery. Other names include local offices of **HEE**—a non-departmental body supporting healthcare training on a national level—or **Local Education Training Boards (LETBs)**. Check which hospitals, practices, and/or workplaces are covered by each deanery (which may also differ between specialties) before submitting preferences during the application process.

Foundation schools Are not places per se, but groups which bring together separate institutions to deliver FP training in a defined geographical area. They include medical schools, local Trusts, and other organizations such as GPs and deaneries. Details of each foundation school and its associated medical school(s) and training locations can be found at https://foundationprogramme.nhs.uk.

Specialty schools Similar to foundation schools, specialty schools are not physical places, but groups with oversight of training in a specialty or group of related specialties in one or more deaneries. They are led by a Head of School who works closely with TPDs, local supervisors, and training committees, as well as relevant Royal Colleges and Faculties. Their role is to manage and deliver training and provide learning opportunities on a regional level. Trainees accepting an offer for specialty training in a specific region automatically become members of the relevant specialty school.

Royal Colleges and Faculties These are professional bodies responsible for training in one or more specialties and/or subspecialties. They are involved in developing curricula and setting standards for assessments (e.g. membership exams) (p. 9), which are then approved by the GMC. They may incorporate, or be advised by, a training board, e.g. the Joint Royal College of Physicians Training Board (JRCPTB), Joint Committee on Surgical Training (JCST), etc. Together, they help design and review curricula and assessments in line with GMC standards, and provide support and guidance to doctors in training. Most are members of the Academy of Medical Royal Colleges (AoMRC) which supports co-ordination across Royal Colleges and Faculties in areas such as setting training standards.

The **General Medical Council (GMC)** became responsible for postgraduate medical education in 2008, taking over from a non-departmental public body called the Postgraduate Medical Education and Training Board (PMETB). It sets standards of training and regularly assesses if these are being met locally and nationally. The GMC primarily functions to maintain the definitive list of doctors registered to practise in the UK. As part of this function, it licenses and revalidates all practising doctors at regular intervals; during training, revalidation occurs as part of ARCP. After CCT, doctors need to revalidate every 5 years. Finally, the GMC sets standards of good medical practice and doctors who fall foul of these can be referred to them. In the most serious cases, doctors may be 'struck off', i.e. removed from the medical register.

Less-than-full-time training

Less-than-full-time training (LTFTT) is on the rise! Contrary to common perception, LTFTT is not limited to only those with young children but is considered for all trainees with 'well-founded individual reasons'. Benefits include more time with children or on other professional activities, support with health problems, and improved work–life balance. Drawbacks include lack of continuity with patients and teams, time constraints, pro rata pay and leave, and longer training time.

Am I eligible?

Those who have young children (until 18 years) or other caring responsibilities or are unable to work full time for health reasons are automatically eligible for LTFTT under a 'Category 1' application.

'Category 2' applications cover other reasons for wanting to train flexibly, and usually involve training opportunities outside medicine, e.g. sports, arts, or other short-term extraordinary responsibilities, e.g. being part of a national committee or training for a religious commitment. Research is not included in this category. Category 2 applications will be considered, but approval is not automatic and is dependent on the needs of the specialty in which the individual is training, and are granted for a year at a time.

More recently, 'Category 3' LTFTT has been piloted, e.g. in emergency medicine, where trainees can choose to work at 50%, 60%, or 80% of full time on the basis of personal choice and needs. Following successful negotiations between the British Medical Association (BMA) and Health Education England (HEE) and NHS Employers, Category 3 is likely to be applicable for all doctors in training in the near future.

How do I apply?

The first step is contacting your foundation programme director (FPD) or training programme director (TPD) to discuss your application. You are then asked to complete an application form, which varies by region. Three months' notice should be given to allow for rota planning. If less notice is given, the application will still be considered, but trainees may have to wait until the next rotation date or until the trust can accommodate the request. Applications to train less than full time (LTFT) due to health reasons will be considered on a case-by-case basis.

What working patterns are available?

LTFT trainees are usually expected to work between 50% (2.5 days) and 80% (4 days) of the full-time equivalent. Fewer sessions are considered in exceptional cases and for a limited time only. Different combinations suit different trainees and specialties; however, the most common working arrangement is a slot-share, with both trainees working 60% (including overlapping for a day). If no slot-share partner is available, working LTFT in a full-time post will be considered. A supernumerary post will be considered if neither of these options are possible but are only arranged in exceptional circumstances.

On-calls are pro rata equivalent of full-time out-of-hours work as a minimum. Trainees are allowed 100% equivalent of on-calls, provided the hours worked do not exceed 40 per week. Working more than pro rata on-call hours does not reduce the length of training.

How is LTFT pay calculated?

As for full-time trainees, basic pay (p. 99) is supplemented by additional payments for out-of-hours work based on intensity of work and unsocial hours. There are further information and worked examples for LTFTT calculations on the BMA website.

LTFT trainees may wish to locum outside their agreed hours. In 2017, the General Medical Council (GMC) released a statement which removed the historical regulatory barrier to LTFT trainees pursuing locum work. However, permission from the postgraduate dean is still required.

How will working LTFT affect my length of training?

Working LTFT will extend the length of training. Training time is calculated based on the percentage of working time equivalent. For example, a trainee working 60% of sessions in a 24-month training programme should expect to take 40 months to complete the training, subject to completion of competences as assessed at annual review of competency progression (ARCP) (p. 95). However, some specialties (e.g. paediatrics) are competency-based and so trainees may be able to complete their training in the same amount of time as full-time trainees.

How does annual leave work?

Bank holidays, study leave, and annual leave are all calculated on a pro rata basis. If a bank holiday falls on a non-working day, the trainee is entitled to a day in lieu, up to the number of bank holidays in their pro rata allowance. Similarly, if a training day occurs on a non-working day, the trainee may attend and take a day in lieu during their normal working days.

What are the challenges of LTFTT?

There are pros and cons, and understanding the implications of LTFTT is important. Whilst it lessens the workload and allows trainees time away from work, it's not necessarily easier, with significant impact on income, length of training, and experience—reduced presence at work may mean feeling less involved with teams and less valued; LTFT trainees can feel looked down on and feel guilty at 'not pulling their weight'. Their ES may not have experience of supervising an LTFT trainee, and this can impact on the quality of training. Trainees may also have difficulty accessing information about how to apply, and even when in post, it can be difficult getting information about contracts and what to expect from employers. Despite these challenges, LTFTT comes with many benefits, including being able to better balance life and work and, for some, it could mean the difference between continuing to train and not.

How can I get the best out of training LTFT?

Once LTFTT is agreed, start planning. Be proactive about how your rota will work; ensure the rota co-ordinator knows that you are working LTFT and which days you work. Organize your working pattern to make the most of the training opportunities, e.g. regular teaching sessions, procedure lists. Contact your ES in advance of starting your post. For those who have not supervised an LTFT trainee before, there is a module available on the HEE e-learning website. Contact your Champion of Flexible Training (see below), and consider joining an online forum to discuss issues with other LTFT trainees and get support.

How to get help

- Most trusts/organizations have a Champion of Flexible Training. Their role is to identify all LTFT trainees in their organization, support their ES, and oversee organizational policy related to LTFTT. They can be contacted for advice and support.
- Each training region also has guidance for trainees planning to work, or working, LTFT which can be accessed on their individual websites.
- BMA and BMA LTFT Forum—extensive information and support for LTFT trainees. Available at: https://www.bma.org.uk/collective-voice/committees/junior-doctors-committee/ltft-forum
- Joint rostering guidance—BMA/NHS Employers. Available at: https://www.bma.org.uk/advice/employment/contracts/junior-doctor-contract/rostering-guidance/roster-design-for-ltft-doctors

▌Doctors' pay

Doctors in training

After a well-publicized 'heated debate' between junior doctors and the Department of Health (DoH), a controversial new contract was implemented in England in 2016. Further amendments were summarized in the 2018 'junior doctor contract refresh'. Scotland, Wales, and Northern Ireland currently remain on the 'old' 2002 contract. Full details can be found at https://www.nhsemployers.org and https://www.bma.org.uk.

Basic pay This is the annual salary before supplements are added (Table 5.1) and tax, student loan, etc. are deducted.

Basic pay under the 2002 contract increases annually, even if trainees are out of programme (OOP) (p. 101). Under the 2016 contract, pay progression is determined by stage of training. This sounds fair until considering less-than-full-time training (LTFTT) (p. 97) or switching careers (p. 22) where pay may stagnate or even reduce.

Supplements

Banding Under the 2002 contract, doctors are paid a 'banding' supplement (usually 40–50% of basic pay), depending on the intensity or frequency of work during antisocial hours. Under the 2016 contract, payment for working antisocial hours is in a collection of separate supplements. In theory, this should be fairer. In reality, most aren't sure what they should be paid, and sometimes neither are Human Resources.

Pay premia (2016 contract) 'Bonuses' of varying amounts awarded to train in oral and maxillofacial surgery (OMFS), general practice (GP), and hard-to-fill specialties, e.g. emergency medicine, psychiatry. Clinical academics may receive pay premia after completing higher degrees. London doctors get a (tiny) supplement to cover higher living costs.

The 2016 contract has measures aiming to ensure doctors are paid for all hours worked:

- **Exception reporting** Doctors submit a formal report when they work beyond contracted hours to receive additional payment or time off in lieu.
- **Rota compliance** Rotas must obey rules about the maximum number of consecutive shifts, hours worked in a week, and minimum periods between shifts.
- **Guardian of Safe Working Hours** Trusts must appoint a named person responsible for overseeing trainees' working patterns.

Locum work Historically, this was extremely lucrative. However, caps have been introduced to limit hourly rates. Trainees must still comply with rules on maximum number of hours and consecutive shifts worked.

Table 5.1 Basic pay for doctors in training

Grade	Basic pay	
	2002 contract	2016 contract
FY1 (NP1)	£23 691–28 899	£28 243
FY2 (NP2)	£31 866–36 034	£32 691
ST/CT1–3 (NP3)	£33 884–44 828	£38 693
ST3–8 (NP3–5)	£33 884–53 280	£49 036–52 036

NP, nodal point.

Source: data from NHS Employers, available at https://www.nhsemployers.org/.
Data is correct at the time of writing.

LTFTT (p. 97) Pay is pro rata, i.e. a percentage of the full-time salary proportionally equivalent to the percentage of full-time work. Additionally, LTFT trainees on the 2016 contract receive an annual supplement of £1000.

Post-Certificate of Completion of Training (CCT) (or equivalent) and non-training doctors

Staff grade and **specialty and associate specialist (SAS) doctors** (p. 19) Basic pay ranges from £40 037 to £74 661, depending on skills and experience, and is open to negotiation with employers.

Consultants New consultants can expect a basic salary of around £79 860, increasing to over £100 000 with 19+ years of experience. Pay is calculated in 4-hour blocks called programmed activities (PAs), with a small on-call supplement. Outstanding or long-serving consultants may receive financially lucrative local or national awards.

General practitioners (GPs) As practices are essentially independent businesses, there are no national pay scales for GPs. Minimum salary for a full-time salaried GP (i.e. one employed by a practice) is £58 808, with no upper limit. Partners (GPs who own all or part of the practice) earn more. Like any business, poor performance could significantly reduce pay, though this is uncommon.

Taking time out

Increasingly, junior doctors are taking a break from training or clinical medicine at some point in their careers. In 2018, only 37.7% of F2s progressed straight into core or specialty training[1]. Time out can feel like a risk, but if well considered, it can be a wonderful and life-defining experience. Reasons for a break include:

- Research
- To explore alternative careers (p. 28)
- Voluntary or paid work overseas (p. 103)
- Simply to have a break or travel
- To enjoy family life.

Does a break affect job prospects?

This depends on the nature and duration of the break. The key question is how the break can be justified at interview or on an application form. Application forms usually ask 'do you have any gaps in your employment history of more than 4 weeks' duration?' The answer isn't scored but may raise questions at interview. Observerships, conferences, courses, and publications can be used to show the educational benefit of a break.

A break can enhance job prospects through standard routes (e.g. research or writing up that long-forgotten case report), but also by less objective measures (e.g. developing a well-rounded and personable doctor). Most consultants fully understand the desire to take a break, providing this has a clear and fulfilled objective. A year spent doing ad hoc locums will likely be viewed more negatively. Certain specialties require additional assessments, documentation, or retraining if the career break is prolonged (usually meaning over 3 years).

Along with career impact, there are logistical issues to consider, e.g.:

- Changes in standard of living if income is reduced
- Practical issues if going abroad (p. 103). For example, what happens to the house, belongings, car, etc.?
- Getting a job/place to live after coming back.

When to take a break

Stages in medicine when it is easiest include:

- **Before university—** gap year!
- **After foundation year 2 (F2)** (the popular so-called 'F3 year')*
- **Between core and higher specialty training (HST)***
- **After HST—** although career pressure might be high.

Doctors in training programmes may take time **out of programme (OOP)** for one of four reasons:

1) **Research** (OOPR) maximum of 3 years: may include doing a higher degree, e.g. PhD, MD
2) **Training** (OOPT): GMC-approved posts in the UK or overseas
3) **Experience** (OOPE): non-GMC-approved clinical posts
4) **Career break** (OOPC): non-clinical job, e.g. industry, or for health issues or domestic responsibilities.

Other than for unexpected health or domestic reasons, trainees must give as much notice as possible for OOP activities to be approved by their training programme director (TPD).

---

[1] UK Foundation Programme Office. F2 Career Destination Report 2018. Available at https://foundationprogramme.nhs.uk/resources/reports/
* It may be necessary to be present for interviews for training posts during years out.

Stress and burnout

Medicine is physically and mentally challenging. It's also been a difficult few years for junior doctors and the pressure and workload on the National Health Service (NHS) continue to increase. Symptoms of burnout include exhaustion, pervasive negativity, and loss of concern for people and work. This may lead to depression and mental health problems, including substance abuse. Recognizing burnout early and seeking help and advice are in the best interests of the doctor, patients, and services. Help is available from a variety of sources, including: supervisors, TPDs, mentors, the Professional Support Unit, pastoral support schemes, counsellors, unions, forums, peers, friends, and family. Taking a break from medicine may be a last resort, but essential for the doctor's well-being.

Working abroad

There are numerous opportunities to work or volunteer overseas, and many find the experience personally and professionally rewarding. Plan well in advance as there are multiple aspects to consider.

Registration and immigration

Doctors practising in any country must register with the appropriate regulatory body. Registration can be a lengthy process and may differ at regional and national levels. Check in advance what documents are required, e.g. visa, job offer, General Medical Council (GMC) letter of good standing, certificates, etc., including certified transcriptions.

Inside the European Economic Area (EEA) The departure of the UK from the European Union (EU) and EEA is likely to bring changes to how UK doctors register. Doctors who are citizens of EEA member states are entitled to full registration in any other member state, provided that's where they completed their medical degree. At time of writing, Brexit negotiations are ongoing, but in future, UK doctors may need additional exams, visas, or registrations.

Outside the EEA Requirements for registration and additional exams or qualifications vary by nation and depend on the duration and type of work (e.g. volunteering, observership, research, clinical practice). Some countries require language exams; even fluent doctors often need experience of the local dialect.

Immigration A complex issue which may also change after Brexit. Check requirements with the relevant high commission or embassy—a tourist visa is not sufficient for work and it is difficult to switch visas after entering a country. If relevant, also check arrangements for travelling with family.

Clinical responsibilities and training

The medical system in each country is unique, with training and career structures differing widely. Prior to taking up any post, confirm what is expected before signing the contract, particularly as UK grades may not be equivalent to those in other countries. For doctors in UK training posts, it may be possible to undertake time out of programme (OOP) (p. 101) overseas, e.g. for research or (sub)specialist experience. For posts overseas to count towards the Certificate of Completion of Training (CCT) (p. 36), prospective approval by the GMC and/or deanery and relevant training board is required.

Medical indemnity Different or additional cover may be required overseas, so check with your indemnity provider before travelling. Legal practice also differs significantly from the UK and it is also worth considering the legal and professional risk of practice overseas.

GMC registration Resigning from the UK register may save money but can mean difficulties re-registering on return to the UK. It is nearly always inadvisable to let registration lapse, but discuss the options with the GMC before leaving.

Finances Check any job offer and contract carefully for how much, how, and when you'll be paid or reimbursed. In addition, consider accommodation, including renting and mortgages, taxes (home and away), living costs, insurance, and pensions.

Finding a job

Foundation year 1 (F1) nearly always has to be done in the UK. Foundation year 2 (F2) in some foundation schools can take place overseas, but only with prospective approval, which can take months to obtain. For more senior doctors, working in low-resource settings and in humanitarian crises can be mutually beneficial for the doctor and the local community. Check medical volunteering websites, e.g. Médecins Sans Frontières (MSF) (p. 222) and Volunteer Services Overseas (VSO) (p. 318), for opportunities and clinical requirements. Word of mouth, recruitment websites, and social media are excellent ways to find work and provide first-hand advice on practical and professional issues.

▌ Discrimination

Discrimination means making distinctions among people, e.g. choosing among doctors based on their qualities. Some forms of discrimination are allowed and even encouraged, e.g. a doctor being chosen for a job based on merit (clinical, academic, etc.). However, many negative forms are unfair, and even illegal. This includes discrimination based on gender, race, pregnancy, disability, religion, sexual orientation, or age, unless there is a justification (e.g. a disability that prevents job performance despite reasonable support).
   Discrimination can take two forms:

- **Direct**, e.g. not giving someone a job because they are female
- **Indirect**, e.g. an unjustified job requirement making it harder for women to apply or succeed.

Medicine is a competitive career with numerous job applications and exams, and there is ample opportunity for unfair discrimination. Discrimination has historically been widespread, e.g. the 'old boy's network' and prejudiced interviewers. Over time, attitudes and application procedures have changed to significantly reduce discrimination. Additionally, allegations of unfair discrimination are taken extremely seriously. However, it would be unrealistic to think discrimination has been eradicated, e.g. international medical graduates and female doctors are still widely under-represented in senior jobs. Sometimes unfair discrimination is more subtle, but nonetheless harmful, e.g. a white trainee being chosen preferentially or more frequently to attend operating lists than their black colleague. It's very important to challenge behaviour if you think you (or a colleague) are being treated less favourably.

What to do if you experience unfair discrimination

Advice If you believe you have been subjected to unfair discrimination, it is a good idea to discuss the matter with someone you trust before you act, e.g. a colleague, your clinical supervisor (CS) or educational supervisor (ES), mentor, or union, e.g. the British Medical Association (BMA).

   Informal complaint You can complain directly to the person or institution you believe has been unfairly discriminatory. This should be made in writing, so you have a record of the issue—note that this is a serious accusation and should not be made lightly.

   Formal complaint Making a formal complaint will begin a legal process to determine if you have been subject to unfair discrimination. Employment tribunals hear claims from people who think their employer has treated them unlawfully—for more information, see https://www.gov.uk/courts-tribunals/employment-tribunal.

Harassment and bullying

Harassment is intimidating, aggressive, or threatening behaviour based on specific characteristic(s) of the victim (e.g. race, gender, sexual orientation, disability, etc.), causing distress, humiliation, or embarrassment. When repetitive, this is bullying, which also occurs without a discriminating cause. Either behaviour may be verbal, physical, or psychological. Acknowledging harassment or bullying can be difficult and it takes courage to raise the issue. The main options for dealing with this are:

- Talking to a colleague, senior, ES, or union
- Confronting the person and asking them to stop behaving in this manner
- Making a written complaint to the member of staff's immediate manager.

Doctors are occasionally subjected to harassment or bullying (and rarely violence, including physical assault and verbal abuse) from members of the public, including patients and families. Do not stay in a situation which makes you feel unsafe, and if necessary, get immediate assistance, e.g. from the security team. Speak to senior staff, e.g. senior doctors, matrons, as soon as possible—the NHS has a 'zero tolerance attitude' towards violence against staff. Workplaces have policies and procedures on how to minimize risk, and report it if staff are affected.

Women in medicine

Increasing numbers of women have gone to medical school over recent decades and now around 50% of doctors are, or identify as, female. However, there is significant variation in the proportion of women at different career stages and between specialties. Around 55–60% of general practitioners (GPs) (p. 13) are women, but they are less likely to be in permanent or management roles. A lower proportion of hospital consultants are women, particularly in surgical specialties, but increasingly trainees are female. Several changes have facilitated the progression and retention of women in medical careers. These include removing the requirement for GPs to work out-of-hours, introduction of the European Working Time Directive (EWTD) limiting work to 48 hours a week, and increasing support for flexible and less-than-full-time (LTFT) work.

Sexism towards women

This can take many forms, including male counterparts being offered more training opportunities, unwanted comments about appearance, and even sexual harassment. Female doctors are frequently mistaken for nurses, allied health professionals, or more junior doctors, particularly when a male professional (not necessarily a doctor) is present. Sadly, it is still not unusual to feel a sense of mistrust develop when a patient realizes the woman taking consent is actually going to be doing the operating. As with all professionals, it is important for women to clearly state their role when speaking to patients and colleagues, which reduces confusion and helps reinforce that not all doctors are men. Over time, as a critical mass of female doctors is reached, and as sexist behaviour is increasingly called out, attitudes and perceptions should change. Some groups are working hard to support female doctors, particularly to redress the lack of women in high-profile, academic, and management positions, including:

- The Medical Women's Federation. Tel: 020 7387 7765. Web: https://www.medical womensfederation.org.uk Twitter: @medicalwomenuk
- Women in Surgery (WinS)—Royal College of Surgeons of England. Web: https://www. rcseng.ac.uk/careers-in-surgery/trainees/foundation-and-core-trainees/women-in-surgery Twitter: @WomenSurgeonsUK
- Women Speakers in Healthcare (WSH). Web: https://www.womenspeakersinhealthcare. co.uk Email: womenspeakersHC@gmail.com Twitter: @womenspeakersHC

Pregnancy and childcare

Pregnancy Occupational health should undertake a risk assessment of the doctor's workplace to identify and mitigate risks to the woman and baby. This may include modifying their role or reducing the frequency of on-calls and night shifts.

Maternity leave This can be taken for up to 52 weeks, starting any time after the 29th week of pregnancy. Discuss the dates for maternity leave with supervisors/employers well in advance (but for obvious reasons, ideally after the first trimester). Employees who have worked in the NHS continuously for at least 1 year are entitled to NHS maternity pay. This is up to 8 weeks full pay, 18 weeks half-pay, then 13 weeks statutory maternity pay or maternity allowance. The final 13 weeks is unpaid.

Returning to work There are courses specifically to help doctors return to work after a break, e.g. the Supported Return to Training (SuppoRTT) programme (Health Education England (HEE)) and the GP Induction and Refresher Scheme. Consider practical issues such as breastfeeding (facilities to express breast milk and freeze it to take home should be available).

Childcare Doctors usually earn enough to pay for part-time childcare, although this is often expensive, particularly at evenings and weekends. If planning to work LTFT, the reduction in pay also needs to be considered. Some workplaces have a crèche or day care on site, but waiting lists are often long.

LTFT training Caring responsibilities, including for childcare, are classed as Category 1 applications, which make doctors automatically eligible to train LTFT (p. 97).

Myths debunked

The myth–reality format appears a lot in Chapter 6 (pp. 110–318) to address misconceptions about individual specialties. Many doctors, from those entering medicine to those retiring, have misbeliefs about medical training and careers. A few of the most common are addressed below.

Myth: **If I take a year out of training, I'll never get the job I want.**

Reality: There is an increasing trend towards doctors taking one or more years out of training (p. 101), usually during natural career breaks, e.g. post-foundation year 2 (F2). Higher trainees are often encouraged to undertake out-of-programme (OOP) activities (p. 101). The trick is to demonstrate personal or professional development during the break—new skills, insights, and experiences are usually rewarded in interviews (even if half the time was actually spent on a beach).

Myth: **There are rota gaps everywhere. It'll be easy to get a job where I want, when I want.**

Reality: True—many Trusts are struggling with unfilled places, and for 'hard-to-fill' regions or specialties, this may not be a myth. However, doctors still need to work hard and be competitive, particularly for popular areas and competitive or niche specialties. Most doctors are likely to find plenty of locum shifts available wherever they work.

Myth: **I will only be a success if I complete training and become a general practitioner (GP) or consultant.**

Reality: This really depends on how you measure success. Each doctor's aims will be different and a career which allows fulfilment of these will be rewarding. Many doctors have very successful careers via alternative routes (pp. 18–33), e.g. as specialty and associate specialist (SAS) doctors (p. 19) or long-term locums (p. 202). The career chapters (pp. 110–318) demonstrate a range of careers which do not follow the standard training pathways in which the right people can be highly successful.

Myth: **Once I'm a consultant or GP, I'm stuck in my role. Forever.**

Reality: After training, a doctor is likely to have at least 30 years left of their career. Boredom or burnout can be a risk for those who do not diversify and expand their repertoire as senior clinicians. Many take on portfolio careers (p. 28) or expand their roles, e.g. through teaching, supervision, academia, etc. There is also the option to switch career pathway (p. 22) or to leave medicine altogether (p. 32).

Myth: **Going into medicine will make me rich.**

Reality: Unlikely. More likely comfortably well off. Remember pay scales are set nationally (p. 99), so if you choose to work in big cities, expect to tighten your belt more than those in rural areas. Add to this ever-increasing student debts. There are other rewards such as job security and job satisfaction. Of course, some doctors do become extremely wealthy, and there are a number of careers which lend themselves to private practice and business opportunities.

Myth: **I don't mind working hard in training—after that it's all golf and pharma-sponsored lunches …**

Reality: Ha!

Myth: **Everyone else knows what they want from their job and how to get there.**

Reality: If that were true, this book wouldn't exist …

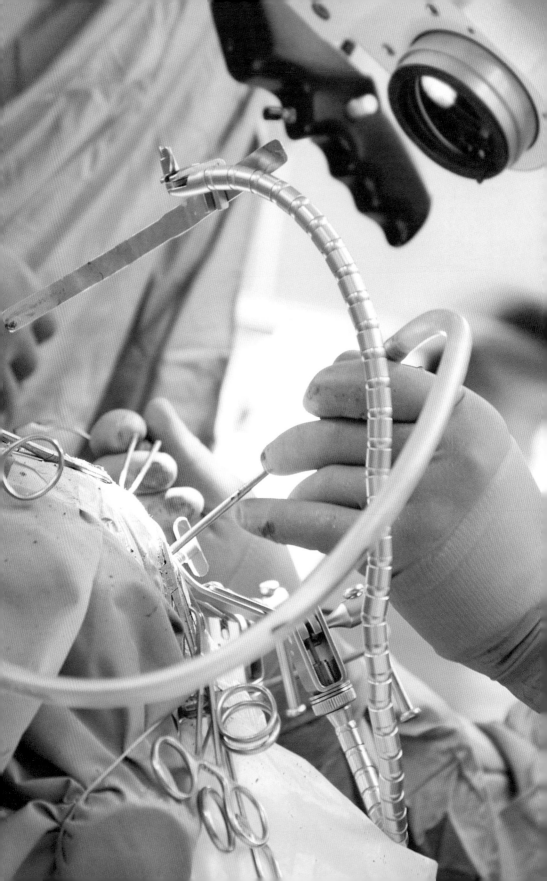

6

Career chapters

Academic medicine

Academic medicine allows doctors to make new and original observations about health and disease, and to change the practice of medicine. Doctors have a privileged position to directly observe and treat diseases. This leads them to recognize patterns and associations, ponder unexplained disease mechanisms, and speculate about novel treatment possibilities. Being equipped with a toolbox of research skills allows the enquiring doctor to test hypotheses of interest that may confirm their ideas. This work might take the form of laboratory work, computational approaches (such as artificial intelligence), or clinical trials. Results will usually be published in a peer-reviewed journal and could lead to a change in clinical practice or policy. Making any contribution to this process can be immensely rewarding.

The patients

A research career is usually developed alongside clinical practice, which can be in any specialty or subspecialty. Clinical contact is essential to identify areas for potential research and its practical application. The 'patients' in research are generally those taking part in a trial or study, either because they are healthy, e.g. control participants, or because they have a condition, medical history, or symptoms relevant to the research.

The work

Academic work usually takes place alongside clinical practice and can occupy 50%+ of the working week. Academic clinicians train in both their specialty and research skills, usually undertaking an additional research degree (e.g. MD or PhD). This develops academic skills for their particular line of research; for example, a dementia researcher might develop in-depth knowledge of brain imaging, whereas a haematologist might focus on laboratory skills. Generic skills will form part of this training: appraisal of scientific publications; data interpretation; and statistical analysis. It is essential that academics are effective communicators—both as scientific writers and speakers—to convey their ideas to funding bodies, colleagues, patients, and the public.

The job

Academic doctors are usually employed by an academic institution (i.e. university) and hold honorary contracts with the health service. Research activities (and sometimes salary!) are typically funded by a fellowship, grant, or collaboration with industry. The job involves designing and executing scientific experiments, networking, leadership and management skills, and public speaking. Academic doctors spend a lot of time collaborating with other researchers, since research is usually carried out by large teams of people with a vast array of complementary skills. Supervising trainees (typically masters or PhD students) is key.

Extras

There is scope for diversification within academic medicine. Academic clinicians may sit on boards which influence strategy. Some might move into industry where they can develop therapies, although this is now also possible through charity and publicly funded drug discovery units. In reality, many have a patchwork of different activities that span different sectors, leading to a diverse and fulfilling career.

For further information

The Academy of Medical Sciences. Tel: 020 3141 3200. Web: https://acmedsci.ac.uk
Email: info@acmedsci.ac.uk Twitter: @acmedsci

National Institute for Health Research (NIHR). Web: https://www.nihr.ac.uk Email: enquiries@nihr.ac.uk Twitter: @NIHRresearch

---

A day in the life ...

08:00 Read journal papers over breakfast

09:00 Assessment of a research participant, including a lumbar puncture required for the study

11:00 Attend a lecture on colleagues' potentially ground-breaking work

13:00 Outpatient clinic

18:00 Skype call with an international collaborator to review progress and talk about strategies to manage problems in a current project

19:00 Home time

22:00 Revise a scientific manuscript based on comments from peer review, or read a PhD student's essay

Myth	Over-ambitious know-it-alls cogitating in ivory towers.
Reality	Medicine is an academic career; it's a privilege to use clinical and academic skills to further knowledge and help patients on a wider scale.
Personality	Highly motivated and competitive risk-taker. Resilient. Versatile. Self-disciplined.
Best aspects	Autonomy. Fast-paced; continuous stimulation. Scope for creative thought. Varied activities from bedside to bench. Teamworking with exceptional individuals. Satisfaction when long-term research projects reach fruition. Opportunity to travel.
Worst aspects	Failure is a core feature; can be extremely uncomfortable for those who excelled in all previous endeavours. Less patient contact. Grant funding is precarious and uncertain. Training is long and may require relocation.
Route	Academic pathways are virtually unique to the individual. Academic training posts (p. 23) are available from foundation to registrar level but are not essential for an academic career. Exams: membership exams and higher degrees (MD/PhD).
Locations	Teaching hospitals; universities.

Life					Work
Quiet On-call					Busy On-call
Boredom					Burnout
Uncompetitive					Competitive
Low salary					High salary

Academic surgery

Academic surgery is the pursuit of advancement and excellence in surgical indications, techniques, and outcomes. It is a multidisciplinary field with interaction between scientists and surgeons—a fusion of basic science and clinical research. There are various training schemes (e.g. those funded by the National Institute for Health Research (NIHR)) in all surgical disciplines nationwide—for foundation doctors, core trainees, and specialty trainees.

The patients

Patients are as described in the core surgical specialty, e.g. plastic surgery, neurosurgery, vascular surgery. Academic surgeons have interests which align with specific aspects of their surgical discipline and these typically evolve during surgical and academic training. Interaction and engagement with patients and family support groups are imperative to realize the clinical significance of research and how it benefits patients.

The work

Academic surgery involves training in both fundamental aspects of health research and surgery, with the ultimate aim of acquiring a higher degree (PhD/MD), alongside specialist training. The NIHR provides a comprehensive scheme of training fellowships for aspiring academic surgeons in foundation and specialty training years. NIHR fellowships allow protected flexible research time during clinical training. Furthermore, NIHR training programmes have built-in formal postgraduate education, as well as training in presentation skills, grant writing, and networking opportunities. Clinical surgical training occurs in parallel within the chosen core specialty.

The job

Academic surgery is usually based in university hospitals within clinical centres of excellence. Academic posts vary with regard to clinical commitments, depending on the individual's choice and the relative demands of the scientific and clinical workloads. During training, achieving a balance which enables the acquisition of both skill sets can be challenging, but with flexibility and protected research time, success is usually possible. Both research and clinical aspects require commitment to teamwork, with close liaison between clinical and academic departments. Inpatients/outpatients and on-call commitments are as per the chosen surgical discipline.

Extras

There is enormous potential for clinical and laboratory research in surgery. For decades, surgery has been considered an art, sometimes at the expense of conducting science. A focus on academic surgery with these NIHR-funded posts has stimulated a tremendous effort from surgeons of all disciplines to engage with academic activities.

For further information

National Institute for Health Research (NIHR). Web: https://www.nihr.ac.uk Email: enquiries@nihr.ac.uk Twitter: @NIHRresearch

Society of Academic and Research Surgery. Web: http://surgicalresearch.org.uk Twitter: @SocSARS

A day in the life ...

07:30   Handover from night doctors

08:00   Inpatient ward round, review tests, prepare patients for surgery

09:00   Theatre list starts

12:00   Review patients postoperatively, finish notes, and hand over to clinical colleagues

12:30   Meeting in the Surgical Trials Unit with a statistician, a methodologist, and members of the research steering group about designing a randomized trial

13:30   Analyse data and draft a publication from a recently concluded study

15:30   Meeting with medical students about a research project they are undertaking

16:00   Teleconference with colleagues in engineering about developing a new surgical device

17:30   Home

Myth	Surgical academics are mythical creatures like unicorns.
Reality	The perfect blend of medical science and bespoke surgery. Demanding clinical work. Long training. Very rewarding work.
Personality	Resilient, adaptable, and compassionate.
Best aspects	Rewarding in both clinical and academic aspects. Pushing the frontiers in surgery; the opportunity to work with pioneering surgeons and scientists; the possibility to make a real advance and improve global healthcare.
Worst aspects	Long training pathway with scientific and clinical exams/assessments, convincing universities and Trusts to commit to, and support, academic surgery.
Route	Academic training post (p. 23); clinical lecturer or postdoctoral post. University lecturer and finally Professor of Surgery. Possible to transfer to academic career path at any stage in career. Exams: membership exams; higher degree, e.g. MD/PhD.
Locations	Tertiary referral NHS Trusts aligned with university hospitals and centres of clinical and academic excellence.

Life					Work
Quiet On-call					Busy On-call
Boredom					Burnout
Uncompetitive					Competitive
Low salary					High salary

Acute internal medicine

Acute internal medicine (AIM) was established in the early 2000s to provide a modern, more efficient way of managing medical patients during the early phase of their hospital journeys. It acts as a conduit between emergency medicine and more specialized medical care, providing rapid high-quality assessment, diagnostics, and management for the whole breadth of medical problems.

The patients

From the 16-year old on their iPad to the 101-year old on their incontinence pad, AIM sees adult patients of all shapes and guises. This leads to huge variety in the type and severity of conditions encountered, ranging from multi-organ dysfunction to patients with minimal clinical needs who can be managed through specialized ambulatory clinics (or even a polite invitation to go home!). Increasingly, acute physicians are becoming liaison medical opinions for allied non-medical specialties; select surgical patients may be admitted under AIM for pre-surgical optimization. Indeed, helping our surgical colleagues cross the minefield of an ECG, chest X-ray, and patient physiology is highly valuable.

The work

As any medical condition can present itself at any time, the work is extremely varied. Day-to-day duties include reviewing and managing the influx of patients admitted to the acute medical unit (AMU). As patients must be moved or discharged in 48–72 hours, patient turnover is rapid. Acute physicians, in addition to being highly skilled generalists, also select an area of medicine in which to specialize to augment their daily work. This can range from practical skills, e.g. ultrasonography, to managerial or educational interests, to extremely specialized roles, e.g. in toxicology or maternal medicine. Some AMUs have a high dependency area which acts as a conduit between ward-based and intensive care, providing additional nursing and medical input, monitoring, and support.

The job

As AIM is a young specialty, acute physicians are generally good-looking, enthusiastic, and dynamic individuals with a drive for change and a lust to improve processes and patient journeys. This makes AIM extremely enjoyable, with a hugely varied scope of work, wide-ranging opportunities for learning and teaching, and interaction with all other medical specialties; there is always something to look forward to (as well as sometimes something to dread!). Generally, time is divided between the AMU and the ambulatory clinic. There is often provision for non-clinical work, teaching, and specialty pursuits, which may occur outside the hospital environment. Time devoted to these aspects of the job depends upon service requirements and your agreed job description—so make sure you argue your case well!

Extras

Because AIM is such a rich seam of opportunities, any doctor who embarks upon a career in the specialty can make of it whatever they choose. There are academic opportunities in research and teaching. Improving and augmenting patient services or setting up clinics pertaining to an area of specialist interest are possible and highly valued. The current drive for moving healthcare into the community means AIM will be in the vanguard for taking secondary health provision into people's homes and GP surgeries, blending seamlessly with pre-hospital medicine to improve care. Really, with AIM, anything is possible.

For further information

The Society for Acute Medicine (SAM). Web: https://www.acutemedicine.org.uk Twitter @acutemedicine

Joint Royal College of Physicians Training Board (JRCPTB). AIM. Web: https://www. jrcptb.org.uk/specialities/acute-medicine

08:00	Catching up on managerial and rota tasks for managing the AMU
08:30	Handover meeting to discuss patients admitted overnight
09:00	AMU ward round with junior doctors to review patients, decide on treatment plans, and identify patients who can be discharged
12:00	Multidisciplinary meeting with the whole acute team, including bed managers and allied health professionals
13:00	Teaching session with junior doctors on an aspect of acute medicine, both for interest and to help fulfil curriculum requirements
14:00	Specialist hot clinic in the ambulatory care department
16:00	Reviewing new admissions and finalizing their managements plans
18:00	Private reading to ensure skills and knowledge are kept up-to-date

Myth	General dogsbodies running a dumping ground for every patient overstaying their welcome in A&E.
Reality	The knight/knightess in shining armour coming to the rescue of their patients and colleagues alike.
Personality	Short attention spans. Also empathic, rational, logical, and decisive. Able to make decisions rapidly and does not buckle under pressure. Often accompanied by a dry sense of humour.
Best aspects	Enormous variety of cases, meaning every day is different. Abundant clinical and academic opportunities. As an expanding specialty, there are ample job opportunities both at home and internationally.
Worst aspects	High intensity, sometimes with little appreciation from patients due to the high turnover rate. As a new and generalized specialty, colleagues may (wrongly) see it as a soft option.
Route	Either internal medicine training (IMT) (p. 44) or acute care common stem–acute medicine (ACCS-AM) (p. 37), then specialty training in AIM (ST3+). Exams: MRCP; SCE in acute medicine.
Numbers	850 consultants, of whom 35% are women.
Locations	Acute hospitals; normally on an AMU or ambulatory emergency care unit; increasing drive for community-placed care.

Life					Work
Quiet On-call					Busy On-call
Boredom					Burnout
Uncompetitive					Competitive
Low salary					High salary

Allergy

Allergy specialists diagnose and treat a wide range of allergic conditions. If you wanted, you could set up shop in Harley Street to see an endless line of glossy-magazine readers who think they might have a 'gluten allergy' and retire at 40. But that's not why you're here, right? The patients who need your help are the people whose lives are impaired or even threatened by their allergies and intolerances, including children with severe reactions to eating peanuts, bee-keepers who've nearly died after their last sting, asthmatics fighting a losing battle with house dust mites, students failing their exams due to awful hay fever, and patients in urgent need of surgery who had anaphylaxis on the table at the last attempt!

The patients

Adults and children with food allergy, drug allergy, venom allergy, anaphylaxis, angio-oedema, and urticaria; asthmatics, rhinitics (noses, allergic, and non-allergic), chronic rhinosinusitics; allergic fungal disease, eczema, and a good smattering of the weird and wonderful and otherwise unexplained. Patients tend to be young (a given as a paediatric allergist, but also generally the case in adult practice) and in full-time education or work. Once other departments get to know you, you'll not infrequently be asked to see their patients with regard to histories of antibiotic and other drug allergies.

The work

The history really does count. You need to be prepared to take time with patients, ingredient lists, drug charts, anaesthetic charts, and old notes to work out what is relevant and potentially causal. If you like talking with patients and detective work, this is a good specialty for you. Beyond skin testing, there's not a lot of procedural work, although some departments work closely with ENT surgeons in combined rhinology (noses again) clinics, in which case you can learn nasal endoscopy and laryngoscopy. You may also work closely with chest physicians in asthma clinics, so an understanding of lung function tests and chest radiology is useful.

The job

The work is largely outpatient-based, with cases for drug and food provocation testing (because sometimes it's the only way to find out!) seen as inpatient day cases. The hours are good. Currently, training is not combined with general medicine, so dry your eyes as you wave a fond farewell to your last on-call!

Extras

The big extras in Allergy are research and teaching. The few training posts in Allergy are at teaching/university-affiliated hospitals where there is plenty of scope for basic science research into the immunology of allergy and asthma (search out your old lab coat), as well as the chance to be involved in clinical research and learn about running clinical trials. Allergy and asthma both are also the subject of much epidemiological and public health research, particularly the intriguing question of why prevalence has increased so dramatically in the past 50 years. As allergy is so common, people need to know about it—GPs, nurses, paediatricians, dermatologists, ENT surgeons, and respiratory physicians—so you may be in demand to teach and speak at meetings and on training days.

> **For further information**
>
> **British Society of Allergy and Clinical Immunology (BSACI).** Tel: 020 7501 3910. Web: https://www.bsaci.org Twitter: @BSACI_Allergy

09:00 Outpatient clinic: 15 patients with a variety of problems across the spectrum of allergic (and sometimes non-allergic) conditions

13:00 Lunch, dictating letters, answering correspondence

14:00 Departmental meeting: discussion of cases for food and drug provocation tests; discussion of cases for allergen immunotherapy ('desensitization')

15:00 Review of ward patient regarding possible penicillin allergy

16:00 Telephone conference with clinical co-investigators on a trial researching a potential new treatment for rhinosinusitis

17:00 Complete dictation, correspondence

18:00 Bicycle home!

Myth	*Is that a specialty? Can you test me for allergies?*
Reality	Allergic disease is incredibly common, potentially fatal, and often badly managed. You can make a big difference to people's lives.
Personality	Patience, a nose for detective work, acceptance that you work in a Cinderella specialty.
Best aspects	Identifying the cause of anaphylactic reactions, especially unexpected or unusual ones (a silk dress on one occasion!).
Worst aspects	Having to disappoint patients who think that 'allergy' must be the cause of their multiple, unexplainable symptoms or their chronic spontaneous urticaria.
Route	Either internal medicine training (IMT) (p. 44) or acute care common stem–acute medicine (ACCS-AM) (p. 37), then specialty training in allergy (ST3+). Exams: MRCP.
Numbers	Approximately 40 consultants, of whom 60% are women.
Locations	Limited to a few large, usually tertiary centres, including in London, Cambridge, Manchester, Leicester, and Southampton.

Life					Work
Quiet On-call					Busy On-call
Boredom					Burnout
Uncompetitive					Competitive
Low salary					High salary

Anaesthetics

Anaesthesia is a diverse, challenging, and humbling specialty. Anaesthetists take responsibility for maintaining life during critical points in a patient's care, across a variety of hospital and pre-hospital settings. Often highly regarded by their medical and surgical colleagues, the arrival of the anaesthetist at an emergency situation is customarily accompanied by an audible sigh of relief from the rest of the emergency team.

The patients

Anaesthetists must be able to draw on a wide knowledge base and tailor their skills to suit a diverse range of scenarios, from the sick neonate through to the centenarian with a fractured neck of femur. Although the patients can be of any age, most children are managed by specialist paediatric anaesthetists. A relatively large proportion of patients whom the anaesthetist encounters are critically ill and require specialist knowledge and skills to support their airway, breathing, and circulation. Communication skills are important, as patients are often anxious about putting their lives into someone else's hands and it's the anaesthetist's responsibility to allay these fears at preoperative assessment and in the anaesthetic room.

The work

Within anaesthesia, there are many subspecialty fields, including intensive care, resuscitation and trauma, obstetrics, paediatrics, cardiothoracics, and pain medicine. Anaesthetists are expected to undertake a range of practical procedures, and much of the work relies on good manual dexterity, spatial awareness, and ability to work with cutting-edge technology. In surgery, anaesthesia is often likened to flying an aircraft—take-off and landing demand high levels of concentration and precise practical skills to ensure a safe flight. However, during surgery, the anaesthetist must remain focused and be able to identify and respond immediately to changes in physiology and biochemistry.

The job

Most of the work takes place in the operating theatre or intensive care unit (ICU). Anaesthetists may also work in outpatient clinics, e.g. pain, surgical pre-assessment. A career in anaesthesia allows the development of working relationships with many other specialists, including surgeons, physicians, obstetricians, radiologists, and allied healthcare professionals. For a theatre to be efficient and safe, all theatre staff need to work closely as a team.

Extras

Due to the sessional nature of the work, it is possible to fit private practice around NHS work. Additionally, other activities, including teaching, research, management, or subspecialist work, can usually be incorporated into the job plan. Other opportunities, such as medico-legal work and providing expertise at events outside of the usual workplace, are also possible, e.g. sporting and crowd events, expedition medicine, pre-hospital care and helicopter medicine, and repatriation of sick nationals who are currently overseas.

For further information

Royal College of Anaesthetists (RCoA). Tel: 020 7092 1500. Web: https://www.rcoa.ac.uk Email: info@rcoa.ac.uk Twitter: @RCoANews

Association of Anaesthetists. Tel: 020 7631 1650. Web: https://anaesthetists.org/ Twitter: @AAGBI

A day in the life ...

07:15 Arrive on the ward to see the patients on today's operating list

08:15 Theatre briefing to introduce the team and run through the surgical and anaesthetic plans

11:00 Called to theatre 5 to help manage a patient with anaphylaxis

13:00 Return to start the afternoon session only to find the next patient has had lunch

13:15 Go to theatre 2 to do an awake fibreoptic intubation for a patient with a dental abscess who can't open their mouth

14:00 On returning to scheduled theatre, join in with a game of 'hunt the swab' as the instrument count is incorrect

17:00 On-call begins—typically involves covering the ICU, obstetrics and labour ward, or emergency theatres

20:00 Lend a hand in obstetric theatres to administer general anaesthesia for a labouring woman with an umbilical cord prolapse who needs an emergency c-section

20:30 Handover to the night team, and head off for a glass of red

Myth	Becomes physically and/or mentally absent once the patient is asleep. Feels time in theatre is best used on crosswords or sorting the tax return.
Reality	A complex and dynamic specialty that requires an advanced knowledge of physiology and pharmacology, with the ability to identify and manage problems rapidly and effectively.
Personality	Diligent, adaptable, composed, good awareness of the situation and one's own limitations. Able to tolerate surgeons.
Best aspects	High level of one-to-one training, being able to concentrate on one patient at a time, and having the skills and training to intervene in a crisis.
Worst aspects	Having to stay alert despite times of low stimulation, not always finishing on time, and running out of coffee.
Route	Core anaesthetics training (p. 39) or acute care common stem (ACCS)-anaesthetics (p. 37), then ST3 in anaesthetics. Exams: FRCA.
Numbers	7400 consultants, of whom 30% are women.
Locations	Nearly always hospital-based, but also found in the pre-hospital setting. In addition to this, there are opportunities to provide medical cover on expeditions and at public events.

Life					Work
Quiet On-call					Busy On-call
Boredom					Burnout
Uncompetitive					Competitive
Low salary					High salary

Armed Forces: Army

The uniformed and civilian medical and dental personnel from all three services (Army, Royal Navy, and Royal Air Force are known collectively as the *Defence Medical Services* (DMS). The role of the DMS is to promote, protect, restore, and maintain the health of service personnel to ensure that they are ready and medically 'fit for task'. Although training and careers in each of the services are similar, there are a number of roles specific to Army doctors.

The patients

An Army doctor could be part of a team working to provide primary healthcare, rehabilitation, occupational medicine, mental healthcare, or specialist medical care to service personnel in the UK or abroad and, in some circumstances, family dependants of service personnel and other entitled civilians. They may also provide some aspects of healthcare to other countries' personnel overseas, in both permanent military bases and within areas of conflict. Their patients will range from recruits with training or sports injuries to those with severe, life-threatening 'battlefield' injuries, and from humanitarian support and preventative healthcare to dealing with serious infectious disease outbreaks e.g. Ebola. The patients can also be your colleagues—those who also dedicate their lives to the armed forces and to their country, and the potential sacrifices that this may entail.

The work

Regular and reserve doctors work alongside civil servants and other supporting units, as well as in the NHS. The role is diverse—working in multi-professional and often multinational teams both in highly staffed base location medical treatment facilities, but also in small, close-knit teams in very austere environments. The role of a unit regimental medical officer (MO) or general duties medical officer (GDMO) has an emphasis on medical force protection, as well as an occupational and pre-hospital care role. Daily work comprises assessment and treatment acute and some chronic conditions, as well as providing advice to the unit chain of command. Key skills include excellent communication and ability to support and motivate those under their command.

The job

At the start of their career, an Army doctor will undertake the Professionally Qualified Officers course at the Royal Military Academy Sandhurst, followed by the DMS training course, learning about diverse subjects from family planning to humanitarian relief. Successful candidates attend the Royal Defence Medical College for an intensive course, including conflict surgery, military psychology, and other Army-specific medical disciplines. As a member of the Armed Forces, the role is not just that of a doctor, but also as an officer and a soldier. Personnel are expected to maintain their military skills and be mentally and physically resilient.

Extras

The Armed Forces can offer undergraduate bursaries and pre-medical school awards following which there will be a minimum service commitment. Although true of the vocation in general, it is not only a special honour and privilege to serve as an Army doctor alongside dedicated and inspirational colleagues, but also to care for patients who are just as inspirational in their response to what often amounts to the most serious injuries and in the most challenging of circumstances.

For further information

HQ Army Medical Services, Camberley. Tel: 0345 600 8080 (Army Careers). Web: https://www.army.mod.uk/who-we-are/corps-regiments-and-units/army-medical-services/royal-army-medical-corps/ Twitter: @RAMCRecruiting

A day in the life ...

08:00 Teaching the emergency department team regarding major incident management

09:00 Ambulatory care clinical shift (minor illness and injury cases)

13:00 Working lunch—checking emails and responding to ePortfolio ticket requests

13:30 Clinical supervisor meeting with military core trainee to review progress

14:30 Meeting regarding upcoming research study

15:00 Checking military emails and responding to diary requests for the next couple of months

15:30 Trust Clinical Standards Sub-Group Meeting as emergency department representative

17:00 Travel to Officers Mess—45-minute drive away

18:00 Mess meeting and evening meal, catch-up with military colleagues

20:30 Return home—finish off PowerPoint slides for next day's teaching session on blast and ballistics

Myth	Glory-hunting gun-toting GPs.
Reality	A demanding and challenging job—both physically and mentally, with a strong team ethos and camaraderie; clinical and academic job satisfaction; diverse opportunities and experience.
Personality	Disciplined outlook; excellent communication and leadership skills, ability to make decisions under pressure, well balanced, and resilient; team player.
Best aspects	Travelling opportunities through overseas deployments and placements; esprit de corps and social life; a platform for expansion beyond core and local medical skills; a secure job and training.
Worst aspects	Disruption due to continually relocating, unpredictability; psychological fatigue—you can see the worst, as well as the best, of humanity and human interaction.
Route	Undergraduate bursaries and cadetship; Royal Military Academy Sandhurst; Royal Defence Medical College; core/GP/specialty training and relevant examinations.
Locations	Mixture of pre-hospital, community, and primary care, rehabilitation facilities, field hospital units, secondary care hospitals, overseas placements, deployed medical treatment facilities.

Life					Work
Quiet On-call					Busy On-call
Boredom					Burnout
Uncompetitive					Competitive
Low salary					High salary

Armed Forces: Royal Air Force Medical Officer

Medical Officers (MOs) in the Royal Air Force (RAF) are mostly GPs but may also be specialists, including general and specialist physicians, anaesthetists, intensivists, emergency medics, general and orthopaedic surgeons, and occupational and public health physicians. RAF doctors provide care to their service population (around 32 000 people, 85% male), provide worldwide aeromedical evacuation for service personnel and entitled persons, and support UK/North Atlantic Treaty Organization (NATO)/United Nations (UN) Operations.

The patients

GPs predominantly care for military personnel living and working on RAF Stations and occasionally their families. Hospital doctors work alongside colleagues in the NHS looking after NHS patients, but also provide expert advice for RAF and Defence medical policy and provide occupationally focused clinical advice for Service personnel seen in the NHS. All RAF doctors can expect to be deployed overseas at some point—patients will be personnel from the UK Armed Forces, its allies, contractors, and occasionally local civilians. In general, military patients are fitter and younger than those usually seen in the NHS.

The work

In addition to caring for patients, RAF doctors develop expertise in aviation medicine and occupational health for military aircrew and the many support occupations which keep aircraft flying. The focus is often on excluding disease and minimizing occupational risk, rather than specifically diagnosing and treating symptoms or disease. GPs, physicians, and anaesthetic intensivists also provide aeromedical evacuation, e.g. from global operational theatres of conflict or returning sick or injured service personnel from overseas bases to the UK. This is a team effort, working alongside RAF personnel, and requires regular military and collective training. Secondary care doctors also train and work in the RAF Hospital Staging Unit and field hospitals, and on board ships, alongside Army and Royal Navy colleagues.

The job

RAF MOs do a wide range of jobs, and although there are fewer specialties available than in the NHS, the job comes with a unique identity and opportunities. GPs normally move station every 2–3 years. Hospital doctors work in the NHS but are employed by the military, so don't move as often—but military tasks are their priority. Deployments (working overseas for up to 6 months) are normally planned and their frequency depends on UK operations. When at home, there are important additional roles, such as strategic aeromedical evacuation, training exercises, or non-medical responsibilities on the station. Whilst the job has the potential to be disruptive to family life, it is highly rewarding, exciting, and comparatively well paid (compared to NHS colleagues of the same grade).

Extras

There are bursaries and cadetships available from year 3 of medical school in the UK. This is in return for a commitment to apply for, or serve, an initial 12-year Term of Service. Participation in sports is strongly encouraged, with unique and amazing opportunities for adventurous training all over the world and experiencing the whole range of military life, including being part of the wider RAF community and learning to fly at University Air Squadrons. There are many (fully funded) research opportunities in the military. For many RAF MOs, many of their closest friends will include other (non-medical) military colleagues. Flexible working has recently become available but is dependent on Service need.

For further information

Royal Air Force Recruitment. Tel: 0345 605 5555. Web: https://www.raf.mod.uk/recruitment Twitter: @RAF_Recruitment

08:00   Arrive at Station Medical Centre (SMC). Hand over airfield cover to duty doctor
08:15   Start morning 'sick parade' (15 minutes per patient)
11:30   Attend Station Executives meeting, representing the health of the workforce
13:00   Circuit training in the Station gym
13:50   Grab a sandwich from the Officers' Mess
14:00   Aircrew medical examinations (30 minutes per patient)
15:30   Seminar with team of medics about being a first responder to an airfield crash
16:00   Finish some paperwork (e.g. sign repeat prescriptions, check test results)
17:00   Training with Station badminton club
18:00   Back to the Officers' Mess to change before dinner

Myth	They fly aeroplanes.
Reality	They fly *in* aeroplanes, looking after patients, and provide care on the ground for aircrew and many others who keep them flying.
Personality	Resilient, enthusiastic, decisive, uncomplaining, able to deal with life's uncertainties, team player.
Best aspects	Opportunity to provide care anywhere in the world and in unique environments; holistic care for patients, their work, and family; expertise in military aviation; strong bonds with other military personnel.
Worst aspects	Exciting jobs can be disruptive to family and relationships; career options are limited; most need to move around the country every few years.
Route	Usually via university bursary or cadetship as a member of a University Air Squadron; sometimes as direct entrant (F1, specialist trainee, or GP/consultant). Training as per NHS specialty, but with additional military responsibilities.
Numbers	280 MOs, of whom 40% are women.
Locations	RAF Stations throughout the UK. Foundation jobs in one of four Joint Hospital Group regions.

Life					Work
Quiet On-call					Busy On-call
Boredom					Burnout
Uncompetitive					Competitive
Low salary					High salary

Armed Forces: Royal Navy Medical Officer

As part of the 'Senior Service', Royal Navy doctors (Medical Officers, MOs) work worldwide on land air and at sea. Those working at sea are predominantly post-F2 General Duties Medical Officers (GDMOs) or GPs, but depending on the mission, medical teams at sea may be augmented by secondary care teams, including emergency medicine (EM) consultants, anaesthetists, trauma and orthopaedic surgeons, and general surgeons, with most specialties available as career pathways within the service.

The patients

Royal Navy GPs and GDMOs primarily provide care for Royal Navy and other service personnel. However, they may be deployed on operations in which they provide urgent care for civilians during humanitarian or environmental crises. Most secondary care MOs train and maintain their skill set in NHS facilities where they provide healthcare for NHS patients as well as bespoke occupational health advice for military cases. Exceptions to this include Royal Navy psychiatrists who work in regional mental health centres.

The work

When deployed at sea or on land, Royal Navy MOs provide primary, occupational, and pre-hospital emergency care, in addition to public healthcare, for a Ship's company. Emergency cases are thankfully uncommon at sea in peacetime; 'battlefield' advanced trauma life support and pre-hospital emergency care courses ensure doctors are prepared for any eventuality. Deployments may be aboard warships or submarines; there are also opportunities to serve in land-based deployments with the Royal Marines and Special Forces. When not deployed overseas, Royal Navy GPs and GDMOs work in primary care centres on military bases as part of multidisciplinary teams, which include civilian GPs, nurses, Royal Navy Medical Assistants, physiotherapists, and pharmacy technicians.

The job

The day job varies widely, depending on specialty and posting. GDMOs and GPs typically deliver primary care in clinics which, when deployed, have the unique feature of a dynamic location. When practising on board, there are also tasks relating to the medical team and the wider Ship's company such as teaching, health promotion, and operational planning. When working on land in medical facilities, Royal Navy GPs fulfil managerial roles akin to practice partnership.

Extras

Medical students can enlist on a Royal Navy cadetship which, at the time of writing, provides a wage and covers tuition fees, with a minimum service commitment attached and a requirement to join the nearest University Royal Naval Unit. Students and doctors of any specialty and grade can join the Royal Navy Reserve whilst maintaining their civilian roles. Depending on career stage and posting, Royal Navy MOs may have the opportunity to complete the Submarine Qualifying Course and earn the 'dolphins' badge, train to be a service scuba diver, or complete the All-Arms Commando Course and earn the coveted green beret.

> **For further information**
>
> **Royal Navy Careers.** Tel: 0345 607 5555. Web: https://www.royalnavy.mod.uk/careers/ (search Medical Officer). Twitter @RNJobsUK, @MedicsNavy

07:45 Starting the day at the Ship's medical centre for 'fresh cases': new problems presenting at sea assessed by the team of medics, nurses, and doctors

08:30 Routine clinic with full scope of primary care and occupational medicine

10:00 Morning break ('stand easy') in the wardroom (Officers' Mess) to catch up with shipmates

11:00 General alarm sounds for a 'Crash on Deck' exercise where the full response to an aircraft crash is practised to train for the real event

12:00 Lunch

14:15 Urgent call to a crew member who has fallen down a lift shaft—they are unconscious and require airway support. The Captain is informed and one of the helicopter crews fly them to hospital escorted by the MO

16:00 Finishing clinical work for the day. The air department has opened the flight deck to visitors, with opportunity for sport

19:00 After dinner, free time with options to watch the sunset, phone home, or relax in the mess. Many doctors use evenings at sea to practise hobbies such as learning the guitar, painting, or postgraduate study

Myth	Untrained appendicectomies and amputations, with rum as anaesthetic.
Reality	Flexible delivery of evidence-based medicine, in any location and circumstances.
Personality	Adaptable, driven doctors with a high degree of initiative and the ability to handle physical and mental adversity. Team players with a strong sense of duty.
Best aspects	Broadening your scope of practice when working at sea, being part of a close-knit team, getting to know your patients, making the most of Armed Forces benefits (such as adventurous training). A very supportive welfare and recovery package in the event of illness or injury and a non-contributing pension scheme unmatched by any other UK employer.
Worst aspects	Periods of uncertainty and some short-notice deployment requirements may occur, although individual circumstances and preferences are balanced with the needs of the service.
Route	University entry (medical cadetship) or direct entry at certain career stages post-graduation. Followed by Initial Officer Training at Britannia Royal Naval College, Dartmouth and the New Entry Medical Officer Course. Following GDMO service, subsequent specialty selection and training to CCT.
Locations	Worldwide.

Life					Work
Quiet On-call					Busy On-call
Boredom					Burnout
Uncompetitive					Competitive
Low salary					High salary

Audiovestibular medicine

Audiovestibular medicine (AVM) deals with the diagnosis, investigation, medical treatment, and rehabilitation of children and adults with hearing and balance disorders. The specialty evolved from better understanding of the medical aetiology of such conditions, few of which are amenable to surgical treatment (e.g. genetic and degenerative causes). Excellent clinical and interpersonal skills are needed as many conditions are complex, disabling, and chronic. Audiovestibular physicians require a strong understanding of the basic science underpinning hearing and balance in order to inform clinical practice. Advances in technology and national initiatives, such as cochlear implants and the Newborn Hearing Screen, have expanded and broadened the specialty in recent years.

The patients

Patients are of all ages, with a variety of hearing and balance problems; typical presentations include hearing loss, tinnitus, dizziness, imbalance, eye movement disorders, and speech problems. You will be referred patients from colleagues in many specialties such as paediatrics, elderly medicine, ENT, and neurology, in addition to direct referrals from GPs. Many patients will experience considerable psychological distress and social difficulties due to the disabling, complex, and chronic nature of their condition.

The work

Some jobs in AVM comprise both paediatric and adult work; others focus on just one. AVM is often a stand-alone specialty, but some audiovestibular physicians work within other departments such as ENT or neurology. The clinical work is varied, and a sound knowledge of both paediatric and adult general medicine is required. In addition to detailed clinical assessment and therapeutic intervention, discussion and counselling surrounding the results of complex audiovestibular investigations form a key component of practice.

The job

AVM is practised in outpatient settings in general hospitals, tertiary centres, or in the community, with no out-of-hours commitments. The specialty lends itself well to less than full-time work. Occasionally, within working hours, you might be called upon to see patients on wards or in A&E by other specialists. Audiovestibular physicians will often be in the position of assisting colleagues in providing a diagnosis and expert management of complex dizzy patients. In paediatric AVM, an important aspect of the role is in the Newborn Hearing Screen programme. Teamworking skills are essential, as AVM physicians work closely with audiologists, vestibular scientists, hearing therapists, psychologists, and speech and language therapists. Close liaison with community health and education professionals is also highly important.

Extras

AVM is a specialty that lends itself to research (both clinical and scientific), as there are many areas still 'unknown' when it comes to the underlying pathology and management of many conditions. Often, an audiovestibular physician joins a department where there has previously not been one and therefore, there are opportunities to develop the service from scratch, which is a challenging, but rewarding experience. Being a small specialty, opportunities for teaching are plenty, both within the specialty and also for allied medical specialties and associated therapists.

For further information

The British Association of Audiovestibular Physicians (BAAP). Web: https://www.baap.org.uk

---

08:30	Pre-clinic multidisciplinary meeting
09:00	Adult/paediatric outpatient clinic; seven patients, including a deaf neonate, a dizzy teenager, and an elderly patient with recurrent falls
12:30	Radiology meeting
13:30	Review of oncology patient with dizziness in protective isolation on the ward
14:00	Dictate letters and other clinical administration
15:00	Cochlear Implant Team Decision Meeting
15:45	Review of interesting and/or unusual audiovestibular test results with audiologists and vestibular scientists
16:00	Management meeting to discuss procurement of new vestibular equipment
16:30	Ad hoc meeting with genetics colleague to discuss co-management of a complex patient with several multisystem problems, including hearing impairment
17:00	Leave work

Myth	'Are you an ENT surgeon or do you just fit hearing aids?'
Reality	Medically trained physicians with a strong understanding of audiovestibular science and its links to general medical and surgical conditions.
Personality	Analytical, empathic, a combination of a technically minded scientist and an emotionally tuned clinician, team player, enjoys working with adults and children.
Best aspects	Having the skill and knowledge to solve clinical problems where others have failed, excellent work–life balance (no on-calls!), working closely with other healthcare and education professionals.
Worst aspects	Constantly having to explain what we do and the value of our service, being a small, less well-known specialty; many clinical areas still under research; limited geographical flexibility.
Route	Entry to specialty training in AVM (ST3+) is via several routes: internal medicine training (IMT) (p. 44) or acute care common stem–acute medicine (ACCS-AM) (p. 37), paediatrics (p. 49), ENT (p. 64), or GP (p. 42). Exams: relevant exam to initial/core training pathway.
Numbers	50 consultants, of whom 55% are women; a significant proportion work less than full time.
Locations	Mixture of hospitals, specialist units, and the community.

Life						Work
Quiet On-call						Busy On-call
Boredom						Burnout
Uncompetitive						Competitive
Low salary						High salary

Aviation and space medicine

Aviation and space medicine is the UK's newest specialty, having been formally recognized by the GMC in 2016. It is primarily focused on understanding the challenges of flight and spaceflight environments, how they affect humans, and how best to protect people against these hazards, not only to survive, but also to perform to the best of their ability in a variety of different conditions. Historically, training in this specialty was limited to military personnel and delivered on an apprenticeship basis. Now there are standardized curriculum competencies that all trainees must achieve to a certain degree.

The patients

Typically pilots, both military and civilian. In addition, passengers, air traffic controllers, drone operators, parachutists, and astronauts all make up the patient population.

The work

The employing sponsor, civilian or military, will determine the focus of clinical work. Military trainees can expect to perform a routine pilot medical examination one day, and deliver G-force training on a human centrifuge or hypoxia awareness training the next day. On other days, they might test a new oxygen system, trial a new piece of flight equipment, consult with industry on purchasing a new aircraft part, or interface with international colleagues on an aerospace medicine dilemma.

A civilian trainee can expect to develop skills needed to make sound and safe aeromedical fitness decisions and to liaise with visiting specialists in varied medical disciplines, including cardiology, psychiatry, radiology, and neurology. They might visit an airfield to supervise a Medical Flight Test or accompany a flight examiner in a commercial flight simulator to assess a pilot's ability to conduct their job. Most days, you will discuss complex medical cases with airline doctors, as well as aeromedical examiners, from the UK and internationally. Trainees also provide important contributions to the development of new regulatory policy and updating existing policy to keep pace with current medical guidelines.

The job

The predominant setting will again depend on the employer but is largely office-based, with emphasis on giving specialist advice. Travel is essential to other facilities which are spread out across the country. Aviation and space medicine physicians often work closely with engineers and industry to ensure equipment meets required human operator specifications.

Extras

First-year trainees undertake the intensive 6-month Diploma in Aerospace Medicine course, run by King's College London, to get a firm grounding in the theory and applied aspects of the subject. There are extensive written exams at the end of the course, hosted by the Faculty of Occupational Medicine. In the UK, there is only a small core of Aviation and Space medicine specialists, so there are opportunities to travel and interact with international partners. Teaching and education are key aspects. Trainees are expected to present at international conferences and on courses. On-call commitments are minimal, limited to aircraft crash accident investigation and aeromedical evacuation advice.

For further information

Royal Aeronautical Society (RAeS). Tel: 020 7670 4300. Web: https://www.aerosociety.com Email: raes@aerosociety.com Twitter: @AeroSociety

UK Space Life and Biomedical Sciences Association (UK Space LABS). Web: http://www.ukspacelabs.co.uk Twitter: @UKSpaceLABS

Next Generation of Aerospace Medicine (group for students and early-career professionals interested in aviation and space medicine). Twitter: @NextGenAsM

08:00 The morning starts with a cup of coffee, looking over emails

09:00 Deliver training to a group of pilots about hypoxia awareness and the dangers of the flight environment

10:30 Review results of a trial of a new piece of flying clothing; consider recommendations to make

12:00 Lunch

13:00 Multidisciplinary team meeting to discuss a specific medical case of a pilot with regard to their fitness to fly

15:00 Prepare a PowerPoint presentation to deliver to a group of engineers the next day

17:30 Home to watch the blockbuster film *The Martian* and criticize all the life support system elements

Myth	Medically trained astronauts.
Reality	Largely an office-based job within a small specialty. Can get geeky!
Personality	Need to be organized and self-motivated to achieve all the curriculum competencies. Enthusiasm about the subject itself is required.
Best aspects	Being an advocate for a pilot and enabling them to return to flying.
Worst aspects	Very small specialty, with few peers. Lots of travelling—currently, having a car and living in the south of England are almost essential. Having to explain what the specialty is at every dinner party!
Route	Specialty training in Aviation and Space Medicine (ST3+) after core training in one of: internal medicine training (IMT) (p. 44), acute care common stem–acute medicine (ACCS-AM) (p. 37), GP (p. 42), or anaesthetics (p. 39). Exams: membership exam relevant to core/initial specialty; Diploma in Aviation Medicine. Training is not NHS-funded, and numbers are extremely limited.
Locations	Include Royal Air Force (RAF) bases and Ministry of Defence (MoD) sites. RAF trainees based at Centre of Aviation Medicine (Bedfordshire); Civil Aviation Authority (CAA) trainees based at Gatwick airport.

Life					Work
Quiet On-call					Busy On-call
Boredom					Burnout
Uncompetitive					Competitive
Low salary					High salary

Bariatric and metabolic surgery

Globally, the problem of obesity has reached epidemic proportions, and bariatric surgery is the most successful and robust treatment available. This new development in gastrointestinal (GI) surgery aims to produce weight loss to treat obesity and its associated disorders. The subspecialty has expanded significantly over the last 20 years, mainly due to advances in minimally invasive surgical techniques, but new operations have also developed, along with the scientific understanding of associated metabolic diseases. Bariatric surgeons must be adept at laparoscopic, endoscopic, open, and emergency surgery, as well as being empathetic with the patient group.

The patients

Adults with body mass index (BMI) ≥35 kg/m^2 and obesity-associated comorbidity (e.g. type 2 diabetes, hypertension, sleep apnoea, osteoarthritis), or with a BMI ≥40 kg/m^2. Patients may be from all ethnicities and socioeconomic groups, and there is no age limit. Centres interested in child and adolescent obesity will operate on teens when surgery is the best option to improve obesity-related health conditions. Postoperative follow-up to monitor weight reduction and morbidity resolution lasts for 2 years, although a surgeon may be involved for some years before and after surgery.

The work

Bariatric surgery is a multidisciplinary team (MDT)-based specialty delivering truly holistic care. The team includes obesity physicians, bariatric nurse specialists, dieticians, exercise therapists, sleep apnoea specialists, anaesthetists, and psychologists. The surgeon's role is focused on deciding a patient's suitability for surgery, preoperative optimization, performing the surgery, and monitoring outcomes. Teamworking with other medical specialties is common. Referrals frequently come from orthopaedic surgeons (e.g. to help patients lose weight prior to joint replacement), neurologists (e.g. for patients with benign intracranial hypertension), respiratory physicians (e.g. to cure sleep apnoea), and renal transplant teams (e.g. to help patients lose weight before renal transplantation). Over 99% of surgery is performed laparoscopically (and most emergency cases) using complex suturing techniques, modern stapling devices, and plenty of fancy gadgets. Bariatric surgeons are the ultimate laparoscopic pros! Operations typically last between 60 and 180 minutes.

The job

One or two days a week will be spent in the operating theatre. Significant time is spent with the MDT, assessing patients in clinic, planning care pathways, and performing investigations. Bariatric surgeons also practise as general surgeons and have regular emergency on-call commitments, clinics, and elective operating lists.

Extras

Academic opportunities are extensive. Bariatric and metabolic surgery is a budding specialty; there is still a lot to understand in terms of how operations work, how to improve them, and the underlying biology of obesity. There is a strong international community active in research, with many opportunities to travel for conferences, surgical masterclasses, and fellowships. Opportunities exist to be involved in public health and the media to raise awareness about bariatric surgery, as well as to advocate for healthcare policies. Private practice is possible but is competitive and has high personal indemnity costs.

For further information

British Obesity and Metabolic Surgery Society (BOMSS). Web: https://bomss.org Email: info@bomss.org.uk Twitter: @bariatricBOMSS

07:30 Consent patients for theatre

08:00 Ward round with team, including bariatric fellow and bariatric nurse specialist

08:30 Morning operating list, including a bariatric surgery case, an antireflux case, and hernia repair. Plenty of time to teach trainee mesh repair and laparoscopic skills

12:00 Medical student bedside teaching

13:00 MDT meeting to discuss new patients and confirm treatment plans

14:30 Endoscopy for one preop patient and one for postoperative surveillance

17:00 Catch up with team for paper ward round and see any unwell patients

17:30 Check through preoperative test results for patients on next week's operating list

18:30 Go home and spend time with family or watch the latest episode of *Grey's Anatomy*!

22:00 Catch up on social media discussions in the international bariatric surgery groups or finish research paper. Tweet the latest RCT results

Myth	'Quick-fix' surgery; the easy option for weight loss by private practice-hungry surgeons with Porsches.
Reality	Lifesaving surgery for chronically ill patients by highly skilled laparoscopic surgeons. The results benefit patients, families, and society as a whole.
Personality	Good listener, multitasker, empathetic, non-judgemental, team player—the friendly surgeon!
Best aspects	Chances to see your work change a person's life, work, and relationships, not just health. Quick outcomes—significant weight loss, often by 6–12 months. No other treatment can cure type 2 diabetes (almost) overnight!
Worst aspects	Dealing with judgement and ignorance towards your patients; having to challenge public, media, and policymaker perceptions of what bariatric surgery is and why it is needed.
Route	Core surgical training (CST), then specialty training in general surgery (p. 61), and declare subspecialty upper GI surgery (benign). Most undergo a bariatric surgery fellowship (UK/international). Exams: MRCS; FRCS.
Numbers	Approximately 160 consultants.
Locations	UK regional centres in teaching hospitals or district general hospitals; some surgeons work full time in the private sector.

Life					Work
Quiet On-call					Busy On-call
Boredom					Burnout
Uncompetitive					Competitive
Low salary					High salary

▌ Cardiology

Cardiology is a fantastic specialty offering an unparalleled breadth of opportunities in which anyone can find their niche. It is undoubtedly demanding, requiring the ability to make and act on decisions quickly, but job satisfaction is immense, from both a diagnostic and therapeutic perspective.

The patients

The spectrum of patients encountered is extremely diverse. Patients presenting with acute coronary syndromes and critical arrhythmias will often be met straight off the ambulance by the cardiologist and taken for urgent lifesaving intervention. Those with chronic heart failure may need advanced medical and device therapy. A growing population of adult patients with complex congenital heart disease require lifelong specialist care, including support during pregnancy. Cardiologists work with patients in theatre, in the intensive care unit (ICU), and across all specialties. Whatever the setting, interaction with the cardiologist will carry huge and lasting significance for each of these patients.

The work

Consultant job plans are variable but typically involve a mixture of general cardiology and a subspecialty (e.g. adult congenital heart disease (ACHD), cardiac imaging, coronary intervention, device therapy, electrophysiology, heart failure, or inherited cardiovascular conditions). Some cardiologists may also have a commitment to the general medical take. One of the great joys of cardiology comes from making a clinical diagnosis and having the tools to confirm it, and indeed often to treat it oneself, e.g. the syncopal patient in whom one diagnoses heart block and inserts a pacemaker, or the patient with acute coronary syndrome on whom one performs coronary angiography and percutaneous coronary intervention. Transthoracic echocardiography is a particularly satisfying and invaluable diagnostic tool that all cardiology registrars learn during their training.

The job

A typical week involves time spent on the wards, in outpatient clinics, at multidisciplinary team (MDT) meetings, and performing procedures or imaging investigations, depending on one's subspecialty. The hours are long; the workload is often unpredictable, and there is usually significant on-call commitment. Cardiologists are constantly in demand, be it a call for help from another specialty, an unexpected finding on a pacemaker check, or an urgent echo required in theatre. Cardiologists work as part of a large MDT, including nurse specialists, cardiac physiologists, and radiographers. There is also a high level of interaction with other specialties, particularly general medicine, cardiac surgery, anaesthetics, and intensive care.

Extras

Cardiology is a highly evidence-based, constantly evolving specialty that traditionally attracts academically minded trainees. The vast majority undertake a higher research degree during training, and many go on to combine clinical and academic work as consultants. There are countless teaching opportunities for cardiologists, both undergraduate and postgraduate, across the broader MDT and in the community. Opportunities for private practice can be lucrative for some.

For further information

British Cardiovascular Society (BCS). Tel: 020 7383 3887. Web: https://www.bcs.com Email: enquiries@bcs.com Twitter: @BritishCardioSo

A day in the life ...

07:45 Arrive, check emails, finish MDT meeting preparation

08:00 MDT meeting—presentation and discussion of ACHD patients with cardiologists, cardiac surgeons, anaesthetist, and obstetrician

09:00 Diagnostic cardiac catheterization list

12:45 Quick lunch on the way to clinic

13:00 Outpatient clinic: 18 patients shared between consultant and registrar, with a mixture of new patients and follow-ups. Arrange for admission of one clinic patient found to be in an arrhythmia that needs urgent cardioversion

17:30 Catch up with ward team—review any concerning results and new admissions

18:30 Home

Myth	Highly competitive specialty, full of big, brash personalities and hard-nosed 'balloonatics' who will destroy you for misinterpreting the ECG.
Reality	Challenging, constantly stimulating specialty, with highly motivated, dedicated colleagues and potential for unparalleled job satisfaction across a range of settings. Don't expect group hugs and high-fives, but when required, support is always on hand.
Personality	Determined, resilient, and hard-working, with the ability to remain calm under pressure. Good practical, communication, and teamworking skills are essential.
Best aspects	The satisfaction of making a clinical diagnosis, confirming it, and treating it yourself. Procedures going well. Never a dull moment.
Worst aspects	Procedures not going well. Being constantly in demand and the unpredictable nature of the work—sometimes a dull moment would be nice.
Route	Internal medicine training (IMT) (p. 44) or acute care common stem–acute medicine (ACCS-AM) (p. 37), followed by specialty training in cardiology (ST3+). Exams: MRCP; European Exam in General Cardiology (previously the Knowledge Based Assessment (KBA)).
Numbers	1700 consultants, of whom 14% are women.
Locations	District general and teaching hospitals, with an expanding role in community services.

Life					Work
Quiet On-call					Busy On-call
Boredom					Burnout
Uncompetitive					Competitive
Low salary					High salary

Cardiothoracic surgery

If you enjoy working under pressure with time constraints and high stakes, then this is the job for you. There are opportunities to cure and improve quality of life in a diverse range of patients and conditions. Although likely to split into pure 'cardiac' and pure 'thoracic' surgery, training remains highly competitive and the work is arduous—increased regulation, scrutiny, and expectation have taken much of the gloss off this specialty. However, for those who can steer through these choppy waters, it is a rewarding and enjoyable career.

The patients

For cardiac surgery, the patients are usually in the 60–80 years age group, predominantly with coronary artery disease and/or degenerative valve disease, often with multiple other comorbidities. They are mostly referred from other hospital specialties rather than by GPs. Congenital cardiac surgery is a formal subspecialty in which surgeons will also repair cardiac defects in babies and children. The thoracic patients are usually referred via the multidisciplinary team (MDT) and the majority of the work deals with lung cancer diagnosis, treatment, or palliation. These patients also have a high incidence of vascular and coronary disease but tend to be slightly younger (50–70 years). All these patients are unique and require a good deal of preparation, so that they will survive an operation. However, this individual preparation is one of the most enjoyable aspects of the job.

The work

Cardiac and thoracic surgeons are only really happy when they are in theatre and away from the other distractions of hospital life (management, dictation, audit, etc.). The range of diseases is varied and complex, but the majority of the work is coronary artery surgery, valve surgery, and intrathoracic malignancy. There is tremendous autonomy due to the responsibility for the patients whilst they are in hospital. Alongside the theatre, there are ward rounds and outpatient clinics. On-calls can be demanding and may be frequent, depending on the size of the unit; common problems include postoperative complications, trauma, and dissecting aneurysms.

The job

Cardiac and thoracic surgeons work as part of a large MDT, including cardiologists, intensivists, anaesthetists, respiratory physicians, general surgeons, vascular surgeons, radiologists, oncologists, and trauma teams. The work is pressurized as the mortality rate is relatively high due to the nature of the surgery and patient population; added to this, there is the spotlight of individual mortality rates being publicized. However, the expectation is that junior consultant surgeons are mentored until they have enough experience and confidence to take on higher-risk cases.

Extras

Alongside standard clinical work, there are many opportunities for research and overseas training. Surgeons can choose to subspecialize in paediatric, transplant, or thoracic surgery, though this is not necessary. There are small amounts of private practice, though less than some other surgical specialties. Less-than-full-time training opportunities are available.

For further information

Society for Cardiothoracic Surgery in Great Britain and Ireland (SCTS). Web: https://www.scts.org Email: sctsadmin@scts.org Twitter: @SCTSUK

07:30	Ward round of postoperative patients on cardiac intensive care unit (CICU)
08:00	Theatre. First case is a 78-year-old man with type 2 diabetes and aortic stenosis requiring an aortic valve replacement
11:30	Leave registrar to close case and inhale some lunch whilst writing case notes
12:00	Start next case—a CABG for a 79-year-old lady with angina
16:30	Finish in theatre
17:00	Ward round on CICU
17:30	Catch up with phone calls, clinic letters, etc.; chat with colleagues
18:00	Sneaky CICU ward round to check juniors have made correct decisions
19:00	Arrive home; pray that patients survive to leave hospital alive
19:03	Stop worrying; bask in the glory of a marvellous and technically skilled job that brings respect from colleagues and admiration from patients
19:04	Start worrying about your performance compared to others in the unit and nationally

Myth	Boys with toys; cracking chests and flying blood.
Reality	Mostly boys with toys, although the number of girls is increasing; challenging and involves surgery that can produce lifesaving results.
Personality	Hard-working, competitive, very good practical skills, degree of OCD, dedicated.
Best aspects	Theatre; working against the clock and getting sick patients through difficult operations never cease to produce a warm glow of satisfaction.
Worst aspects	Government targets and public expectation.
Route	Run-through training in cardiothoracic surgery from ST1 or entry at ST3 after core surgical training (CST) (p. 61). Exams: MRCS; FRCS (Cardiothoracic Surgery)
Numbers	375 consultants in England, of whom 9% are women.
Locations	Mostly teaching hospitals, with a few district general hospitals.

Life					Work
Quiet On-call					Busy On-call
Boredom					Burnout
Uncompetitive					Competitive
Low salary					High salary

Chemical pathology

Chemical pathology (also known as clinical biochemistry) is a specialty with great variety. There are four main facets, which form the basis of all posts, although these vary in extent from post to post. These are: clinical, laboratory (service commitments), laboratory (research), and teaching. There is the potential for considerable flexibility within the specialty, which is very advantageous. The five clinical modules of the metabolic medicine subspecialty (p. 226) include diabetes, lipid disorders, metabolic bone and renal stone, nutrition, and adult inborn errors of metabolism.

The patients
Patients can be of either sex, range from young to old, and be of any ethnicity. Clinic patients tend to be adult, unless specifically paediatric-trained. There is good continuity of care, with many patients being followed up over their lifetimes. Often the diseases encountered require chronic management (e.g. diabetes). However, clinical interventions can make potentially significant beneficial changes to patients in all aspects of the specialty. Interesting cases tend to be either endocrine-related or inborn errors of metabolism. Difficult cases tend to involve patients who have chronically poorly controlled conditions (such as diabetes).

The work
The main role of chemical pathologists is to be a laboratory consultant, with day-to-day responsibilities for the running of the clinical biochemistry laboratory. This typically entails working with, and managing, biomedical and clinical scientists, as well as liaising with appropriate medical staff; this maintains quality and ensures that appropriate investigation of patients is performed. Most doctors trained in the subspecialty of metabolic medicine are trained in the main specialty of chemical pathology. Common clinics performed are diabetic and lipid clinics. Other clinics related to the modules of metabolic medicine are an alternative, and it is not uncommon to see chemical pathologists involved in endocrine work and associated clinics.

The job
Typically, there are 1–3 outpatient clinics per week, and 1–2 nutrition rounds per week. Management meetings may occupy a few hours. Otherwise the rest of the time is devoted to laboratory time (either research or chemical pathology). The specialty has close connections with the diabetic and endocrinology teams, and the clinic work reflects this. Some clinics (e.g. adult inborn errors of metabolism) are specialist and tend to be in large centres. In the laboratory, there is very much a multidisciplinary ethos, with much work being done in collaboration with the clinical and biomedical scientists. On-calls tend to be from home and it's unusual to be called in. Phone calls tend not to be that frequent but sometimes can take a couple of hours to sort out. On the whole, the job does allow significant autonomy.

Extras
The specialty is incredibly varied and flexible. It offers a good variety of clinical mix. There are good opportunities for teaching and biochemical research (a research project is currently a requirement for FRCPath). Flexible training and working are practical and well established. Private work tends to be limited.

For further information

The Association of Clinical Pathologists. Tel: 01273 775 700. Web: https://pathologists.org.uk/specialities/chemical-pathology/ Email: info@pathologists.org.uk Twitter: @ACP_Pathologist

The Royal College of Pathologists (RCPath). Tel: 020 7451 6700. Web: https://www.rcpath.org Email: info@rcpath.org Twitter: @RCPath

---

09:00 Outpatient clinic—could be diabetic, lipid, nutrition, metabolic bone/renal stone, or adult inborn errors of metabolism

13:00 Lunchtime meeting, e.g. grand round or journal club

14:00 Laboratory work, including assessing biochemistry results that have just been obtained. Can also involve interpretation of complex test results and discussion with hospital doctors and GPs

15:30 Teaching junior doctors about biochemistry tests and how they're performed

16:30 Finish writing a review article for a well-respected journal

18:00 Home after another satisfying and varied day at work!

Myth	Lab-based boffin.
Reality	Academically minded doctor, often based in the lab, but with regular patient contact.
Personality	Leadership skills, team player, an enquiring mind, good communication skills.
Best aspects	Great variety of work, with interesting case mix.
Worst aspects	Always bureaucracy!
Route	Run-through training in chemical pathology (ST1+) (p. 52). Exams: FRCPath (Clinical Biochemistry); MRCP if subspecializing in metabolic medicine (ST3+) (p. 226).
Locations	Hospital laboratory and clinics. Can be found in any hospital, although some hospital laboratories are run by clinical scientists.

Life					Work
Quiet On-call					Busy On-call
Boredom					Burnout
Uncompetitive					Competitive
Low salary					High salary

▊ Clinical genetics

Clinical genetics is a rapidly evolving specialty driven by recent advances in genomics. Geneticists are physicians who bridge the gap between laboratory and clinical medicine. Clinical diagnostic ability remains a core aspect, but are complemented by new technologies to make genetic diagnoses. Contrary to popular belief, geneticists are practising clinicians who see patients in their own right, and thus excellent communication skills are essential. In the near future, there are likely to be therapeutic options for an increasing number of genetic conditions; geneticists are likely to be involved in clinical trials to evaluate their efficacy and risks. Advising families regarding reproductive risks and surveillance for genetic conditions is also an important aspect.

The patients

The specialty deals with the diagnosis and management of genetic disorders affecting both children and adults, and even prenatally. Clinical geneticists work with families; by definition, they see patients of all ages, making diagnoses and considering associated risks for the whole family. They are experts in diagnosing a wide range of conditions, including rare diseases and inherited cancer syndromes, so the job provides immense variety for doctors who enjoy many different specialties. Paediatrics is an important aspect of genetics—many referrals come from paediatricians requesting diagnostic assistance for children with complex conditions or interpretation of results from genetic investigations.

The work

The clinical genetics service is predominantly outpatient-based and is delivered in clinics at individual Clinical Genetics Centres, hosted by an NHS Trust. They also provide outreach services, e.g. in DGHs and Fetal Medicine Centres, as part of a managed network of genomic disease and inherited cancer services. Direct inpatient assessments are also provided in, but not limited to, neonatal and paediatric intensive care units (ICUs) and neurology services to support genomic testing and phenotypic assessment. Clinical geneticists spend a lot of time 'working up' patients before clinic, understanding the presenting phenotype, and often spend significant time writing detailed letters explaining complex conditions. Genetic testing is done at ever increasing speeds—timely results can be valuable in urgent fetal diagnosis, or when diagnosis may alter acute management. Interpretation of genomic results is complex and geneticists play a key role in this process, making clinical judgements as to whether a patient's phenotype is explained by a genetic variant.

The job

Clinical genetics is ideal for physicians wanting flexibility and autonomy, but requires close attention to detail and strong communication skills. Less-than-full-time working is common, and on-call commitment is minimal. Multidisciplinary work is a key aspect of the role—geneticists liaise closely with laboratory scientists and other clinicians within an MDT setting to establish diagnoses. There is much scope for subspecialization within a particular clinical area, e.g. neurogenetics, cardiac genetics, prenatal diagnosis, or cancer.

Extras

There are significant opportunities for providing genomic education to medical students, healthcare professionals, and patients. Many geneticists have a clinical area of particular interest and form networks with patient support groups and specialist clinicians in that field. Participation in research, e.g. recruiting patients for studies, and undertaking personal research and/or a higher research degree are actively encouraged.

For further information

The British Society for Genetic Medicine (BSGM). Tel: 020 3925 3675. Web: https://www. bsgm.org.uk Email: membership@bsgm.org.uk Twitter: @BritSocGenMed

Clinical Genetics Society, London (constituent group of BSGM). Web: https://www.clingensoc.org

---

08:45	Genetics meeting (weekly) with clinical and laboratory colleagues discussing diagnostically or ethically challenging cases and genetic testing options
09:15	MDT meeting to discuss genomic results and whether variants are pathogenic or normal genetic variation
10:00	Emails and admin—responding to queries, requesting genetic tests
10:30	Clinic prep, including reviewing referrals and researching potential diagnoses
12:30	Lunchtime meeting discussing service improvement
13:30	Paediatric dysmorphology clinic: five patients with complex undiagnosed conditions
17:15	Head home for dinner, family/life activities
19:30	Spend an hour reading about newly identified gene, writing slides for genomic teaching

Myth	Geeky science nerds, creating incomprehensible reports of jumbled numbers and letters.
Reality	Conscientious communicators who are skilled at clinical examination and enjoy explaining genetic diagnoses to patients and families.
Personality	Hard-working and thorough, with a close eye for detail and an ability to apply logic to genomic data; adaptable as new technologies are integrated into genomic testing.
Best aspects	Ample opportunity to develop specialist interests and expertise in a flexible and family-friendly job; clinical contact with whole families.
Worst aspects	Giving bad news and dealing with grief in upsetting situations; the frustrations of 'false positive diagnoses' that may occur due to over-interpretation of normal genetic variations.
Route	Either internal medicine training (IMT) (p. 44) or acute care common stem–acute medicine (ACCS-AM) (p. 37), or paediatrics level 1 training (p. 49), then specialty training in clinical genetics (ST3+). Exams: MRCP or MRCPCH; Certificate Examination of Clinical Genetics. Note: entry criteria set to broaden to include additional specialties, e.g. obstetrics and gynaecology (O&G) (p. 47) and GP (p. 42).
Numbers	270 consultants, of whom 65% are women.
Locations	Genomic Medicine Centres in tertiary hospitals; outreach clinics in DGHs.
Life	Work
Quiet On-call	Busy On-call
Boredom	Burnout
Uncompetitive	Competitive
Low salary	High salary

Clinical neurophysiology

Clinical neurophysiology primarily deals with the diagnosis of patients presenting with a wide range of disorders that affect the nervous system and muscles. Beyond the importance of accurate diagnosis and appropriate treatment (e.g. of different types of epilepsy and peripheral neuropathies), it also provides a window to understand the human brain and its disorders. While it is a stand-alone specialty in the UK, it has strong links with neurology.

The patients

Patients may be referred as inpatients or to the clinic, and come with a wide range of acute or chronic central and peripheral nervous system disorders of varying severity and type, typically at the peak of their symptoms. Patients can be of any age, from premature neonates to elderly citizens, and in any state of consciousness, from lucid and co-operative to confused or comatose. Therefore, whilst the duration of direct care with patients may be short and mostly limited to those with neuromuscular disorders, excellent communication skills and an empathetic approach are required as many are vulnerable with severe or intractable conditions such as motor neuron disease.

The work

Clinical neurophysiologists are usually asked to examine a clinical hypothesis, but often it is their intervention that will solve a diagnostic conundrum or make a significant breakthrough. Their opinion is based on the clinical interpretation of neurophysiological studies in the light of pertinent clinical information, often through direct clinical examination of patients, using specialist tests such as electromyography (EMG) or electroencephalography (EEG). A more direct involvement with patients' treatment and care is possible through specialized procedures such as EMG-guided botulinum toxin for spasticity and dystonia and, in future, emerging transcranial magnetic stimulation for some types of epilepsy. Close liaison with fellow consultants or other specialists, e.g. neuroradiologists, is mandatory for correct interpretation of results, accurate diagnosis, and optimization of patients' care, as well as being interesting, educational, and ultimately rewarding for all parties.

The job

The specialty is hospital-based and consultant-led, but supported by clinical physiologists who have a technical background. The range of diagnostic tests provided is wide, often focusing on an area to meet specific hospital or service needs. Acute video EEG in the intensive care unit (ICU), diagnostic video telemetry, overnight sleep video EEG studies, and home video telemetry are examples of specialized diagnostics developed alongside acute or sleep medicine or an epilepsy centre. Many consultants develop an interest in a subspecialty, usually neuromuscular diseases or epilepsy, and some conduct specialist clinics.

Extras

The specialty is known for its potential for clinical research—from sophisticated nerve and muscle hyperexcitability studies in channelopathies, all the way through the complexities of epilepsy diagnosis, to the study of neurocognition and consciousness in coma. Often in association with imaging techniques, such as functional magnetic resonance imaging (fMRI), consultants can develop their particular interests and have a rewarding academic career alongside their clinical practice. Teaching is often actively pursued.

For further information

British Society for Clinical Neurophysiology. Web: https://www.bscn.org.uk

---

08:30 Departmental meeting with fellow consultants and physiologists to plan the day

09:00 Clinic which may be one of outpatient EMG, EEG reporting, or epilepsy clinic

13:00 Ward round of patients undergoing telemetry

14:00 Inpatient EMG or EEG recordings in the ICU

16:00 Multidisciplinary diagnostic meeting to discuss challenging cases

17:00 Time for clinical research (opportunities also before 08:30 for the devotees ...). Reporting the last urgent EEG of the day and liaising with the treating team

20:00 Peaceful evening, bar occasional calls from the telemetry unit (when on-call)

Myth	Non-clinical specialty and therefore not as important; provides only diagnostic support.
Reality	Although rarely concerned with day-to-day patient management, daily consultations and clinical examination of patients are the norm.
Personality	Clinician with a vivid interest in neurophysiology and pathophysiology, a penchant for technology, and attention to meaningful detail; empathetic, particularly in the EMG lab, team player, an eye for research.
Best aspects	Being in the position to make accurate diagnosis, multidisciplinary approach in clinical practice; clinical research
Worst aspects	Not knowing the outcome of other consultants' patients. Risk of boredom when not developing own special interests or research
Route	Internal medicine training (IMT) (p. 44), acute care common stem–acute medicine (ACCS-AM) (p. 37), or paediatric level 1 training (p. 49), followed by specialty training in clinical neurophysiology (ST3+). Exams: MRCP or MRCPCH.
Numbers	150 consultants, of whom 25% are women.
Locations	Mostly tertiary centres and teaching hospitals; some district general hospitals.

Life					Work
Quiet On-call					Busy On-call
Boredom					Burnout
Uncompetitive					Competitive
Low salary					High salary

Clinical oncology

Clinical oncologists specialize in non-surgical management of cancer, by using radiotherapy along with an array of systemic therapies (chemotherapy, hormone therapy, and biological therapies). The specialty is unique to the UK, compared to most of the world, where 'radiation oncologists' do not administer systemic therapies. Clinical oncology is a rewarding discipline that requires a high level of independent thought and analysis, as well as strong interpersonal skills. There is an opportunity to be involved in fascinating technical innovations in radiotherapy and research into improving treatments.

The patients

The incidence of cancer is rising—whilst it predominantly affects people in later years of life, it can affect any age group. Patients can present at various stages of the disease, with diagnosis in early stages offering potential cure, whilst in later stages, treatment is aimed at prolongation of life and symptom control. Treatment can be demanding due to toxic side effects and may not be suitable for less fit patients—treatment in such cases focuses on a palliative approach. The diagnosis of cancer and its treatment is stressful for both the patient and their families. It is therefore important to involve them in decision-making about their care and provide ongoing support.

The work

By the time a patient is seen by a clinical oncologist, they are already aware of the diagnosis. In the first consultation, they are given information on suitable treatment options. This could be radiotherapy alone, systemic therapies alone, or a combination of both or none. Close follow-up is integral to patient care in order to assess the effectiveness of therapy and to assess and alleviate the side effects resulting from the treatment and those related to the cancer.

The job

As both modalities of treatment (radiotherapy and systemic) can be delivered to otherwise ambulatory patients, the majority of clinical work is outpatient-based. However, some patients are admitted to hospital, for management of either treatment toxicities or symptoms from the disease. There is a dedicated session or two per week for technical planning of radiotherapy. On-call commitments are sociable and often carried out from home, with advice provided via telephone, but this is changing due to the introduction of acute oncology services. Clinical oncologists work as part of a multidisciplinary team (MDT) consisting of surgeons, radiologists, pathologists, medical oncologists, and clinical nurse specialists to facilitate holistic patient care right from their diagnosis and through continuing care.

Extras

There are plenty of research opportunities and the chance to be part of constantly improving radiation technology and exciting new systemic therapies. There is strong support from government, patient groups, and charities that help with funding. There are opportunities galore to be involved in teaching and gaining higher qualifications. There is an opportunity to undertake private practice.

For further information

The Royal College of Radiologists (RCR). Tel: 020 7405 1282. Web: https://www.rcr.ac.uk
Email: enquiries@rcr.ac.uk Twitter: @RCRadiologists

08:30 Lymphoma multidisciplinary meeting, discussing patients who need radiotherapy and reviewing those on treatment

10:00 Outpatient clinic; patients include two new referrals with a diagnosis of germ cell tumour

12:30 Call from chemotherapy suite to see a patient who had reacted adversely to a drug

13:00 Paperwork and lunch

13:30 Pop up to the ward to see a patient admitted with infection post-chemotherapy

14:00 Radiotherapy planning of a case of prostate cancer and plan discussion with physicist

16:00 Call from a clinical nurse specialist about an inpatient with lymphoma now diagnosed with relapse in the brain. Attend the ward to see the patient and discuss palliative radiotherapy

17:00 Head home for an evening out with the family

Myth	Techie doctors who just do radiotherapy.
Reality	Very much clinically focused, but with application of radiation technology to enhance and improve the treatment of cancer.
Personality	Caring, compassionate, empathetic, motivating, strong interpersonal skills, and a flair for research.
Best aspects	Opportunity to help patients during life-changing illness, working as part of an MDT, possessing unique skills of therapeutic application of radiation and being part of rapidly advancing and exciting research.
Worst aspects	Can be emotionally draining, limited resources.
Route	Internal medicine training (IMT) (p. 44), acute care common stem–acute medicine (ACCS-AM) (p. 37), then specialty training in clinical oncology (ST3+). Exams: MRCP; FRCR in clinical oncology.
Numbers	930 consultants, of whom 50% are women.
Locations	Radiotherapy is delivered only in specialist centres but may have clinics in peripheral cancer units.

Life					Work
Quiet On-call					Busy On-call
Boredom					Burnout
Uncompetitive					Competitive
Low salary					High salary

Clinical pharmacology and therapeutics

Clinical pharmacology and therapeutics (CP&T) covers the whole gamut of medicine and therapeutics, from anaesthesia to virology and from abacavir to zuclopenthixol. One day you're treating seriously ill patients, the next you're researching anticancer drugs at the bench or in a clinical trial. On other days, you're giving a keynote lecture at an international conference or editing a major influential textbook. Many clinical pharmacologists are academics. Some are consultant physicians in busy teaching hospitals. Some work in pharmaceutical companies, and some are involved in drug regulation (e.g. Medicines and Healthcare products Regulatory Agency (MHRA). The range of opportunities is enormous!

The patients

Patients may be of any age and with any medical problem. Clinical pharmacologists may be general physicians or specialists, e.g. in paediatrics, infectious diseases, endocrinology, or psychiatry. Occasionally, they are asked to review a patient with a pharmacological problem (e.g. a drug allergy) or to advise on a legal case (e.g. as an expert witness on drug therapy in coroner's court). Those working in drug companies may be running clinical trials or involved in pharmacovigilance (see Pharmaceutical medicine, p. 264).

The work

CP&T is exceptionally diverse. It includes: patient care in general or specialty medicine, advising colleagues on the management of their patients; teaching a range of colleagues about practical drug therapy; formulating drug policy both locally and nationally; editing and writing important text (e.g. the *British National Formulary* (*BNF*) and *BNF for Children*); and doing research (bench work, clinical research, or thought experiments; often all three). All prescribers need to know about the effects of medicines and their appropriate uses, and clinical pharmacologists have an important role to play in educating them and troubleshooting their problems. They are also essential in helping the NHS get the best out of available medicines in an effective and affordable way.

The job

Many clinical pharmacologists are university academics and divide their time among the above activities. Some are employed by the NHS as hospital consultants and spend about half their time doing inpatient and outpatient clinical medicine, alongside research. Others are employed by regulatory or national bodies such as NICE.

Extras

Meetings of the British Pharmacological Society, the Clinical Pharmacology Colloquium, and other UK groups are among the best that you will attend anywhere. Successful academics often have opportunities to travel to meetings overseas and collaborate on an international level. Consultancies with pharmaceutical companies can be very interesting, educative, and remunerative, as can medico-legal work. There are excellent opportunities to contribute to the development of international formularies and guidelines, helping to optimize the management of patients in different circumstances around the world, ranging from collaborations with expert societies on subspecialty topics through to work with the World Health Organization (WHO) focusing on resource-poor settings.

> **For further information**
>
> **British Pharmacological Society.** Tel: 020 7239 0171. Web: https://www.bps.ac.uk Twitter: @BritPharmSoc

A week in the life ...

MON Research; dealing with proofs of the next issue of the *BNF*

TUE A.M. Ward round, 25 acutely ill patients with a wide range of medical conditions

TUE P.M. Chair local Drug and Therapeutics Committee; advise colleagues on designing a pharmacokinetic study of a new drug for prostate cancer

WED A.M. NICE Technology Appraisal Committee: management of metastatic colo-rectal cancer

WED P.M. NICE Technology Appraisal Committee: a new treatment for multiple sclerosis

THU A.M. Write papers, edit international encyclopaedia on adverse drug reactions

THU P.M. General medical grand round; radiology meeting; student case presentations

FRI A.M. Ward round/teaching

FRI P.M. Research; applied pharmacology in the King's Arms with PhD students

Weekend (optional) Editing, preparation for committees/consultancies

Myth	A moribund discipline. Unexciting, poorly paid work.
Reality	The discipline is expanding. There are many diverse activities, constantly surprising and challenging. Consultancies and legal work can be lucrative.
Personality	Wide interests. Good communicator. Sensitive when advising colleagues. For research: curiosity, good logical and analytical skills, perseverance.
Best aspects	Enormous variety; no two days are alike. Travel, if you want; the world is your oyster. Opportunities to influence national and international policy.
Worst aspects	Research bureaucracy (e.g. grant applications); NHS bureaucracy.
Route	Numerous routes into specialty training in clinical pharmacology and therapeutics (ST3+), including internal medicine training (IMT) (p. 44); acute care common stem–acute medicine (ACCS-AM) or emergency medicine (ACCS-EM) (p. 37); paediatrics (p. 49); GP (p. 42); and core anaesthetics training (p. 39). Can dual-CCT with some medical specialties.
Numbers	70 consultants in hospitals; many opportunities in drug companies and posts in regulatory authorities.
Locations	Academic/NHS (CP&T is usually a joint university- and NHS hospital-based specialty); pharmaceutical companies; regulatory authorities.

Life — Work
Quiet On-call — Busy On-call
Boredom — Burnout
Uncompetitive — Competitive
Low salary — High salary

Dermatology

Dermatology is a broad discipline—it offers the opportunity to be a polymath with mastery over an enormous range of diagnoses overlapping multiple specialties. Alternatively, within subspecialty areas, dermatologists can be skin cancer surgeons, paediatricians, or immunologists or have expertise in complex systemic treatments. As skin is visible, many patients present to their GP at a threshold lower than in many systemic diseases, which leads to much of dermatology management being undertaken by GPs. This, in turn, means that consultants have a close working relationship with primary care professionals such as teachers, supervisors, and providers of support tools such as teledermatology. Dermatology consultant training numbers have fallen behind the number of posts in the last 10 years, such that around 200 (>20%) of dermatology consultant posts in the UK are not currently filled.

The patients

Patients may be of any age, including children, depending on the chosen area(s) of practice. Referrals to dermatology fall into two main groups—in most centres, the largest group are those who have a mark or lump on their skin which might be skin cancer. Many of these people require review in under 2 weeks, which creates a high throughput. The other group are those with inflammatory skin disorders, including eczema and psoriasis. Ten years ago, the latter group was the larger of the two, but with increasing age of the population and the aim to provide a diagnosis earlier in the evolution of skin cancer, there has been an increase in the numbers referred for assessment.

The work

The primary emphasis is on diagnosis and establishing the significance of the diagnosis to the patient. Diagnostic skills with close clinical assessment, e.g. dermoscopy and skin biopsy, are central to daily work. All dermatologists will have basic skin surgery skills to enable performance of diagnostic biopsies and small skin excisions. A large number will further develop these skills and provide a skin cancer treatment service for all but the largest of skin cancers. Both medical and oncological dermatology practice is typically undertaken within multidisciplinary teams (MDTs) sharing care with other medical or surgical specialties.

The job

The vast majority of the work is undertaken in hospital-based outpatient clinics. Some dermatologists also support or run community services. Out-of-hours requirements are limited, but availability for advice or shared care of complex patients with life-threatening diagnoses, such as toxic epidermal necrolysis, remains important. Review of patients admitted to other specialties with coincident skin problems is common and your contribution can often enable earlier discharge.

Extras

All dermatologists are teachers, educating undergraduate and postgraduate learners in a variety of disciplines and specialties. Most dermatologists will choose an area of specialist expertise, which might evolve within the consultant post or be developed as a trainee. Less-than-full-time training is available and there is a high proportion of women entering dermatology training. Private practice is common and lucrative.

For further information

British Association of Dermatologists (BAD). Tel: 020 7383 0266. Web: https://www.bad.org.uk Email: admin@bad.org.uk Twitter: @HealthySkin4All

---

08:30	Meet with the nursing and support team, and prepare for clinic
09:00	Dermatology clinic with registrar, specialist nurse, and maybe students; 20 patients with various conditions from acne to cutaneous sarcoidosis. Two urgent biopsies at the end of clinic
13:30	Review ward referral with possible drug rash
14:10	Discuss cancer referrals with manager over lunch
14:35	Respond to emails, then attend skin cancer MDT meeting to discuss results and treatment options
16:30	Review phototherapy patients in light treatment area
17:00	Advise a colleague calling from the ICU about a patient with skin desquamation
17:45	Dictate notes from the morning's MDT and clinic, and check patient results
19:00	Provide teledermatology service to primary care
19:30	Go home

Myth	It's a soft option—the 'dermaholiday'.
Reality	There is an enormous and unmeetable workload, with high patient expectation.
Personality	Careful, interested in detail, good listener, and a brain that likes to work with images and colour. Manual dexterity useful for surgery.
Best aspects	Most treatments make a considerable difference to patients' lives. Skin surgery provides a wonderful opportunity to get to know the patients and theatre staff. The breadth of patient groups is stimulating.
Worst aspects	Too little time for each patient, such that there is not enough time to provide the level of care you might want. Big lack of capacity.
Route	Core training in medicine (either internal medicine training (IMT)) (p. 44) or acute care common stem–acute medicine (ACCS-AM) (p. 37) or paediatrics level 1 training (p. 49), then specialty training in dermatology (ST3+). Exams: MRCP or MRCPCH; SCE in Dermatology.
Numbers	850 consultants, of whom 60% are women.
Locations	Tertiary, teaching, and district general hospitals. Some community clinics.

Life						Work
Quiet On-call						Busy On-call
Boredom						Burnout
Uncompetitive						Competitive
Low salary						High salary

▌ Diving and hyperbaric medicine

Diving medicine involves the management of disorders related to the undersea environment. The closely allied field of hyperbaric medicine encompasses the medical use of pressures higher than atmospheric pressure, predominantly to administer oxygen. Both require an appreciation and understanding of a broad range of associated specialties, including aspects of occupational and respiratory medicine, toxicology, anaesthetics, psychology, and general practice. An interest in extreme environments and physiology and an enquiring mind, open to subtlety and diagnostic conundrums, are ideal attributes.

The patients

Diving casualties, most commonly injured in the recreational or commercial sectors, can range from the 'walking wounded' to the extremely unwell. Due to the myriad manifestations of diving-related disease, a sizeable number of patients represent diagnostic dilemmas, and a paucity of useful investigations requires the practitioner to develop good and integrated clinical acumen. Patients requiring hyperbaric oxygen therapy may be critically ill (e.g. with necrotizing soft tissue infection or severe carbon monoxide poisoning) or have a chronic condition, e.g. diabetic foot ulcer. Other patients may be well rather than ill, requiring surveillance-style medicals to work or assessment of whether a medical condition is compatible with safe diving.

The work

Diving medicine is a particular subset of occupational medicine, whilst hyperbaric medicine involves treatment of a seemingly disparate group of conditions which can respond well to pressure/oxygen, or more usually to a combination of both. The work is therefore varied but requires a high degree of diagnostic skill, together with an ability to manage expectations in a potentially vulnerable group of patients. Clinical duties may involve: fitness to dive assessments in a commercial or recreational setting for the well and those with medical conditions; evaluation and treatment of diving casualties; prescribing and overseeing chamber recompression therapy; and quite often teaching about all of the above.

The job

Most doctors in the field work in close proximity to a hyperbaric chamber, sited in or near a hospital. The chamber team can be small, so good teamwork and communication are vital. Access to, and judicious use of, other clinicians and selected investigations is useful to whittle down the wide range of differential diagnoses in diving cases. A flexible and constructive attitude to problem-solving is highly desirable. Out-of-hours work and on-call commitments vary widely according to the team size, but a sick diver may require intensive management for many hours.

Extras

Research will become an increasingly important aspect, to enlarge the evidence base upon which future funding is contingent. International conferences tend to take place in exotic locations where diving is an option. Teaching opportunities abound as diving medicine is exciting and the physiology of extreme pressures compelling. Hyperbaric medicine is far more widespread in other regions of Europe, Australasia, and North America; sabbatical and exchange posts are thus more widely available overseas, including to UK doctors.

For further information

The British Hyperbaric Association. Web: http://www.hyperbaric.org.uk Twitter: @UKHyperbaric

European Underwater and Baromedical Society. Web: http://www.eubs.org

Undersea and Hyperbaric Medical Society (USA). Web: https://www.uhms.org
Email: uhms@uhms.org

08:00 Arrive, deal with overnight emails/referrals, review patients before hyperbaric treatments commence

09:00 Clinic for commercial/recreational diving assessments; review patients after hyperbaric treatment

12:00 Lunch with team, often involving ad hoc educational session

13:30 Clinic or teaching session (commercial diver training or medical/physiology students)

16:30 Finish off admin, catch up on emails/referrals

17:30 Home

18:30 Lecture to local dive club on diving diseases and prevention

20:00 Give advice over phone to a concerned diver with possible decompression illness

Myth	Pioneering explorer participating in remote azure sea expeditions.
Reality	Clinic-based diagnostician with interest in gases, pressures, and extreme environments.
Personality	Empathetic, keen clinical acumen, conscientious, independent thinker, but a good team player.
Best aspects	Diversity of emergency patient presentations, satisfaction of effective treatment, flexibility of career path, team camaraderie.
Worst aspects	Occupational health assessments for divers can become mundane; constant fear of funding inadequacy; danger of professional isolation and deskilling in niche specialty with small teams.
Route	Highly idiosyncratic, but usually based in anaesthesia, respiratory medicine, or general practice, with some postgraduate training in diving medicine.
Locations	Specialist unit, often based in/near hospital.

Life						Work
Quiet On-call						Busy On-call
Boredom						Burnout
Uncompetitive						Competitive
Low salary						High salary

Ear, nose, and throat (ENT or otolaryngology)

ENT surgeons have a huge impact on patients' lives by restoring senses (hearing, smell, and taste), improving function (voice and balance), treating life-threatening conditions (airway pathology and head and neck cancer), and improving cosmesis (facial plastic surgery). There are four principal subspecialties (otology, rhinology/facial plastics, head and neck surgery, and paediatric ENT), each requiring different surgical skills and utilizing different surgical technology. The day-to-day work is mainly outpatient-based and there is a large medical component to keep the academically orientated surgeon very busy.

The patients

ENT is 'cradle-to-grave' treating patients of all ages with both medical and surgical problems, e.g. elderly patients with skin and upper aerodigestive cancers, young adults with nasal polyps and thyroid disease, and premature neonates who cannot breathe or were born with a hearing loss. Over 30% of ENT patients are children and most of the patients are medically fit and usually quite happy!

The work

Most conditions are managed with minor procedures or medications in the outpatient setting. Only around 20–30% require surgery; cases range from the straightforward, such as putting in grommets, to the highly specialized, such as reconstructing a child's trachea, all in the same operating list. ENT is at the forefront of medical innovation, utilizing a wide range of technology such as endoscopes, microscopes, lasers and robotics during surgery, and devices such as implantable hearing aids and prosthetic ears.

The job

ENT surgeons can practise in district general hospitals (DGHs), as well as in tertiary centres, depending on the complexity of the work they want to perform. Most of the work is outpatient-based and a consultant typically carries out 3–4 outpatient clinics per week and two operating lists. They work closely with a number of other professionals such as audiologists, speech and language therapists, dieticians, and other specialties, e.g. plastic surgery, oncology. Whilst there is probably more clinic work than other surgical specialties, the intensity of ward work and on-call is generally less. It is unusual for a consultant to be called in the hospital at night, but when they are, it is usually for something life-threatening such as acute stridor or a major haemorrhage.

Extras

Most ENT surgeons subspecialize, and many go on fellowship at home or abroad after their training. This may be a year in a tertiary unit in Australia, an observership in Europe, or an 'ear camp' in Africa. This is hugely encouraged and is a fantastic life experience. Less-than-full-time training is increasing and usually well supported. There is ample private practice and medico-legal work for those who would like it.

For further information

ENT UK, c/o Royal College of Surgeons, London. Tel: 020 7404 8373. Web: https://www.entuk.org Email: entuk@entuk.org Twitter: @ENT_UK

Association of Otolaryngologists in Training (AOT). Web: https://aotent.org Email: aotent@gmail.com Twitter: @socialmediaAOT

07:45	Take informed consent from the five patients on the operating list
08:20	Meet with the entire surgical team in the anaesthetic room for a surgical briefing and discussion of the morning cases followed by a large coffee and a pastry
09:00	Start of operating list. Cases include inserting grommets for a young child, removing the tonsils of an older child, and endoscopic sinus surgery in an adult.
13:00	Lunchtime and then on to clinic. Whip through 15 patients, book three patients for an operation, and chat through interesting cases with the registrar and fellow
17:00	Go back to review the patients from the morning operating list who thankfully are all well and about to be discharged home
17:45	Arrive home to see the kids
21:00	Called in to review and operate on a man who has been stabbed in the neck. The wound needed exploring in theatre, but luckily no major injury
23:00	In bed getting some zzzzzzzzzz!

Myth	It's all snot, wax, and phlegm!
Reality	An exciting mix of medicine and cutting-edge surgery, making a profound difference to patients' lives.
Personality	Precision, dedication, and innovation. Calm and decisive under pressure, as ENT emergencies can get very serious very quickly.
Best aspects	Challenging surgery, lots of subspecialties, great work–life balance, few emergencies.
Worst aspects	Heavy demand for services; competitive entry into the specialty.
Route	Core surgical training (CST) (p. 61), followed by specialty training in ENT (ST3+) (p. 64). Exams: MRCS (ENT); FRCS (ENT).
Numbers	750 consultants, of whom 15% are women.
Locations	Hospital-based specialty available in most hospitals.

Life					Work
Quiet On-call					Busy On-call
Boredom					Burnout
Uncompetitive					Competitive
Low salary					High salary

Elderly medicine

Elderly care medicine (also known as geriatric medicine) is a multidisciplinary, holistic specialty that aims to optimize the health and well-being of older people. The specialty is person-centred rather than disease-focused, and specialists often treat patients with the same disease quite differently, depending on their preferences, coexisting illnesses, and life expectancy. It is the largest hospital specialty, yet still rapidly expanding as health systems recognize that the care of frail older people has become their core business.

The patients

Elderly care physicians look after some very fit centenarians, but also many frail older people, most of whom have several different, and sometimes competing, problems. The patients are full of stories and wisdom; they have a wealth of life experience and are often pragmatic about the challenges that they face. Patients may rely on their families or friends and neighbours for support and advocacy, so communication with caregivers is vital. Some patients have curable diseases and get better. Many more have multiple long-term conditions that need careful management. Others will be towards the end of their lives, including some who need palliative care.

The work

Older people may not always present typically. An increasing tendency to fall may require medications to be stopped but may sometimes be the sign of a serious illness such as infection, kidney failure, or even cancer. Unpicking this is part of the skill of elderly care medicine. A key part of the role is to advocate for older people, ensuring they are not denied access to the best treatments that younger patients receive. The other side of the coin is avoiding protocolized treatment that may cause harm in a frail patient. Sometimes the answer isn't clear, and it takes wisdom and good communication skills to choose the right course of action. A wise elderly care physician will have a good working knowledge of evidence-based treatments for particular conditions, yet also realize when those treatments are not suitable for individual patients.

The job

There is a rich variety of work, from seeing acutely unwell patients in the emergency department and wards to seeing patients in specialist clinics or proactively in domiciliary settings. The specialty is very much team-orientated and requires close co-operation with nurses, therapists, and pharmacists. Being an elderly care physician involves knowing a little bit about everything, but a lot about something—some subspecialize in areas as diverse as acute or emergency care, surgical liaison, stroke medicine, movement disorders, or community geriatrics. Depending upon location, on-call commitments may be confined to older patients or, more commonly, to general and acute medicine where older people still make up a significant proportion of the population.

Extras

Elderly care physicians are often found performing a variety of non-clinical activities such as medical education, management, quality improvement, and research. They are also well represented in health policy, with several figures from the specialty having prominent roles within national bodies. Private practice is not common; most geriatricians derive enough variety and job satisfaction from NHS work.

For further information

British Geriatrics Society (BGS). Tel: 020 7608 1369. Web: https://www.bgs.org.uk/ Email: enquiries@bgs.org.uk Twitter: @GeriSoc

JRCPTB Geriatric Medicine information. Web: https://www.jrcptb.org.uk/specialties/geriatric-medicine

A day in the life ...

08:00 Answer emails and admin. Look through online notes for new patients before ward round

09:00 Safety huddle with ward staff, highlighting priority-review patients and determining plans to reduce risk of falls and pressure injuries to skin

09:15 Start ward round accompanied by junior doctor and a medical student, incorporate teaching for both

12:00 Ward multidisciplinary team (MDT) meeting to discuss plans, including discharge plans

12:30 Lunchtime departmental teaching session

13:00 Outpatient clinic: 12 patients, a mix of new and follow-up patients

16:00 Return to ward to speak to relatives and answer any queries from junior doctors

17:00 Review clinic and discharge letters, complete junior doctor ePortfolio assessment tickets

Myth	Jack of all trades, master of none; there's nothing that can be done anyway.
Reality	Holistic doctors advocating for older people and managing complex problems and decisions; highly skilled in determining when treatment burdens outweigh the benefits.
Personality	Hardworking, positive, energetic, and caring; highly developed communication skills.
Best aspects	Variety of patients, as well as of team members, work pace, settings, and skills.
Worst aspects	Perceptions of the specialty, although this is changing.
Route	Internal medicine training (IMT) (p. 44) or acute care common stem–acute medicine (ACCS-AM) (p. 37), then specialty training in geriatric medicine (ST3+). Exams: MRCP; SCE in Geriatric Medicine.
Numbers	1700 consultants, of whom 40% are women.
Locations	Hospital-based, from district general hospitals to teaching hospitals; community-based care is increasing.

Life						Work
Quiet On-call						Busy On-call
Boredom						Burnout
Uncompetitive						Competitive
Low salary						High salary

Emergency medicine

Emergency medicine (EM) is the only hospital specialty that is required to deal with every patient presentation, across all ages and severities of illness. Patients present with anything and everything, requiring quick-thinking, adaptable, and broadly skilled clinicians. The emergency physician is what the public think a doctor is—someone who can cope with any medical problem—and you have the benefit of knowing that everything you learn may at some point be useful to your practice. EM is an exciting job that is endlessly interesting—for proof, just look at the number of compelling TV shows based on emergency care!

The patients

Patients attend emergency departments (EDs) for the widest range of reasons. Some come in by ambulance and may be critically unwell or victims of major trauma; others will walk in off the street and may attend just because they have run out of medication or because they simply don't know where else to seek help. Patient cohorts vary substantially between departments, particularly between major trauma centres and acute hospitals. In line with population needs, EDs see a high proportion of geriatric and paediatric patients, and bear witness to a many of the consequences of social deprivation.

The work

EDs are the gateway to the hospital for the majority of inpatient services and are given priority access to much of the hospital's resources—more can often be done in the first 4 hours than in the next 4 days. EM is now a predominantly medical specialty despite its surgical origins. Emergency physicians are risk managers whose primary job is to work out who is at risk and to take immediate steps to mitigate this where necessary. For those not at immediate risk, emergency physicians facilitate safe discharge, with timely follow-up where necessary, protecting inpatient specialties from a tide of unnecessary admissions.

The job

EM is practised in the ED, split into zones, including majors, minors, paediatrics, and resus—there may be contribution to clinics and ambulatory care too. EM is usually one of the few disciplines to work a shift-based system rather than a traditional 9–5 with oncall commitment, mapped to a peak-hours staffing model to meet patient demand. As such, there is high out-of-hours working commitment, but also scheduled non-clinical time (e.g. for education, research, audit) at all levels. Emergency care is very much a team sport—emergency physicians will work with clinicians from nearly all specialties, advanced and emergency nurse practitioners, and allied health professionals, often providing clinical oversight and co-ordination to deliver the best possible care for patients.

Extras

There is little private practice in EM, but consultant job planning makes for excellent flexibility and easily accommodates portfolio careers. Shift work easily accommodates less-than-full-time training and working. As trained systems thinkers who are embroiled daily in hospital performance, emergency physicians are well placed to work with and in healthcare management. Emergency physicians are excellent candidates for humanitarian and global health work, with a skill set that lends itself well to both postgraduate and undergraduate medical education. EM also offers subspecialty training in paediatric (p. 156) and pre-hospital EM (p. 158), and dual training in intensive care medicine (p. 200).

For further information

The Royal College of Emergency Medicine (RCEM). Tel: 020 7404 1999. Web: https://www.rcem.ac.uk Twitter: @RCollEM

A day in the life ...

14:00 Departmental clinical governance meeting, including review of new sedation policy and audit of previous performance

16:00 Departmental handover, discussion of high-risk, complex, or interesting patients

16:30 Ward round of observation unit, to decide whether to discharge or refer patients

17:10 Attend and run a trauma call for a 40-year-old cyclist vs car. Co-ordinate investigations, arrange follow-up under trauma and orthopaedics

18:00 Move to majors; discuss and review patients with junior trainees

18:30 Discuss safeguarding concerns with nursing staff around patient admitted with possible neglect from a nursing home, liaise with local social work team

19:00 Continue reviewing patients, including a 4-year-old child with breathing difficulties and a woman with a possible stroke

20:30 A much needed break!

21:00 Return to floor, this time to minors to manage waiting time, review several patients

22:00 Departmental handover to night team, then review more paediatric patients

00:00 Leave department and go home

Myth	Non-stop adrenaline-fuelled major trauma and cardiac arrest calls.
Reality	High-stakes risk management, requiring excellent clinical oversight and resource co-ordination skills.
Personality	Generalist with a wide range of clinical interests, calm under pressure, able to switch between tasks quickly, with a good dose of pragmatism and practical ability.
Best aspects	Always going home thinking you've made a difference doing something worthwhile. Never bored; usually have the best medical stories and occasionally actually save a life.
Worst aspects	High risk of burnout, high proportion of unsocial hours, occasional feelings of fighting 'the system'; limited capacity to follow up patients.
Route	Acute care common stem–emergency medicine (ACCS-EM) (p. 37) either run-through from ST1 or uncoupled with reapplication to specialty training in EM (ST4+). DRE-EM (ST3+ see p. 37) after core surgical training (CST) (p. 61) or acute care common stem–acute medicine (ACCS-AM) or ACCS-anaesthetics (p. 37). Exams: FRCEM.
Numbers	1800 consultants, of whom 55% are women.
Locations	Major trauma centres, trauma units, and acute hospitals.

Life					Work
Quiet On-call					Busy On-call
Boredom					Burnout
Uncompetitive					Competitive
Low salary					High salary

Emergency medicine: paediatric

Paediatric emergency medicine (PEM) is a subspecialty of both emergency medicine (EM) (p. 154) and paediatrics (p. 256). It offers the opportunity to care for patients with a huge variety of clinical presentations, ranging from minor injury to severe and life-threatening medical conditions and trauma. It is therefore the ideal specialty for the child-orientated doctor with a passion for variety and fast-paced clinical work. PEM doctors work within a close-knit team that includes nurses, doctors, and other professionals to offer high-quality care in an emergency department (ED) treating both adults and children, or a dedicated paediatric ED.

The patients

Most PEM specialists care for children from birth to 16 years old, through the most varied period of life. The PEM physician is a true generalist, and there is no such thing as an average day. Viral illnesses are common and although you may see several cases in a shift, every clinical encounter is potentially exciting, challenging, or thought-provoking. The variety of presentations means becoming a combination of GP, general paediatrician, and resuscitationist, which allows doctors to holistically manage the large number of complex and undifferentiated patients that come through the ED.

The work

The work is, above all other things, fun. Children have an infectious enthusiasm which makes for a joyful (and usually very loud) working environment, and their underlying physiology often allows them to bounce back from illness in a way adults simply don't. A PEM physician has to have the flexibility to switch rapidly from managing minor ailments as a solo practitioner to managing severe illness with a large MDT. The PEM team is close-knit and helps when managing cases that can be distressing or stressful. Clinical work is hands-on and can involve a degree of creativity and lateral thinking, seldom needed in adult practice, in order to achieve a satisfactory examination on a wriggling child, communicate with a patient with learning difficulties, or gain the trust of an anxious parent. PEM requires frequent use of practical skills, including sedation, fracture manipulation, and wound closure.

The job

Although training posts are relatively competitive, there is a paucity of PEM consultants. All departments treating children should have a PEM consultant and although there are increasing numbers, this standard is still not met in many hospitals. PEM doctors work within the ED on the general shift-based rota. Like both of its parent specialties, PEM has a relatively high rate of burnout due to the constant nature of the work, sick patients, and the high proportion of out-of-hours commitments. This is well recognized, and most clinicians regularly reflect on their emotional health and the subspecialty benefits from a supportive culture.

Extras

Among PEM clinicians, there is a lot of enthusiasm for teaching and research. Many utilize their generalist skills to vary their clinical work, including operating in the adult department (if from an EM background), paediatric decision unit, and paediatric intensive care unit, working in safeguarding, or deploying with humanitarian medical teams. Opportunities for private work are limited.

For further information

The Royal College of Emergency Medicine (RCEM). Tel: 020 7404 1999. Web: https://www.rcem.ac.uk Twitter: @RCollEM

The Royal College of Paediatrics and Child Health (RCPCH). Tel: 020 7092 6000. Web: https://www.rcpch.ac.uk Email: enquiries@rcpch.ac.uk Twitter: @RCPCHtweets

12:00	Start shift and take handover
13:00	Departmental teaching for junior doctors on paediatric elbow X-ray interpretation
14:00	Sedate a child for fracture manipulation
15:00	See patients on the shop floor, including a child with possible appendicitis and a teenager having an asthma attack
16:00	Multidisciplinary safeguarding meeting
17:00	Discuss management plan for a patient with a paediatric consultant
18:00	Lead resuscitation team for a paediatric trauma
19:00	Huddle with nurses and managers to manage crowded department
20:00	Supervise junior doctor performing a lumbar puncture on a baby with fever
21:00	Home to try and get the soundtrack of *Frozen* out of your head

Myths	Jack of all trades, master of none. It's all about the resus.
Reality	Fast-paced, high-variety clinical work in a fun and enthusiastic patient group.
Personality	Able to think quickly and multitask. Able to analyse risk and weigh this up to facilitate safe discharge or admission.
Best aspects	Working in great teams, with a supportive network of specialists. Wide variety of clinical skills in a patient group that frightens a lot of other clinicians. A blossoming specialty, with lots of opportunities for teaching and development.
Worst aspects	Shift work late into career. High risk of burnout. Occasional harrowing cases that can impact on you emotionally. Lots of Baby Shark on repeat.
Route	EM training as per adult EM (p. 37), with subspecialty training in PEM (ST5+ or post-CCT), or paediatric run-through training (ST1+) (p. 49), then ST6+ PEM Grid Training. Exams: exams relevant to core/initial specialty; FRCEM.
Numbers	Approximately 75 PEM consultants, and 45 general paediatricians with a subspecialty interest in PEM.
Locations	Hospitals providing emergency services, including major trauma centres and tertiary, teaching, and district general hospitals.

Life						Work
Quiet On-call						Busy On-call
Boredom						Burnout
Uncompetitive						Competitive
Low salary						High salary

Emergency medicine: pre-hospital emergency medicine

Pre-hospital Emergency Medicine (PHEM) is one of the most difficult, but rewarding jobs there is. All patients will stretch you to your limits, through a combination of medical, technical, and non-technical challenges.

The patients

Patients may be suffering from minor illnesses through to life-threatening emergencies, e.g. polytrauma from a road traffic collision, life-threatening asthma, or a fitting child. Interventions required are therefore just as varied and can be minor, e.g. providing medications, through to pre-hospital anaesthesia or even surgical procedures such as thoracotomy. More often than not, the patients are critically unwell, with relatively limited survival, and whilst the duration of contact with all patients is short, it is intense, powerful, and often literally lifesaving.

The work

PHEM is about providing a level of care normally found in an emergency department (ED) resuscitation room or critical care setting, but before the patient reaches hospital. It usually involves treating patients at the scene of the incident, which can vary from a patient's home to the middle of a field or the centre of a busy motorway. Getting to your patients and then transferring them to hospital typically involve transport which can include travelling by road or even flying, although the back of a helicopter is a very small place, especially for a very sick patient! Your team therefore usually includes a critical care paramedic (and pilots!) who join first responders (usually various members of the ambulance service) at the scene. PHEM relies on good medical knowledge, in conjunction with vital technical and non-technical skills, e.g. communication skills, leadership, and crew resource management, to get the best outcome for the patient.

The job

It is, in some ways, perfect—almost total autonomy and no clinics, ward rounds, or work that could be considered 'routine'. PHEM has developed from voluntary emergency pre-hospital care and is now an approved subspecialty for both EM (p. 154) and anaesthetics (p. 118). It is a specialty that is continually developing and will continue to advance in terms of the skills and resources that can be provided on the pre-hospital scene. The job is a challenging one, usually providing care to the most critically ill, under physically challenging conditions, with limited resources in an unfamiliar environment, but it provides an amazing opportunity to deliver extreme levels of care to the most critically unwell patients in a timely fashion and to a very high standard.

Extras

There are plenty of opportunities for teaching which is often stimulating and fun. There is great overlap with expedition medicine (p. 162), offering exciting travel opportunities. Meeting with peers can be stimulating, and the opportunity for research is increasing but can be practically and ethically difficult. Oh, and did we mention there are helicopters?

For further information

The Intercollegiate Board for Training in Pre-Hospital Emergency Medicine, Edinburgh. Web: http://www.ibtphem.org.uk Twitter: @rcsed.ac.uk

The Faculty of Pre-Hospital Care of the Royal College of Surgeons of Edinburgh, Edinburgh. Web: https://fphc.rcsed.ac.uk Twitter: @FPHCEd

---

08:00 Arrive at base site. Cup of coffee with team

08:30 Check over response vehicles and equipment, fixing any issues immediately

10:53 Call comes in, reporting a five-car pile-up on the motorway 2 minutes ago

11:06 Arrive at scene via hard shoulder with flashing lights and sirens on; quick triage: one not breathing (RIP), one in respiratory distress, six walking wounded. Start primary assessment on patient with respiratory distress

11:25 Needle decompression of tension pneumothorax; ambulance arrives; work with paramedics to stabilize the patient and treat the injuries and shock of the others

12:30 Accompany patient with pneumothorax to ED

12:50 Hand over to ED team

13:30 Back to base site for lunch

14:30 Weekly team meeting with other members of the critical care team to discuss previous cases; identify what went well and areas to improve

19:30 Hand over to night team—thankfully a quiet day!

Myth	Wears underwear over flame-resistant trousers; has considered adding a cape.
Reality	Being cold, wet, and dirty in a ditch at night, feeling lonely whilst making lifesaving clinical decisions.
Personality	Calm, confident team player who knows their strengths and weaknesses, willingness to learn, problem-solving skills.
Best aspects	Feeling you may have made a difference, if only by being present and supporting your colleagues in the other emergency services.
Worst aspects	Being cold, wet, and dirty in a ditch; misconceptions of the job and the handover being ignored by ED staff.
Route	Training in either EM (p. 37), anaesthetics (p. 39), acute medicine (p. 44), or intensive care medicine (p. 39), then subspecialty training in PHEM (ST5+) as out of programme (OOP) (p. 101) or blended with training in parent specialty. Exams: exams required by parent specialty; Diploma and Fellowship of Immediate Medical Care.
Locations	Anywhere, anytime, in any weather.

Life						Work
Quiet On-call						Busy On-call
Boredom						Burnout
Uncompetitive						Competitive
Low salary						High salary

Endocrinology and diabetes

Clinical work in endocrinology and diabetes is immensely varied. The majority of specialists manage both endocrine conditions and diabetes, although they are quite distinct fields—endocrinology is the specialty that looks after patients with hormonal conditions; diabetes is more self-explanatory. Both specialties involve working in partnership with patients themselves and as part of a large multidisciplinary team (MDT). One of the best aspects of the specialty is multidisciplinary working, which enables the provision of holistic and comprehensive care from diagnosis and throughout patients' lives.

The patients

Many patients referred are complicated and often have undiagnosed problems affecting multiple aspects of their life. For example, a patient with thyroid disease might complain of changes to their hair, nails, skin, bowels, periods, weight, mood, heart, and head! The endocrinologist often feels like a detective, trying to pull all of these symptoms together to finally get to the bottom of the problem, with which the patient has often been struggling for many years. Patients with diabetes can be of any age, although children are more likely to present with type 1 diabetes which needs insulin straight away, whilst older patients might have type 1 or type 2. Patients with endocrine conditions can also be of any age, but the majority are young adults and overall, most endocrine conditions are more common in women.

The work

Most work is done in the outpatient (or community) clinic where specialists review new and follow-up patients, taking a history, examining them, then requesting and reviewing various test results. Most patients can be diagnosed and treated without ever hitting a hospital bed. Most endocrinology and diabetes specialists also specialize in general internal medicine (GIM) and also look after acutely unwell medical patients. This means that specialists can also see patients with an amazing range of problems during their inpatient stay, as well as patients with diabetes or endocrine conditions requiring hospital-based care.

The job

Endocrinologists spend most of their time in clinics and their offices going through subsequent results. They also attend regular meetings with the MDT, e.g. to discuss imaging with radiologists, surgeons, and ophthalmologists in endocrinological cases, or to discuss patients with particularly challenging diabetes with the whole team, including specialist nurses, other physicians, and psychologists. Both types of MDT meetings are there to help decide on the very best management advice to give individual patients. Depending on the size and expertise of the hospital, endocrinologists may also spend time on the wards, looking after patients with complications of their endocrine condition or needing general medical care.

Extras

Endocrinology is a very academic specialty, with numerous opportunities for research and teaching. Most endocrinologists will undertake research at the start of their training, and many choose to continue this throughout their clinical career. Many also have links to patient support groups and charities, as patient involvement and education are so crucial for people living with chronic conditions. Private practice is also fairly common in endocrinology, and there is plenty of extra work, e.g. acting as an expert witness and writing reports, for those interested. Less-than-full-time training and working is also very well established.

For further information

Society for Endocrinology. Web: https://www.endocrinology.org Twitter: @Soc_Endo

Association of British Clinical Diabetologists (ABCD). Web: https://abcd.care Email: info@abcd.care Twitter: @ABCDiab

A day in the life ...

08:00 Pituitary MDT confirming treatment plans for patients, based on their scans and results, and discussion with neurosurgeons, radiologist, and pathologist

09:00 General endocrinology clinic; four new patients with a variety of conditions and several follow-up patients considered 'old favourites'

13:00 Lunch during post-clinic meeting discussing interesting cases with other consultants and trainees

14:00 Clinical admin, including reviewing results, letters to patients, and GPs

16:00 Pop to the ward to review a patient under the care of another team who has just been picked up as having an abnormal thyroid result

16:30 Back to the office to write a brief review of a paper which has been submitted to an endocrine journal, and do some work on a presentation for next week

17:30 Head home for tea with the kids!

Myth	Incredibly clever doctors ordering innumerable incomprehensible investigations.
Reality	Academically interesting specialty putting all the pieces together using a thorough history and appropriate investigations; your friendly local biochemist helps with the complicated tests!
Personality	Open-minded, curious generalists with good communication and diagnostic skills; attention to detail and excellent teamworking skills.
Best aspects	Variety of patients; close working with patients and lots of other specialties; having a huge impact on people's lives—helping people have babies and actually making the blind see is hard to beat!
Worst aspects	General medical on-call can be hard. Finding it difficult to add much to the care of complex multimorbid patients during prolonged admissions.
Route	Either internal medicine training (IMT) (p. 44) or acute care common stem–acute medicine (ACCS-AM) (p. 37), then specialty training in endocrinology and diabetes (ST3+). Exams: MRCP; SCE in Endocrinology and Diabetes.
Numbers	1350 consultants, of whom 35% are women.
Locations	Hospital-based; clinics in community or GP surgeries, especially for diabetes.

Life					Work
Quiet On-call					Busy On-call
Boredom					Burnout
Uncompetitive					Competitive
Low salary					High salary

Expedition medicine

Expedition medicine can be as exotic, wild, or adventurous as you like, and every day is unique. Opportunities are increasing as the market for challenging experiences develops. You have the privilege of calling your travels 'work', whilst making your international debut as photographer, counsellor, teacher, latrine-digger, and chef.

The patients

The spectrum is vast. Your clientele could be extreme athletes breaking records, disabled ex-servicemen, young people from inner cities, or middle-aged men in Lycra. It depends entirely on the expedition, so ultimately the choice is yours. Expeditioners may be from any country, may speak a variety of languages, and include other team members such as local guides and porters, event leaders, and further support crew.

The work

The work begins with pre-expedition preparation: assessing potential participants' health, advising on suitable vaccinations, assembling medical kit, and researching the expedition environment. Once away, you may see everything, from blisters and diarrhoea to altitude sickness and major trauma. Managing patients in unfamiliar and remote environments demands good clinical and communication skills, as imaging and diagnostic facilities are rarely available. The majority of problems can be dealt with using simple treatments such as dressings, antibiotics, and analgesia, although emergency evacuation is occasionally required. A key component of the work is psychological, supporting the group and managing their expectations in unfamiliar surroundings. Developing experience in working outdoors, risk assessment, evacuation planning, and kit selection is essential, and roles may require specialist adventure sports skills, e.g. diving, kayaking, climbing, etc.

The job

The job may be in any environment, anywhere in the world. Many doctors are sole practitioners but may be supported by medical colleagues, nurses, or allied health professionals either in person or remotely. Expedition medics are on-call 24/7, as expeditioners can become patients at any time of the day or night. The medico-legal position can be complex, so it is essential to have personal indemnity cover for any role taken on.

Extras

Watching wildlife from your boat in the Antarctic, sleeping under the stars in the desert, or waking to the noise of the jungle from your hammock. There is scope to get involved with charity projects, try new sports, and do original research, alongside a wide range of conferences and teaching opportunities.

For further information

Adventure Medic. Web: https://www.theadventuremedic.com Email: contact@theadventuremedic.com Twitter: @adventure_medic

---

02:00	Climb out of your tent for an alpine start on a mountain summit. Feel grateful the weather's improved after having to call off the summit yesterday
02:10	Check in with everyone; make sure they are fed, warm, and ready to climb
02:30	Position yourself at the back of the group, keeping an eye on the team
07:00	Share incredible sunrise views from the peak
09:00	Review a climber complaining of headache and nausea—a possible case of altitude sickness. Arrange for a porter to accompany them back to base camp
11:00	Back to base camp to debrief climbers and then run an ad hoc clinic
12:00	Enjoy the vistas, check the facilities are hygienic, enjoy time with the group, help around the camp
21:00	Bedtime after some awe-inspiring stargazing

Myth	It's a holiday.
Reality	Preparation galore, high levels of responsibility, always ready for the unexpected.
Personality	Sociable team player, detailed planner, situationally aware, physically fit, adaptable, good communicator and leader, responsible, aware of own and others' limits.
Best aspects	Sharing life's highs and lows with fascinating people in incredible destinations. Calling 'once-in-a-lifetime experiences' your day job!
Worst aspects	On-call 24/7, being a surrogate leader/parent, having to make unpopular decisions that may conflict with the group's expectations.
Route	Roles are available from F2 onwards. An expedition medicine course and emergency medicine (EM) experience are often minimum requirements. GP) (p. 42) and EM (p. 37) training are the easiest paths to follow, in parallel with expedition medicine work.
Locations	Worldwide!

Life					Work

Quiet On-call					Busy On-call

Boredom					Burnout

Uncompetitive					Competitive

Low salary					High salary

Fertility medicine

Reproductive medicine is a wide-ranging field covering anything that affects fertility, from girls born without a uterus right through to management of the menopause. This field is expanding as many women delay having children. *In vitro* fertilization (IVF) has been around for 40 years, but other treatments such as ovulation induction and reproductive surgery are still used.

The patients

The majority of patients are couples of reproductive age who have been trying to conceive for some time. Many just need reassurance that normal fertility can take time, maybe even years. However, modern families come in all shapes and sizes. Fertility specialists see same-sex couples, single women, and egg and sperm donors. Fertility preservation may also be an option, e.g. for those about to start chemotherapy which will damage their fertility, or even for social reasons. Some patients don't have a fertility problem at all, but instead use preimplantation genetic diagnosis (PGD) to prevent transmission of genetic problems to their children.

The work

A varied mix of medicine and practical procedures. Investigation requires detailed knowledge of reproductive endocrinology and andrology, and liaison with other medical specialties. Procedures include ultrasound scanning, egg collection, embryo transfer, and laparoscopic surgery. Fertility is a highly emotive topic and treatment is not just about getting pregnant, but also about providing support throughout the fertility journey. Work is within a team of doctors, embryologists, fertility nurses, and administrative staff. Only a few emergencies exist such as severe ovarian hyperstimulation syndrome, but each day presents itself with many ethical dilemmas.

The job

Fertility medicine can be practised in primary and secondary care, but IVF requires a lab and licence from the Human Fertilisation and Embryology Authority (HFEA). In the UK, about half of clinics are in the NHS, but increasingly treatment is being provided by the private sector, as now about 60% of IVF cycles are funded by patients themselves.

Extras

Despite the National Institute of Health and Care Excellence (NICE) guidance, the NHS doesn't fund the majority of fertility treatment, so private practice is commonplace. Arrangements include working for a private fertility clinic or seeing self-funded patients in NHS clinics. Fertility stories regularly appear in the media and so there is the opportunity to participate. As a relatively new specialty, research is essential to improve outcomes for patients. Most consultants will have done a higher degree (MD or PhD) and continue to participate in research studies.

For further information

British Fertility Society, Middlesex. Tel: 020 3725 5849. Web: https://www.britishfertility society.org.uk Email: bfs@profileproductions.co.uk Twitter: @BritFertSoc

---

07:30 Ultrasound scanning. Patients having monitoring of ovarian stimulation for IVF treatment

09:00 Oocyte retrieval. Several short procedures under sedation to collect eggs for treatment

11:30 Embryo transfer. Short procedures to put back an embryo 5 days after egg collection

12:00 Oncology patient—a young woman diagnosed last week with breast cancer to discuss fertility preservation

13:30 Fertility clinic. A mixture of couples just referred for fertility treatment and those who have had several unsuccessful cycles

19:00 Patient information evening. Give a talk on treatment for same-sex couples

Myth	A licence to print money.
Reality	Ethical dilemmas, intense emotive consultations.
Personality	Easy-going and not embarrassed to talk about sex; aptitude for practical procedures.
Best aspects	Creating families.
Worst aspects	Managing patient expectations.
Route	Specialty training in obstetrics and gynaecology (O&G) (ST1+) (p. 47), then subspecialty training in reproductive medicine (ST6+). Exams: MRCOG.
Locations	Clinics and theatres, either in the NHS or in private facilities.

Life					Work
Quiet On-call					Busy On-call
Boredom					Burnout
Uncompetitive					Competitive
Low salary					High salary

Forensic medicine

Forensic medicine can be described as A&E (police custody) on steroids (the detainees) with proper bodyguards (the police). Add to that images of violent, drunk patients or those high on drugs, murderers, mass demonstrators, shootings, drug dealers and terrorists. This is medical jurisprudence or legal medicine where *clinical medicine and science meet the law*. Forensic medicine encompasses a range of different specialists, but this chapter only describes the work of forensic physicians (FP) (previously called police surgeon or forensic medical examiner (FME)) who cover general forensic medicine (GFM) in police custodies. Custody healthcare in Scotland is commissioned by NHS Scotland, but in England and Wales, it is a mixture of direct police (London) and private contractors.

The patients

Include those arrested in police custody, alleged drink drivers in hospitals, injured police officers, victims of physical or sexual assaults (both children and adults), torture victims and even alleged terrorist suspects. Most are male (85%) and between 18 and 44 years (74%). A survey of detainees found 38% had mental health conditions, 33% used drugs and 66% alcohol, and 24% had sustained injuries[1]. Detainees can be held for 24–36 hours in custody, under the Police and Criminal Evidence Act 1984, so most interactions and care provisions are brief, with little follow-up and no ward rounds, bleeps, clinics, or discharge letters! Most detainees would not wish their GPs to receive a letter stating they have been in police custody. Sexual assault examinations are undertaken in specialized sexual assault referral centres (SARCs) which combine police and NHS resources such as genitourinary medicine (GUM) and paediatrics. Some forces include this with GFM work.

The work

The FP has a dual role: to provide healthcare to detainees and to support the criminal justice system. This can present interesting medico-legal and ethical conflicts. The FP may be asked to declare if a detainee is fit to be detained, interviewed, or charged, prescribe or administer medications, assess and record in the correct forensic manner and treat injuries, assess and manage drug/alcohol intoxication or withdrawal, and assess for mental health conditions or learning difficulties. They may be required to take forensic samples for drink/drug drive cases or other forensic samples or, in very rare cases, to lead or perform emergency medical interventions. Remuneration is usually by the hour, with pay ranging from £40 to £70 per hour. Workload is also variable, depending on the time of the day, the day, and the urban areas covered.

The job

The primary workplace is a police custody suite, but FPs may be called to attend A&E to take blood for drink/drug drive cases, attend suspicious death scenes, attend court/inquest, or provide statements. As many contracts are zero hour and there are shifts available around the clock, there is opportunity to work part-time or develop a portfolio career. There are fewer jobs as most forces/providers are going down the nurse-led route.

Extras

Opportunities exist for providing expert reports once your knowledge and credibility develop. As this is relatively uncharted territory, research and audit potentials are huge, e.g. in areas such as violence reduction, TB epidemiology, mental health, learning disabilities, cases of female genital mutilation, and human trafficking, etc.

For further information

The Faculty of Forensic and Legal Medicine of the Royal College of Physicians. Web: https://fflm.ac.uk Email: forensic.medicine@fflm.ac.uk Twitter: @FFLMUK

---

[1] Health Needs Assessments of Detainees in Metropolitan Police Service (2015). Therapeutic Solutions Ltd. Accessible at: https://www.england.nhs.uk/commissioning/wp-content/uploads/sites/12/2016/01/nhs-mps-hna-rep-sept-15.pdf

06:30 Start shift. Review outstanding calls from night FP, including one to administer insulin

07:00 Arrival at Custody Suite A—log on police computer and medical systems. Insulin administered; alcohol-dependent with mild shakes reviewed

09:00 Quick cup of coffee and chat with police sergeant

10:00 Call to another police station; detainee is exhibiting paranoia. Liaison and diversion practitioner contacted

11:00 Drug addict requesting your attention assaulted—not clinically withdrawing

12:00 Called back to Custody Suite A. Three detainees to review: an epileptic patient, a drug addict, and two police officers with injuries

14:00 Called to attend sudden death in housing estate

15:30 Finally arrived—nightmare finding address and traffic building up

17:00 Back to Custody Suite B for another detainee review. Also confirmed previous detainee has been sectioned. As usual, no mental health beds available

18:30 Home

Myth	This is like CSI, with high-profile murder cases daily (Quincy/Dangerfield for the older readers).
Reality	High levels of independence. Work in the police environments is very safe and chaperoned. You should remain/provide evidence independent of the police and be accountable to the criminal justice system.
Personality	Strong, confident, open-minded, independent, especially if you need to challenge the police.
Best aspects	Independent nature of work; pay (tax rebates), flexibility (leave/work), freedom after work, with no follow-ups. Respect shown by the police and seeing reality, e.g. cases on news.
Worst aspects	Disruptive last-minute call to attend court/inquest; detainees demanding drugs, challenging barristers, a death in custody.
Route	Most jobs available to post-F2 doctors. Emergency medicine (EM) and psychiatry experience helpful. Usual requirements include an introductory course, vetting, insurance/indemnity (which can be high, but offset by tax rebates), safeguarding, and Immediate Life Support.
Locations	Police stations/custodies, sexual assault centres, hospitals scenes of death, magistrate/crown/coroners court.
Life	Work
Quiet On-call	Busy On-call
Boredom	Burnout
Uncompetitive	Competitive
Low salary	High salary

Forensic pathology

Forensic pathology involves the investigation of deaths with medico-legal elements to ascertain the cause of death and assist in identification of the deceased (if not known) and the recovery of evidence from the body. In the UK, training in forensic pathology requires initial histopathology training before specialty training in forensic histopathology, which is a CCT specialty in its own right. The forensic pathologist is part of a wider team that includes the Coroner (or Procurator Fiscal in Scotland), the police, crime scene investigators, specialist pathologists (neuropathology, paediatric pathology), clinicians, and other experts, including ballistics, anthropology, and entomology.

The patients

The majority are deceased with circumstances around their deaths being unnatural, suspicious of homicide, in custody, or involved in complex medico-legal cases, as well as 'routine' postmortem cases. Forensic pathologists may be required to examine the deaths of both adults and children; some specialize in paediatric forensic pathology. There are occasions when a forensic pathologist is required to examine, assess, and give an opinion on injuries in the living.

The work

Forensic pathology is a varied specialty that requires an enquiring mind—whether examining a scene, reviewing circumstances relating to a death, going through medical notes, or reading witness statements. Dexterity is needed for the postmortem examination itself, as well as a methodical approach, with attention to detail in documenting and recording the findings. There is increasing specialization and forensic pathologists can have specific areas of interest, e.g. forensic neuropathology and human rights abuses. Good communication skills are vital to ensure efficient flow of information between different departments. Presenting evidence in court can be daunting, but specialist expert witness training is provided.

The job

Training is currently limited to a handful of departments which are usually based in either NHS Trusts or university departments. In England and Wales, forensic pathologists are on a Home Office register and although independent practitioners, they are grouped into practice areas to provide 24/7 cover. Under the Scottish system, consultant forensic pathologists are located in NHS or university departments covering designated geographical locations. In Northern Ireland, they are employed by the State Pathologist's Department. A forensic pathologist can be requested to investigate a wide variety of deaths, not just homicides, so discussion with colleagues and other experts is essential.

Extras

A range of teaching opportunities, whether formal or informal, are available. Individual forensic pathologists can offer their services to perform second 'independent' postmortem examinations on behalf of the legal defence team. At present, the research associated with forensic pathology in the UK is not as prolific as other specialties, but the national and international meetings are excellent forums to highlight areas of innovation or more unusual cases. Whilst the role of a forensic pathologist may not be as glamorous as portrayed on TV, there are opportunities to be involved with the media.

> **For further information**
>
> **The Royal College of Pathologists (RCPath).** Tel: 020 7451 6700. Web: https://www.rcpath.org Email: info@rcpath.org Twitter: @RCPath

A day in the life ...

08:00 Routine Coroner's cases at city or hospital mortuary

10:00 Review of histology and toxicology to complete postmortem reports

12:00 Coronial inquest—explanation of autopsy findings and conclusions

13:30 Lunchtime forensic meeting with forensic trainees and Home Office pathologists

14:30 Continue with completing postmortem reports

15:00 Call from the police to attend the scene of a suspicious death

17:00 Start Home Office postmortem examination

19:00 Home time

20:00 Prepare for upcoming crown court case

Myth	*Silent Witness*-style death investigators who inevitably find the obscure, but vital, clue to ensure justice is served. Every time.
Reality	A physically and mentally demanding role where you may not have all the answers.
Personality	Inquisitive (really just nosy), disciplined, thorough, flexible, and resilient.
Best aspects	Variety; every day is a learning day.
Worst aspects	Regional differences in standards of death investigation and facilities.
Route	Specialty training in histopathology (ST1+) (p. 52), followed by specialty training in forensic histopathology (ST3+). Exams: FRCPath.
Numbers	Around 70, of whom <30% are women.
Locations	Hospital and city mortuaries, courts, histopathology departments, universities, and independent offices.

Life						Work
Quiet On-call						Busy On-call
Boredom						Burnout
Uncompetitive						Competitive
Low salary						High salary

Gastroenterology

Gastroenterologists are physicians who investigate and treat patients with gastrointestinal (GI) disorders, including diseases of the bowel, liver, pancreas, and biliary tree. Gastroenterology is truly one of the most widely varied medical specialties, offering an interesting blend of cognitive and practical skills to manage all forms of pathology, from infections to neoplasia. Moreover, there are now effective treatments, if not cures, for many of the conditions encountered. This combination of varied practice and good rates of treatment success makes working as a gastroenterologist genuinely rewarding.

The patients

Around one in six patients presenting to the acute medical take have a GI problem. These commonly include GI bleeding, abdominal pain, deranged liver function, and jaundice. The various complications of chronic alcoholism are also usually cared for by gastroenterologists, which can present significant clinical and ethical challenges. Many GI conditions require long-term follow-up in outpatient clinic—patients are usually divided by subspecialty, often along the lines of luminal disease (of the GI tract itself) or solid organ disease (hepatopancreatobiliary (HPB) medicine). Many of these groups encountered are young patients (e.g. inflammatory bowel disease (IBD)), with a great deal to be gained from the increasing number of effective treatments now available.

The work

The variation in daily workload is what draws many gastroenterologists to the specialty. In addition to routine upper and lower GI endoscopy, there is a wide range of specific endoscopic skills which can be acquired, e.g. to treat gallstones or benign and malignant oesophageal pathologies. In addition, there is frequent need for urgent endoscopy to control upper GI haemorrhage, which has good success rates and often (though not always) gives a sense of instant gratification to the endoscopist.

The job

Most patients are managed in outpatient clinics and endoscopy lists, but the job also includes inpatient care. In addition, most gastroenterologists take part in the acute general medical on-call, alongside a 24-hour emergency endoscopy on-call rota. Being a gastroenterologist is a very sociable job, requiring effective teamworking and communication with surgeons, radiologists, clinical nurse specialists (who are quickly becoming invaluable members of many gastroenterology services), and endoscopy nurses (who are often highly skilled in many endoscopic techniques). Whilst the multifaceted nature of the job keeps it interesting, varied, and challenging, it can also mean that days can be busy and occasionally long.

Extras

Opportunities in the UK and abroad exist for trainees to take time out of programme (OOP) for research, subspecialty training, and/or to gain practical experience of advanced endoscopic skills. An additional year of subspecialty training is now part of the specialist curriculum for trainees wishing to become liver specialists, and it's possible that a similar approach will be adopted for subspecialty training in nutrition, IBD, and interventional endoscopy. Gastroenterology lends itself well to private practice where there is scope for consulting, as well as for procedural work, and less-than-full-time training is well established.

For further information

British Society of Gastroenterology (BSG). Tel: 020 7935 3150. Web: https://www.bsg.org.uk Twitter: @BritSocGastro

---

08:00 Journal club

08:30 MDT meeting and discussion of inpatients

09:00 General gastroenterology outpatient clinic (mix of hepatology, luminal disease, and HPB)

12:00 Review ward referrals from other teams and selected inpatients

13:00 Journal club with lunch

13:45 Endoscopy list: eight patients, mixture of upper and lower GI cases

14:15 Give telephone advice to colleagues in ED, GP and other specialties between procedures

16:30 Additional emergency endoscopy to treat an upper GI bleed

17:30 Admin: sign letters, reply to emails, call patients with results that require action, etc.

18:00 Home

Myth	Wannabe surgeons, limited to endoscopic views of poorly prepped bowels.
Reality	So much more than just endoscopy. Variation keeps you on your toes but can feel less fun being pulled between ward, endoscopy unit, and clinic.
Personality	Seekers of instant gratification with at least a hint of the cerebral. Generally, a jovial and friendly bunch.
Best aspects	Gaining endoscopic skills which can directly and immediately benefit patients. Everyone (even those most long in the tooth) enjoys stopping a bleed!
Worst aspects	Struggling to treat functional bowel disorders without being able to offer appropriate psychological support. And poor bowel prep.
Route	Internal medicine training (IMT) (p. 44) or acute care common stem–acute medicine (ACCS-AM) (p. 37), then specialty training in gastroenterology (ST3+). Exams: MRCP; European Specialty Examination in Gastroenterology and Hepatology.
Locations	Secondary and tertiary centres, as well as private medical clinics and endoscopy suites.
Numbers	1400 consultants, of whom 20% are women.

Life					Work
Quiet On-call					Busy On-call
Boredom					Burnout
Uncompetitive					Competitive
Low salary					High salary

General practice

General practice (GP) is a challenging but rewarding career, offering the chance to develop and use diverse skills as part of the primary care team. GP offers the chance to be a truly all-round doctor providing continuity of care to patients in the community. Generalism is a specialty in its own right. The job requires a vast breadth of knowledge, along with the skill to know when and where to seek further advice. In this way, GPs act as gatekeepers to the rest of the health service. GPs are now working in primary care networks (PCNs), typically covering 30 000–50 000 patients. The aim of the networks is to bring practices together, to work at scale, and to support and develop local services based on local patient needs.

The patients

GPs care for patients and their families from birth until death (and sometimes beyond)! They see anyone and everyone, and patient mix can include the homeless, refugees, commuters, the very young, and the very old, as well as the worried well. Looking after several members of the same family can raise confidentiality issues but also offers valuable insight. Patients often form strong bonds with their family doctor, which can be both rewarding and frustrating.

The work

Includes clinical medicine/surgery, ENT, gynaecology, urology, dermatology, paediatrics, endocrinology, psychiatry, palliative care, social problems, and health promotion (and much more). One of the major challenges is having no idea what the patient is going to present with. A good GP will get to grips with the problem within 7–10 minutes, without access to any immediate tests, and formulate an appropriate plan with the patient; the process is then repeated again and again up to 40–50 times a day. The diversity is endless. One minute you might be dealing with a child with eczema, and the next you may be called upon to resuscitate a collapsed diabetic with a suspected heart attack or a patient who has become psychotic in the waiting room.

The job

Many GPs become partners within a practice and are jointly responsible for running the practice as a business (usually partly delegated to a practice manager). Others work as a salaried GP without the management responsibilities, but with a similar clinical workload. GPs mainly work alone during surgery times, but with support from other practice team members (partners, nurses, etc.). They form part of a wider multidisciplinary team (MDT), including district nurses, health visitors, and other community professionals. Some GPs carry out minor operations and procedures. Many GPs are now taking on management roles with the local Clinical Commissioning Group (CCG). GPs are leading the electronic revolution in the NHS's bid to get rid of all paper. Many jobs, from consulting to prescribing, are now done electronically, making technophobia something of a disadvantage.

Extras

Good opportunities for part-time/flexible hours and portfolio careers. Option to subspecialize and become a GP with extended roles or 'GPwER' (p. 182). Becoming a partner offers the chance to 'buy in' to the business and premises, which remains a good long-term investment. There are multiple research opportunities for the interested, but there is no obligation for those who are not. There is also the chance to train future doctors and GPs by becoming an F2 supervisor or a GP trainer.

> **For further information**
>
> **Royal College of General Practitioners (RCGP).** Tel: 020 3188 7400. Web: https://www.rcgp.org.uk Email: info@rcgp.org.uk Twitter: @rcgp

A day in the life ...

08:00 Paperwork: checking/actioning results, reading letters, insurance reports

09:00 Morning surgery: 7- to 10-minute consultations, followed by phone calls; consultations include earache, depression, urinary frequency, and diabetic review

12:30 MDT meeting with district nurses, community matrons, and palliative care nurses discussing patients who have complex needs or require review

13:30 Home visits: agree to post a letter for one housebound patient who just needed a chat; visit to a nursing home to see two residents; call 999 for a middle-aged woman with unexpected sepsis due to pneumonia

14:30 Afternoon surgery: 22 patients, runs late after sending child with appendicitis to A&E

18:00 Phone calls to patients, including medication queries, and fielding complaints about the unavailability of appointments

18:30 Surgery closes, hand over responsibility to out-of-hours service; sign prescriptions, dictate letters, check/action results, and read hospital letters

19:30 Home to dinner/relax with family, followed by a quick log on via a practice laptop to finish looking at results/letters from earlier

Myth	'Just' a GP—failed hospital doctors who stay in one job until they retire.
Reality	Becoming a GP is an active choice for most; a GP is jack of all trades and master of many; many start as salaried doctors and move around until they find a practice that suits them.
Personality	Calm, open, logical, good listening skills, non-confrontational, able to deal with uncertainty, a business mind helps.
Best aspects	Seeing the same patients over and over again; getting to know patients as people and seeing their homes and families; wide diversity of presentations; optional out-of-hours.
Worst aspects	Seeing the same patients over and over again! Increasing workload due to rising patient expectation and transfer of work from secondary to primary care.
Route	Run-through GP specialty training (ST1+) (p. 42). Exams: MRCGP.
Numbers	48 000 GPs, of whom 55% are women.
Locations	Anywhere from city to countryside; practice-based with home visits, and possible to do some hospital sessions.

Life						Work
Quiet On-call						Busy On-call
Boredom						Burnout
Uncompetitive						Competitive
Low salary						High salary

General practice: academic

Many GPs seek portfolio careers (p. 28), which allow them to engage in salaried activities beyond providing direct clinical care. For GPs interested in research and teaching, an academic career provides day-to-day variety, as well as opportunities to influence clinical care in a wider context. Many combine clinical sessions with weekly academic activities, including undergraduate or postgraduate teaching or developing and leading research.

The patients

Most academic GPs have regular NHS clinical sessions within their week and provide long-term care to a cohort of patients. Many find their academic activities can feed into this, with opportunities to enhance an already rich skill set. They have the opportunity for increased patient contact through involvement in organized teaching or involving patients in developing medical curricula. Being in a privileged position to identify and address clinical gaps and areas for improvement, academic GPs can also provide research leadership by selecting and co-ordinating clinical studies in their practice. Additional patient contact comes from involving patients and the public in the development of new scientific proposals.

The work

This is diverse and will appeal to those who like variety. Those with teaching responsibilities may be at the forefront of organizing and providing integrated undergraduate community-based teaching, as well as having wider involvement in formal postgraduate training at regional and national levels. For others, engaging in programmes of research provides an opportunity to focus on specific clinical areas of research relevant to primary care, e.g. chronic disease management or childhood infections. Senior academic GPs may become principle investigators of research. Given the critical role that primary care plays in supporting the NHS, much of the research generated by academic GPs has the potential to be taken up at a wider NHS policy and clinical guidance level.

The job

The division of time between direct and indirect clinical activities is often based on individual circumstances and choice. Posts are usually linked to university departments where there is involvement with other members of the primary care research team, including statisticians, information specialists, health service researchers, and clinical tutors from other specialties. As the appeal of becoming an academic GP has increased over the last few years, so have job opportunities. Many university departments show commitment to the most productive senior academic GPs by offering them positions as senior lecturers or professors.

Extras

Achieving the balance between being a good GP and a successful academic can be a challenge. Nevertheless, most find a balance that suits them and take advantage of a range of significant opportunities and potential rewards. In addition to outputs such as publications and local curricular development, there are increasingly opportunities to work with the media, influence national health policy or educational curricula, travel, and network with other academics. After qualification, there are opportunities to apply for further fellowships, usually leading to a higher degree, e.g. PhD. Pay depends on seniority—the most senior academic GP will earn salaries comparable to that of a hospital consultant.

For further information

The Society for Academic Primary Care (SAPC). Web: https://sapc.ac.uk/ Email: office@sapc.ac.uk Twitter: @sapcacuk

---

08:30	Start work in academic department, answering emails
09:00	Educational meeting to discuss curriculum content
10:00	Research planning meeting within department
11:00	Work on current research project
13:00	Travel to general practice (lunch in car)
13:30	Review clinical post, results, and prescription requests
14:00	Begin clinic
17:00	Review any patients requesting a same-day appointment
17:30	Finish clinic and ensure all relevant referral letters or requests have been completed
18:30	Home for dinner and spend time with family
21:00	Work on home laptop to complete research grant/publication or answer further academic-related emails

Myth	GPs sitting in ivory towers, avoiding clinical practice.
Reality	A challenging job that involves striking a balance between clinical care and academic activity.
Personality	Organized, dedicated, able to balance time well, capable of switching work environments within the same week and still excel, team player.
Best aspects	Variety, flexibility, opportunities to improve clinical care or medical education in a wider context, lifelong training, leadership opportunities.
Worst aspects	Being able to get the balance right between clinical and academic time; funding applications.
Route	(Specialized) Foundation training, followed by academic clinical fellowship (ACF) (p. 23) which integrates GP specialty training (p. 42) with protected academic time. Exams: MRCGP.
Numbers	Around 200 academic GPs (6% of the medical academic workforce).
Locations	Teaching hospitals, universities, and surrounding general practices.

Life						Work
Quiet On-call						Busy On-call
Boredom						Burnout
Uncompetitive						Competitive
Low salary						High salary

General practice in rural settings

GPs are the first point of contact for most patients, particularly in a rural setting. The nearest hospital could be over an hour away or require a flight or ferry journey to get there. Because of this, a rural GP becomes part of the community and may need more acute medical knowledge and skills than a city GP. GPs deal with patients from birth to death (and their families before and after these events). Rurality brings its own challenges, from hardy farmers who don't present until they are very unwell to areas of significant deprivation and lack of employment. However, it also brings opportunities to hone a diverse range of skills.

The patients

GPs see patients of all ages, with a variety of undifferentiated problems. Getting to know your patients is a benefit of general practice, which can be very helpful in contextualizing and assessing the severity of problems. Skills in paediatrics to geriatrics and everything in between are required. Managing family members and their concerns, whilst also navigating the minefield of confidentiality, particularly in small communities, is a skill in itself—but one you develop, alongside being able to build a family tree and work out how people in the community are related!

The work

GPs consult in the surgery or practice, on the phone, and in people's homes. In a rural area, this can involve travelling through miles of beautiful scenery and farm tracks where the post code is next to useless. Patients can book appointments in advance, and a triage system prioritizes patients requiring more urgent review. GPs are involved in managing physical and mental health in the context of the patient's social circumstances. GPs make referrals to secondary care when more specialist input is required. Working more rurally with district general hospitals (DGHs), you get to know consultants and they get to know you. This makes it easier to pick up the phone and ask for advice, but also means your reputation is very important—but this can only serve to make you a better doctor and a more polite human being.

The job

Each practice is run slightly differently but does the same job and provides similar care to patients. In general, surgeries are run as small businesses, with GPs as partners/business owners, allowing more autonomy over how the practice is run. This sounds scary but can add to job satisfaction, because change is within your power. All patients have 10-minute consultations, but each GP will develop their own style of consulting which suits them and their patients. Out-of-hours work is an optional extra, for which GPs are paid per hour or are managed between GPs working in a practice, particularly the more rural ones.

Extras

GPs can develop areas of special interest, known as extended roles (p. 182), such as minor surgery and sexual health, and may run specific clinics in the practice. Rural GP surgeries often take and train medical students and trainees. This gives plenty of opportunities for learning and education. DGHs often offer opportunities to work in special-interest secondary care for a session or two a week. GPs work as part of a multidisciplinary team (MDT) and this is expanding as the service develops.

> **For further information**
>
> **Royal College of General Practitioners (RCGP).** Tel: 020 3188 7400. Web: https://www.rcgp.org.uk Email: info@rcgp.org.uk Twitter: @rcgp
>
> **RCGP Rural Forum.** Tel: 020 3188 7400. Web: https://www.rcgp.org.uk/rcgp-near-you/faculties/rural-forum.aspx Twitter: @RuralForumRCGP

07:30   Early morning surgery, approximately every 2–3 weeks

08:15   Partnership business meeting discussing issues affecting the practice

09:25   Morning phone triage clinic as doctor on-call with advanced nurse practitioner

11:00   Meet with other GPs for coffee and prescription signing, morning debrief

11:30   Morning clinic for emergency and urgent cases

12:30   Drive to home visit(s)

13:30   Drive back before lunch and dealing with letters, results, and referrals

14:30   Afternoon routine clinic, simultaneously supervising a trainee

17:00   Evening emergency clinic

18:00   Doors close, calls over to NHS 24 (111 in England), paperwork

18:45   Home for dinner

Myth	Prescribing bedrest to farmers before heading off to play golf.
Reality	Busy days with a wide variety of simple and complex problems, short appointments, and large numbers of patients. Sometimes emotionally draining, but very rewarding.
Personality	A people person with good communication skills and empathy; able to draw boundaries and share decision-making with patients. Emotionally resilient; knowledgeable and good problem-solving skills.
Best aspects	Getting to know patients and their circumstances, working in a good team, variety of problems and presentations. Autonomy and flexibility, e.g. in location, working hours.
Worst aspects	Patients not taking responsibility for their health, complaints, high patient expectations, high volume of paperwork, and increasingly defensive medicine. Lack of phone signal.
Route	Run-through GP specialty training (ST1+) (p. 42). Exams: MRCGP.
Locations	Primary care settings in (often isolated) geographical areas with low population densities, e.g. Scottish Highlands. Ability to drive essential.

Life					Work
Quiet On-call					Busy On-call
Boredom					Burnout
Uncompetitive					Competitive
Low salary					High salary

General practice in secure environments

Primary care in secure environments encompasses the delivery of services in settings that include prisons, young offenders' institutions, immigration removal centres, secure children's homes, and medium- and high-secure hospitals. It is by virtue of the patient's detention that they are not able to access wider NHS primary care services, and there-fore, GPs are commissioned to deliver services into these settings. Importantly, treatment of these patients needs to be non-judgemental and delivered to what is equivalent to that available in the wider community, irrespective of patients' circumstances and any offence committed. This specific objective requires attention to the particular practical, ethical, and medical issues affecting the appropriate delivery of care for patients, many of whom are among the most vulnerable and underserved members of our society.

The patients

The health needs of detained patients are known to be higher than those of the general population. This results from a range of factors, including high levels of substance and alcohol misuse, mental health issues, and an increased prevalence of infectious diseases. They are also less likely to access long-term condition management normally addressed in the pri-mary care setting. A significant proportion of patients in immigration removal centres may have been exposed to torture in their country of origin. It is often thought that working with offenders and detainees could be considered more 'risky' or hostile, but the collective ex-perience of GPs working in these settings demonstrates they are generally extremely safe.

The work

GPs need to work effectively in what can be quite an enclosed and isolating environ-ment. Examples of the more challenging aspects of practice include making decisions about if and when a patient needs transfer to hospital; a patient who is self-harming or suicidal; food and fluid refusal; advance statements; and issues of consent and mental capacity. GPs in these settings work with a wide range of primary (nursing, optometry, dental, physiotherapy, etc.) and secondary care services (mental health, sexual health, etc.) and this must be done in conjunction with the staff who are responsible for ensuring the security of the establishment. This type of work requires taking into consideration a wide range of specific guidance, as well as being able to think 'on your feet' about how to solve individual difficulties as they arise. It is useful to have additional skills, including experience of emergency medicine, minor surgery, substance misuse, and mental health.

The job

Frequently, GPs working in secure environments work elsewhere in the wider community and the skills obtained from working in these settings are transferrable to wider prac-tice. Prescribing in secure environments requires special consideration towards 'safer pre-scribing', as many medications can be sought for their effect and 'currency' if diverted.

Extras

It's truly a rewarding specialty. The vast majority of patients seen in these settings will, of course, be released back into the community—carefully addressing their needs plays an important part in helping to address wider health inequalities in the community. Flexible working is possible.

For further information

Royal College of General Practitioners (RCGP) Secure Environments Group. Web: https://www.rcgp.org.uk/clinical-and-research/about/special-interest-groups/secure-environments-group.aspx Email: seg@rcgp.org.uk Twitter: @RCGPSecureEnvi1

08:30 Arrive at the gate, leaving mobile phone and any prejudice behind; collect keys and head to the medical centre

09:00 Start of morning clinic: ten patients booked in, a mix of straightforward and complex problems

12:00 Lunch

13:00 Team meeting to discuss complex cases

13:45 Head to 'segregation' to see the patients who are currently residing there

14:00 Start of afternoon clinic: eight patients booked in

16:00 Clinic finishes. Review a patient on the wing who has been unwell

16:30 Time to finish admin and complete outstanding tasks

18:00 (Optional) evening reception clinic

Myth	Every patient is Hannibal Lecter.
Reality	An extremely rewarding role; working at the cutting edge of an ever-evolving field of practice, with a strong team philosophy.
Personality	Caring, compassionate, able to handle complex medical issues, empathy mixed with a degree of toughness, well balanced, team player. Able to set boundaries with demanding patients.
Best aspects	Genuine gratitude from patients; opportunity to make a difference to someone's life, often to those who have been let down by society; emphasis on teamwork; no home visits (!).
Worst aspects	Some patents can be chaotic and/or demanding and that can make consulting within the usual framework of GP consultation models a challenge!
Route	Run-through GP specialty training (ST1+) (p. 42). Exams: MRCGP. Apply directly to service provider (often a private/independent company).
Locations	Prisons and young offenders institutions (Category A, B, C, and D), immigration removal centres, secure children's homes, secure training centres, medium- and high-secure hospitals.

Life					Work
Quiet On-call					Busy On-call
Boredom					Burnout
Uncompetitive					Competitive
Low salary					High salary

General practice: private practice

Most cities in the UK have a small number of GPs who practise partially or fully outside of the NHS—London, in particular, has a concentration in the Harley Street area, alongside their specialist colleagues. The introduction of online remote consultations has increased the awareness and scope of private general practice. Many patients who use these services for the first time are surprised how available, user-friendly, and helpful they are.

The patients

Patients are of all ages and come from all social groups, but whilst the elderly, mentally ill, and disabled can rarely afford ongoing private care, they do consult for one-off illnesses or second opinions. Some patients use only private services and the typical patient is a young person who works in the city centre and does not want to take time off to see their local GP. Lack of rapid access to NHS services is the main driver of patients into private GP services. Overseas patients often use these services, and so a range of language skills in the clinical and administrative staff is useful. There is no long-term commitment from the patient other than paying for a one-off consultation.

The work

Similar to the NHS, but in general terms less stressful—longer consultation times and around 20–30 patients per day. Some private GPs offer home visits and a 24-hour service, but there is no obligation to do so. Weekends are busy, as are Bank Holidays, as access to other services is limited. Serious and challenging illnesses can present as walk-in patients and there is open access to pathology and imaging services, including magnetic resonance imaging (MRI), and ultrasound scanning. Referral to private secondary care is frequent and private GPs have a local network of specialists and private hospitals to enable this. Ability to understand how to run a small business is helpful. Some doctors work full-time in private general practice, especially if they have a particular subspecialty, e.g. cosmetic work or sexual health. NHS GPs are kept informed of treatments given in private practice.

The job

Many NHS GPs opt to do occasional sessions for private employers or online FaceTime-type providers. Usually it is paid at a modest hourly rate (actually less than NHS locum work), but some private providers offer share-of-profit schemes too. Private sessions work well as part of a portfolio career (p. 28), but it is important to ensure that indemnity insurers will cover these sessions and this can be expensive. The patients are pleasant and often (perhaps surprisingly) less demanding than NHS patients, making it relatively easy to agree with them on management and care plans. The Care Quality Commission (CQC) do inspect private doctors in the same way as NHS doctors. Appraisal and revalidation are exactly the same and must include the full scope of work, including private work.

Extras

The Independent Doctors Federation (IDF) organizes meetings and appraisals, and has a Responsible Officer (RO) for those with no NHS connection. Corporate work often brings extras such as theatre tickets or networking/concert opportunities.

For further information

Independent Doctors Federation (IDF). Tel: 020 3696 4080. Web: https://www.idf.uk.net Email: info@idf.uk.net Twitter: @idf_uk

---

07:00	Arrive. Check and email pathology and imaging reports that came in from doctors/nurses overnight
07:30	Deal with incoming emails from overnight
08:00	Clinic starts
10:00	Phone call to discuss with theatre company manager regarding fitness of an actor
10:15	Visit to local hotel to see a guest taken ill
11:00	Back to clinic
13:00	Break
13:15	Management and medical policy meeting with colleagues
14:00	Afternoon clinic
16:00	Hospital visits to see patients under shared care with secondary care consultants
18:00	Final clinical session
20:00	Chase up and email lab and imaging reports from all doctors/nurses from the day
20:30	Home to watch a blockbuster film and try to spot any actors seen in clinic

Myth	Dealing with demanding dowager duchesses with poodles.
Reality	Varied, challenging acute medicine, with exciting moments.
Personality	Affability, availability, flexible, but not reckless.
Best aspects	Interesting patients both clinically and personally.
Worst aspects	Seven days a week in touch with office and an email/mobile phone addiction.
Route	Run-through GP specialty training (ST1+) (p. 42). Exams: MRCGP. After CCT apply directly to private GP services, or maybe even start your own.
Numbers	Approximately 600 full-time private GPs, countless sessional doctors.
Locations	Clinics in cities and some country areas; some opportunity to work from home.
Life	Work
Quiet On-call	Busy On-call
Boredom	Burnout
Uncompetitive	Competitive
Low salary	High salary

GP with extended roles

About 5 years after qualifying as a GP (p. 172), you might think about this role. There are two directions in which you could go—firstly, providing a specialist clinic as part of your week, e.g. respiratory, dermatology, cardiology, drug and alcohol, and more. This option was previously described as being a 'clinical assistant' to a specialist in their clinic. The title evolved to GP with special interest (GPwSI, pronounced gypsy) and, more recently, GP with an extended role (GPwER) where you have your own service and more autonomy. Secondly, GPs can become a specialty 'Clinical Champion', working at population level, doing quality improvement, designing or commissioning services, teaching, and integrating with specialist colleagues, rather than doing what they do. Many do a bit of crossover between both paths.

The patients

GPwERs will usually see people with a specific health issue that needs more time and expertise to be sure of the diagnosis when it isn't clear-cut, and set up management plans that your primary care colleagues can then follow. Sometimes people need a special test or procedure that wouldn't be done in a usual GP surgery such as spirometry or skin biopsy. The patients usually come from GP surgeries in your local area. Some GPs have an extended role in frailty medicine and will go to local residential and nursing homes, rather than have the patients coming to them.

The work

Depending on the chosen specialty, GPwERs might need to see people with diabetes who need to start insulin or are poorly controlled, complex or elderly heart failure, or chronic obstructive pulmonary disease (COPD), asthma, undifferentiated cough, or breathlessness where the diagnosis is proving difficult or the management is complex. The dermatology GPwER is different in that they will see a very broad spectrum of disease with which colleagues might be struggling. The GP 'Clinical Champion' role tends to involve more in the way of data crunching, writing pathways and business plans, education, and lobbying and meeting with colleagues, commissioners, and patients to improve services.

The job

GPs work in sessions (i.e. a morning or an afternoon), up to ten sessions per week. In general, most GPwERs tend to do a day or two a week (i.e. 1–4 sessions) in their other or additional role. They might work from their own practice, a population hub, or a hospital setting, or go to the patient's residence. They often work with other professionals such as specialist (consultant) physicians, but also with nurses, physiotherapists, and pharmacists who may have extended specialist roles themselves. In this way, they all bring their own unique professional lens to the problem.

Extras

The role is constantly developing and shifting, meaning many can end up writing a job description unique to them. Just because a GPwER post doesn't exist currently doesn't mean it shouldn't; for example, a gap was identified in providing smoking cessation services in the UK and a GPwER post was created to fill it, resulting in an interesting and impactful career. You need to check out if you need extra medical indemnity in your role, and need to be registered as doing this work with your local GP performers list and show development in this area in your appraisal.

For further information

RCGP General Practitioners with Extended Roles. Web: https://www.rcgp.org.uk/training-exams/practice/general-practitioners-with-extended-roles.aspx Email: gpwer@rcgp.org.uk

A day in the life ...

08:00 Checking emails and referrals. Primary care colleagues asking advice, commissioners asking about a service design, patient charity asking if you will do a talk to a patient group

09:00 Morning surgery—your day job

12:00 Home visits for your own practice

13:30 Meeting at a local community hub with specialist physician, nurse, physiotherapist, pharmacist, and GP colleagues to design a new diagnostic and treatment algorithm

14:30 GPwER clinic in a community health and social care hub

18:30 Evening teaching meeting with primary care colleagues

20:30 Checking results, emails, and letters online from home

Myth	Eternally frustrated wannabe specialist.
Reality	Can take a while to get everyone to trust you know what you are doing.
Personality	Entrepreneurs, passionate about issues, political, like teams and being a leader.
Best aspects	Being able to make it the job you want it to be; huge scope and variety.
Worst aspects	Standing out from GP colleagues, whilst being a GP, can bring its challenges.
Route	Run-through GP specialty training (ST1+) (p. 42). Exams: MRCGP. Then take a few years to decide what really inspires you. Do a Diploma or Master's if there is one, but if not, start networking, join a society, build a portfolio, and write about it.
Locations	Online, GP surgeries, community hubs, hospitals, people's homes, and other primary and secondary care settings.

Life					Work
Quiet On-call					Busy On-call
Boredom					Burnout
Uncompetitive					Competitive
Low salary					High salary

General surgery

If you are looking for a specialty which is dynamic and challenging and offers endless variation, then look no further than general surgery. General surgery encompasses several subspecialties and surgical procedures on some of the most vital organ systems. Historically, it is the specialty from which all other surgical specialties have been derived and is now subdivided into lower gastrointestinal (GI) surgery (distal small bowel, colon, rectum, anus), upper GI surgery (oesophagus, stomach, proximal small bowel), hepatobiliary surgery (liver, biliary system, pancreas), and breast and endocrine surgery (e.g. thyroid, adrenal glands). Other smaller subspecialties include transplant surgery (p. 306) and the new, but rapidly expanding areas of bariatric (p. 130) and emergency surgery. The options available to someone entering a career in general surgery are truly unrivalled.

The patients

In most hospitals without a dedicated paediatric surgical service, the general surgeon will be expected to look after patients from 3 years upwards for emergency cases and from 16 years upwards for elective cases. The general surgeon will be expected to communicate equally adeptly with a 10-year-old girl who has acute appendicitis and with a 90-year-old man who has to be given the devastating news that he has bowel cancer. General surgeons can have brief encounters with some patients (e.g. day case elective repair of a straightforward hernia) or forge lasting relationships which last a lifetime (e.g. cancer or inflammatory bowel disease patients). The diversity of the patients and their illnesses will always give the general surgeon variety and be richly rewarding.

The work

The work can be roughly divided into planned vs emergency surgery. Planned operations, major or minor, can be life-changing for the patient (e.g. cancer resections, hernia repairs, cholecystectomies). The general surgeon finds satisfaction in mastering a wide array of skills to improve the lives of the patients going 'under the knife'. Emergency surgery requires fast decision-making under pressure, as sometimes a matter of minutes could mean the difference between life and death for the patient. General surgeons are required to work closely with the emergency department (ED), theatre, anaesthetists, and intensive care unit (ICU) to ensure the best possible outcomes for patients.

The job

Each week, there will be 2–3 outpatient clinics, 1–2 days of operating, a session or two of endoscopy (for upper and lower GI surgery), and daily ward rounds of inpatients. General surgeons attend multidisciplinary team (MDT) meetings for malignant and benign conditions relevant to their subspecialty. Most are on-call once per week, covering the emergency cases for a 24-hour period. The team consists of consultants, specialty trainees, and more junior doctors rotating through that area in their foundation and core training. The work is aided by specialist nurses in the relevant fields.

Extras

Research and publication opportunities are aplenty, with many trainees taking time out of programme (OOP) to complete higher degrees. Consultants commonly have private practice to supplement their income.

For further information

Association of Surgeons of Great Britain and Ireland. Tel: 020 7973 0300. Web: https://www.asgbi.org.uk Twitter: @asgbi

---

08:00 Ward round of acute admissions and postoperative patients on wards and the ICU

08:30 Outpatient clinic: 15–20 patients with a variety of pathologies, e.g. hernias, haemorrhoids, gallstones, bowel cancer

12:30 Lower GI cancer MDT meeting with lunch

13:30 Operating list: one laparoscopic colectomy followed by a hernia repair

17:30 Review of postoperative patients, assess if any can go home tonight

18:00 Home unless on-call or doing private practice

Myth	Jack of all trades, 'barber surgeons' who lance boils.
Reality	Diverse, rewarding area of practice, with opportunities for subspecialization.
Personality	Calm under pressure, teamworker, leadership skills, decisive, assertive, good practical skills, resilient, good time management.
Best aspects	Curing by operation, seeing the immediate effect of operations on patients. Performing life-changing surgery. Mastery of skills.
Worst aspects	Serious complications, with serious outcomes inevitable. Long, gruelling on-call shifts having impact on life outside of work. Stress levels high.
Route	Core surgical training (CST) (p. 61), followed by specialty training in general surgery (ST3+). Exams: MRCS; FRCS.
Numbers	2450 consultants in England, of whom 16% are women.
Locations	Hospital-based, present in most hospitals.

Life						Work
Quiet On-call						Busy On-call
Boredom						Burnout
Uncompetitive						Competitive
Low salary						High salary

Genitourinary medicine

Since the introduction of the Venereal Disease Regulations in 1916, which tasked local authorities to provide confidential clinics to treat sexually transmitted infections (STIs), sexual health clinics have become an integral part of the UK's health system. Genitourinary medicine (GUM) is a medical specialty dedicated to the diagnosis and management of STIs, including HIV. It is a dynamic, wide-ranging, and rapidly developing area of medicine which sees patients of all ages, ethnicities, and sexualities. Clinicians contemplating a career in GUM must be interested in people, infections, and public health and, above all, have excellent communication skills.

The patients

Sexual health clinics mostly see young patients (<35 years) who are otherwise fit and well. Specific services are often provided for men who have sex with men (MSM), transgender people, and commercial sex workers. In the UK, MSM and people of black African ethnicity make up the majority of people living with HIV (PLWH). With the life expectancy of PLWH nearing the normal life expectancy, our HIV cohort are increasingly older. Specialists care for PLWH throughout their life, from starting antiretroviral medications, dealing with drug resistance and interactions, to management of chronic comorbidities such as cardiovascular and bone health. The HIV component of GUM provides opportunities to form life-long working relationships, in contrast to the rapid turnover of general sexual health clinics.

The work

GUM is a diverse specialty. It encompasses gynaecology, dermatology, sexual dysfunction, sexual assault, adolescent health, public health, microbiology, and virology. Few specialties can boast including so many aspects of medicine! With many sexual health clinics now integrated with contraception services, advanced contraception skills are often required. Over 30% of PLWH are women, so prenatal counselling, prevention of mother-to-child transmission, and women's health are key parts of the job. Acute medicine skills are used caring for sick patients admitted with opportunistic infections such as tuberculosis. Public health efforts to prevent spread of infection, test, treat, and educate is core business for GUM clinicians.

The job

GUM is predominantly an outpatient specialty, working in sexual health and HIV clinics. Sexual health clinics are much like working in an emergency department (ED), except with more talking about sex! On-call work is usually non-residential, although it may include more general medical work in the future. GUM is a multidisciplinary specialty and good patient care relies on a close rapport with allied health professionals. Consultations are often sensitive and personal. Excellent communication skills and the ability to be non-judgemental and empathize with people are key traits if considering GUM as a career.

Extras

Research is an integral part of GUM and trainees are encouraged to participate in research. Teaching is strongly encouraged and there are many opportunities to teach undergraduates, postgraduates, and allied health professionals. Many clinicians develop subspecialty interests e.g. in genital dermatology, specialist HIV, or sexual assault. Being a relatively small specialty, there are many opportunities to get involved in regional and national committees.

For further information

British Association for Sexual Health and HIV (BASHH). Tel: 01625 664 523. Web: https://www.bashh.org Email: admin@bashh.org Twitter: @BASHH_UK

British HIV Association (BHIVA). Tel: 01462 530 070. Web: https://www.bhiva.org Twitter: @BritishHIVAssoc

09:00 HIV multidisciplinary meeting discussing the medical, social, and psychological needs of patients

10:00 Ward round of HIV inpatients

12:00 Teaching session with emergency medicine doctors regarding HIV testing

13:00 General GUM clinic

16:00 Sexual health walk-in clinic

20:00 Home and start of non-residential on-call

22:00 Phone call from medical admissions regarding management of a patient with acute breathlessness and hypoxia with known HIV and a low CD4 count

02:00 Phone call from ED asking for advice regarding starting a patient on post-exposure prophylaxis following unprotected sex with a PLWH

Myth	A simple specialty; gossip enthusiasts talking about sex and swabbing … 'things'.
Reality	A dynamic, multifaceted, rapidly developing specialty which has many areas in which develop subspecialty interests.
Personality	Excellent communication skills, open-mindedness, non-judgemental attitude, empathy, and a sense of fun!
Best aspects	The ability to talk to anyone and everyone about personal, sensitive issues. Making a difference to people during difficult situations e.g. patients newly diagnosed with HIV.
Worst aspects	Seeing the stigma that PLWH still suffer, as well as the missed opportunities for HIV testing in patients who have been presenting to other specialties.
Route	Internal medicine training (IMT) (p. 44) or acute care common stem–acute medicine (ACCS-AM) (p. 37), then specialty training in GUM (ST3+). Exams: MRCP; there are several GUM-related diplomas.
Numbers	430 GUM consultants, of whom 62% are women; further 30 HIV/AIDS specialists.
Locations	Predominantly an outpatient specialty in clinics, based either in hospitals or in the community.
Life		Work
Quiet On-call		Busy On-call
Boredom		Burnout
Uncompetitive		Competitive
Low salary		High salary

Gynaecological oncology

Gynaecological oncology involves the treatment of women with cancers of the vulva, cervix, uterus, and ovary/fallopian tube/peritoneum. It is a broad surgical specialty and many consultants also perform upper abdominal, gastrointestinal (GI), and plastic surgery, or work with other teams to achieve optimal oncological clearance. There is also a close-knit multidisciplinary team (MDT) working outside of theatre, involving clinical and medical oncologists, palliative care specialists, and cancer psychologists, because these diseases and their treatments directly affect fertility, sexuality, femininity, and body image.

The patients

Exclusively female and often elderly, obese, socially excluded, vulnerable, and in need of psychological support, although this varies, depending on cancer site. Younger patients present a unique set of emotive challenges regarding the impact that their cancer treatment may have on fertility and hormonal status. Strong communication skills are therefore essential. Gynaeoncologists see their patients regularly throughout an entire cancer journey, usually spanning several years. This leads to excellent continuity of care and high levels of satisfaction for both parties, with patients frequently being cured.

The work

The work is varied as the four cancer sites affect different demographics and have different causes, treatments, and prognoses. The majority of the cancers are of the ovary, endometrium, or cervix, and less commonly the vagina, vulva, or placenta. Genetic counselling, fertility-sparing surgery, minimally invasive surgery, strenuous multicavity ovarian debulking operations, and massive pelvic exenterative procedures all make for a stimulating mix of work. The primary role of the gynaeoncologist is to perform complicated surgery (often 3–4 hours in duration), whilst limiting damage to other pelvic organs.

The job

Gynaecological oncology is subspecialized and centralized to cancer centres. Job plans typically include clinics (colposcopy, gynaecological oncology, joint clinics with oncologists), MDT meetings, a whole-day operating session, and an on-call session covering postoperative patients and occasional admissions. Gynaeoncologists in major cancer centres are unlikely to be involved in benign gynaecological work and general obstetrics and gynaecology (O&G) on-call.

Extras

Most gynaeoncologists are involved in research and a research output is mandatory in centres with a fellowship programme. Large-volume private cancer practice is infrequent outside of London, but a general gynaecological private practice for the motivated is possible, given the skill set of gynaeoncologists.

For further information

Royal College of Obstetricians and Gynaecologists (RCOG). Tel: 020 7772 6200. Web: https://www.rcog.org.uk Twitter: @RCObsGyn

British Gynaecological Cancer Society (BGCS). Web: https://www.bgcs.org.uk Email: administrator@bgcs.org.uk Twitter: @BGCS_org

08:30	Review an inpatient admitted as an emergency under the surgeons—a new diagnosis of ovarian cancer. Discuss plan with patient and family
09:00	Clinic: 11 patients; a mix of new referrals with recent diagnoses of cancer, patients returning for results and plans, long-term follow-ups, and one 2-week wait patient
12:30	Time with secretary to plan lists, answer queries, write to patients, and review results
13:30	MDT meeting discussing diagnoses and treatment plans
16:00	Ward round of day 2 postop patients; a radical vulvectomy and a primary radical ovarian debulking surgery
17:00	Management meeting to discuss cancer targets
18:00	Post-MDT admin
19:00	Home!

Myth	Gynaecologists who couldn't cut it in obstetrics, performing futile extensive surgery.
Reality	Highly trained surgical oncologists who cure or significantly help most patients. Talented obstetricians who dislike obstetrics and night work.
Personality	Surgical boldness and high standards without the personality issues that accompany this in other specialties. Superior soft skills, stamina, and commitment
Best aspects	Highly motivated, tight-knit community nationally and internationally. A life outside of work is usually possible.
Worst aspects	Surgical complications. Cinderella specialty.
Route	Specialty training in O&G (ST1+) (p. 47), then subspecialty training in gynaecological oncology (ST6+). Exams: MRCOG.
Numbers	Approximately 200 consultants, of whom 30% are women.
Locations	Cancer centres, mostly in teaching hospitals.

Life					Work
Quiet On-call					Busy On-call
Boredom					Burnout
Uncompetitive					Competitive
Low salary					High salary

Haematology

Haematology is a diverse and unique specialty, combining clinical and laboratory work to manage blood disorders. Malignant haematology includes treating myeloid, lymphoid, and plasma cell dyscrasia and transplantation. Non-malignant haematology includes laboratory work, transfusion, haemostasis and thrombosis, haemophilia, and haemoglobinopathies. Haematologists usually have the opportunity to develop strong relationships with patients with chronic, complex, and often incurable disease. The specialty is somewhat demanding and intense but can be extremely rewarding. There are several new and exciting treatments and therapeutic techniques, which also enables combining academia with a clinical career.

The patients

Those with malignant disease, such as leukaemia or lymphoma, will be referred from either the GP or other hospital disciplines. At presentation, they will be scared and unwell, with family members asking lots of probing questions. Patients can be young or old, with both needing careful explanation about diagnosis, prognosis, and treatment options. Patients with non-malignant disease such as haemophilia or haemoglobinopathy usually transition from the paediatric service. These patients have chronic life-long conditions which require continuous input. Haematologists are actually involved in the care of (practically) every hospital patient by being responsible for laboratories in which routine blood tests are analysed; when needed, they also report blood films and bone marrow biopsies.

The work

It is an exciting time for haematology, with a plethora of new diagnostic techniques and therapeutic targets. The work can encompass a complete patient journey—from finding an abnormal blood film in the pile of reports to performing and reporting the bone marrow biopsy, explaining the diagnosis to the patient and their family, and finally prescribing them chemotherapy. After all this, the haematologist will have a special bond with their patient as they progress through treatment. In malignant haematology, there are emerging techniques such as patient-specific cell therapies, cancer vaccinations, and improved off-the-shelf biological agents. The non-malignant side is also showing exciting results with gene therapy for haemophilia and new long-acting factor replacement therapies.

The job

The job of a haematologist working in a tertiary hospital is often superspecialized in a particular area, e.g. lymphoma or transfusion. Alternatively, they may focus on laboratory work, microscopy, analysing mutations, or counting chromosomes. Many jobs concentrate on patient-centred work with ward rounds, ward consultations, and clinics. In contrast, haematologists in district general hospitals (DGHs) usually have a very varied workload which includes laboratory work, a large outpatient and ambulatory component, and advising other specialties, e.g. general physicians and intensive care.

Extras

Haematology is an academic field with a lot of interest in clinical trials and research. Many complete higher degrees (MD or PhD) during training, and there are numerous conferences around the world to share experiences, learn, and travel. Further experience in specialist areas can be gained as out of programme (OOP) or post-CCT fellowships. Some consultants choose to do a bit of private practice. Flexible training and working are well established, and there are opportunities to work abroad.

For further information

The Royal College of Pathologists (RCPath). Tel: 020 7451 6700. Web: https://www.rcpath.org Email: info@rcpath.org Twitter: @RCPath

A day in the life …

08:00 Journal club discussing an article on a new treatment for lymphoma

09:00 Ward round of haematology inpatients

11:00 Ward consults and review referrals from other specialties

12:00 MDT meeting to discuss new diagnoses and complex patients, with lunch

14:00 Bone marrow biopsy of inpatient

15:00 Blood film reporting

16:00 Meeting laboratory team to authorize flow cytometry reports

16:30 Clinical trials meeting

17:30 Urgent haematology day unit review

18:00 Home for a break before taking phone calls overnight (screened by haematology advanced nurse practitioner)

23:00 Code red massive haemorrhage emergency call—advise treating clinicians and authorize release of a lot of blood products

Myth	Easy specialty hiding behind a microscope; more interested in clotting cascades than patients.
Reality	Very demanding specialty with high levels of contact with sick patients requiring intense care and psychological support.
Personality	Empathetic, caring, interested in laboratory work, with a keen eye for attention to detail … Yes, that usually means a bit type A.
Best aspects	Patient continuity and building strong relationships with patients and families; research and development means that the specialty is exciting and constantly stimulating.
Worst aspects	Some malignant and stem cell transplant work can be emotionally draining. Weekend workload can be heavy in tertiary centres.
Route	Either internal medicine training (IMT) (p. 44) or acute care common stem–acute medicine (ACCS-AM) (p. 37), or paediatric level 1 training (p. 49), then specialty training in haematology (ST3+). Exams: MRCP or MRCPCH; FRCPath.
Numbers	1075 consultants, of whom 45% are women.
Locations	Practically all hospitals have a haematology department.

Life — Work

Quiet On-call — Busy On-call

Boredom — Burnout

Uncompetitive — Competitive

Low salary — High salary

Hand surgery

Hand surgery is an interesting and varied career that involves seeing patients in clinics, on the wards, and in the emergency department (ED). It also involves operating on them in a theatre setting. There are opportunities to be a hand surgeon in the field of plastic surgery (p. 266) or trauma and orthopaedic surgery (T&O) (p. 308 and p. 250). In T&O, there is a lot more involvement in fixing the bones of the hand and also the wrist. In plastic surgery, there is more opportunity to perform microsurgery.

The patients

Patients are a mixture of traumatic and elective cases. Trauma patients have, by definition, sustained an injury to the bones and/or soft tissues of the hand or wrist—they need treating as a matter of urgency to repair the damaged structures and prevent chronic pain and loss of function. Elective patients, e.g. carpal tunnel syndrome, ganglion cysts, etc., are referred by their GP or from another specialty and will normally be added to a waiting list for their surgery to be done. Some patients don't require surgery and can be managed with hand therapy, splints, or injections. Many patients can be managed as ambulatory day cases and a lot of patients have their surgery performed awake under local or regional anaesthesia.

The job

The job consists of a mixture of outpatient clinics, fracture clinics, elective theatre lists, trauma lists, and ward rounds. Surgeons are also called to the ED or fracture clinic to review patients with acute injuries. There is an on-call rota which may involve being on-call for all trauma or only for hand injuries, depending on the unit. Hand surgery involves managing a wide variety of different conditions and the surgery involves using many different techniques and treating many different structures. Examples range from using plates and screws to fix fractures or fuse joints to using very small sutures under magnification to repair damaged digital nerves.

The work

Hand surgeons work closely with a wide multidisciplinary team (MDT) which includes anaesthetists, nurses, operating department practitioners, healthcare assistants, occupational therapists, physiotherapists, plaster technicians, radiographers, and radiologists. It also involves having a good working relationship with the patient as they need to know what to expect and what they need to do to get a good result. It is a very rewarding job, with most patients having good outcomes and regaining better use of their hand following treatment, which may make a life-changing difference, e.g. if a person is able to return to work or resume their hobbies.

Extras

As it is a specialist area, most hand surgery is performed in university teaching hospitals. There are therefore plenty of opportunities to become involved in undergraduate and post-graduate education and teaching, and there are also opportunities to be involved in research, quality improvement, and audit. Private practice is available for those who want it.

For further information

The British Society for Surgery of the Hand (BSSH). Tel: 020 7831 5162. Web: https://www.bssh.ac.uk/ Email: secretariat@bssh.ac.uk Twitter: @BSSHand

---

08:00	Trauma MDT meeting reviewing radiology and deciding on treatment plans
08:30	Review ward patients
09:00	Fracture clinic, review 25 new and follow-up patients with fractures and soft tissue hand injuries
12:30	Teaching medical students hand anatomy
13:30	Theatre team briefing
13:40	Operating list; diverse range of patients and conditions
17:30	Theatre debrief
17:45	Review of postop patients
18:30	Home time for a well-deserved night off

Myth	Bored surgeons endlessly releasing carpal tunnels.
Reality	Highly skilled subspecialized surgeons who take a holistic approach to care and management.
Personality	Caring, empathetic, team player, and team leader; good technical ability, precision, and attention to detail.
Best aspects	Seeing patients get better, satisfaction of performing surgery.
Worst aspects	Busy on-calls.
Route	Core surgical training (CST) (p. 61), then specialty training in T&O surgery or plastic surgery, followed by advanced training or fellowship in hand surgery. Exams: MRCS; FRCS.
Locations	Trauma centres, large teaching hospitals, and some district general hospitals.

Life					Work
Quiet On-call					Busy On-call
Boredom					Burnout
Uncompetitive					Competitive
Low salary					High salary

Histopathology

Histopathology is an exciting and diverse diagnostic specialty involving the examination of tissue and fluid samples. Pathology is at the heart of all medical and surgical specialties. Histopathologists are medical detectives identifying the cause of illness. Macroscopic and microscopic examination of biopsies and surgical specimens is necessary to provide diagnoses, allowing the histopathologist to guide treatment and management within the context of a multidisciplinary team (MDT). In the dawning era of truly personalized medicine, histopathologists are at the forefront of areas such as molecular testing and digital pathology, which help to guide targeted therapy. This is an advancing specialty, with scope to make a significant difference to patients through involvement in translational research.

The patients

Most histopathologists do not have any patient contact, although in some centres, they perform fine-needle aspirations and take biopsies in outpatient clinics. However, they are essential to the diagnostic process, determining whether patients have benign or malignant disease and guiding further investigations. They play a vital role in the management of cancer by determining tumour subtypes and prognostic features, including tumour stage, grade, and completeness of excision. They also provide information about mutations and other molecular characteristics of tumours and disease. Histopathologists who perform autopsies have a valuable role in determining the cause of death and understanding the mechanisms of disease, and also assist families who are coming to terms with the loss of a relative. Many are also qualified medical examiners working closely with other clinicians and patients' families to review patient deaths.

The work

Almost all medical and surgical specialties require input from a histopathologist. Biopsies, tissue resections, or fluid samples are sent to the histopathologist who reviews the sections microscopically (using a microscope or a digital platform) and determines the diagnosis. Immunohistochemical stains or molecular tests may assist with this. They are an essential component of the MDT, working closely with physicians, surgeons, radiologists, and oncologists to determine the correct management strategy of each patient. For those performing autopsies, they identify the cause of death and work closely with the coroner's office and participate in inquests.

The job

Histopathology is a hospital-based specialty. Some time will be spent in the lab providing macroscopic descriptions of specimens and selecting sections of tissue to review microscopically. Each week, specialists will participate in one or more MDT meeting, and will regularly provide phone advice to other clinicians. Time will be spent in the mortuary for those performing autopsies, and digital autopsy (a non-invasive procedure using imaging techniques) is available in some centres. There is a strong team basis, consisting of consultants, trainees, biomedical scientists, electron microscopists, clinical scientists, and administrative staff. On-call commitments are generally minimal but depend on subspecialty. Those working in a tertiary referral centre or teaching hospital setting may be specialized within one area, e.g. haematopathology.

Extras

Lots of opportunities for teaching medical students and trainees (dependent on location). There is a huge research component for those who are interested in academia, although this is not a necessity. Private practice is an option from the first day as a consultant.

For further information

The Royal College of Pathologists (RCPath). Tel: 020 7451 6700. Web: https://www.rcpath.org Email: info@rcpath.org Twitter: @RCPath

07:30 Begin autopsy in the mortuary

09:00 MDT meeting to discuss diagnoses and treatment options

10:00 Cut up/macroscopic review of specimens in the lab

11:00 Microscopic review of cases and construction of reports

13:00 Call to deal with urgent frozen section from theatre

13:30 Teaching junior trainees/medical students

14:30 Microscopic review of cytology cases

15:30 Supervision of cases with trainees then review cases for next MDT meeting

18:00 Home for supper. Evening spent making plans for a teaching course, marking, and digital pathology reporting

20:00 Call from renal physicians about urgent kidney biopsy

Myth	Death-obsessed body snatchers who are best left alone in the mortuary.
Reality	Busy and demanding specialty with a lot of responsibility to provide the correct diagnosis. Strongly team-based. The vast majority of work helping living patients (only 3–5% is autopsy related).
Personality	Team player, personable, inquisitive, able to communicate well (written and verbal), organized, enthusiastic, enjoys medical detective work, teaching, and research.
Best aspects	Very satisfying to know that the report you produce provides the patient with a definitive diagnosis, allowing the correct treatment to be implemented, often after other investigations have been unsuccessful.
Worst aspects	Very busy and demanding, with a huge case load which is ever increasing!
Route	Run-through specialty training in histopathology (ST1+) (p. 52). Exams: FRCPath; optional exams in autopsy training and cervical cytopathology.
Numbers	1450 consultants, of whom 48% are women.
Locations	Hospitals (district general hospitals, teaching hospitals), laboratory, mortuary, office-based, coroner's court.

Life					Work
Quiet On-call					Busy On-call
Boredom					Burnout
Uncompetitive					Competitive
Low salary					High salary

Immunology

(Clinical) immunology is both a clinical and laboratory specialty. The main clinical areas are allergy and immunotherapy, immune deficiencies (primary and secondary), and auto-immunity (which paradoxically features in many cases of immunodeficiency). In this rapidly evolving and expanding specialty, novel tests and treatments are aplenty, including genetic markers and biological treatments. A particular field of interest can potentially direct your future career, with some clinical immunologists practising in specialist areas such as HIV, transplantation, or rheumatology, in addition to their mainstream work. Clinical immunologists run diagnostic laboratory services alongside clinical practice. The laboratory component involves understanding and interpreting tests, clinician liaison, and regular multidisciplinary meetings. A good understanding of laboratory medicine is extremely helpful in practising as a clinician.

The patients

An increasing cohort of patients with immune deficiencies are developing with improved diagnosis of primary immunodeficiency and with increasing use of biological treatments and other immune suppressants, resulting in secondary immunodeficiencies. These patients are generally very complex with chronic problems, and with whom a strong clinical relationship is often created. The allergy patients are relatively well, young individuals who often require only one visit. Additionally, clinics often see patients with rare auto-immune disease such as vasculitis, cryoglobulinaemia, immunoglobulin G4 (IgG4)-related disease, among others.

The work

This is a mixture of overseeing laboratory work and delivering outpatient clinics, but minimal inpatient care. The day case workload is ever increasing with the need to deliver immuno-therapies (e.g. immunoglobulin, immunosuppressants, biologics). Consultation of the literature on putative treatments in unusual situations forms part of the work in caring for patients with rare and complex syndromes. Interpretation of laboratory testing on behalf of other clinicians is also an important part of routine work.

The job

There is usually no on-call commitment, although phone call advice may be required. This may depend on local working practices (e.g. transplantation or HIV medicine might require shared cover). Clinical immunologists typically work in medical school centres with an on-site diagnostic laboratory. Both clinical and laboratory work necessitates good communication skills with a wide range of medical and laboratory specialists. The immunology team is usually small, with 2–3 consultants, 1–3 registrars, and 1–2 specialist nurses, and a team of ten or more laboratory scientists, so working relationships are generally close.

Extras

Clinical immunology is an academic specialty and lends itself to research, either clinical or basic science, with trainees often undertaking a PhD or an MD. There are several immunology conferences nationally and internationally. Flexible working, private practice (particularly allergy), or working with pharmaceutical companies are very possible.

> ### For further information
>
> **British Society for Allergy and Clinical Immunology (BSACI).** Tel: 020 7501 3910. Web: https://www.bsaci.org Twitter: @BSACI_Allergy

A day in the life ...

08:00 Attend medical grand round

09:00 Outpatient clinic: ten patients, six of whom are allergy, three well-known immuno-deficient patients, and one patient with vasculitis

12:30 Discuss the plans for the allergy challenge clinic and the immunodeficiency day case infusion patients with the specialist immunology nurses

12:45 Go for a 30-minute lunch with the specialist immunology nurses and registrars

13:15 Return to the office, and check everything is OK in the lab. Phone several GPs and clinicians about test results, including a positive antineutrophil cytoplasmic antibody (ANCA) and a suspected myeloma case

14:00 Review letters from yesterday's clinic, authorize some new/unusual lab complement and lymphocyte flow cytometry data

15:00 Look up the latest research on the possible management of a patient you saw that morning with a rare autoimmune (non-sarcoid lung granulomas) complication of their immunodeficiency

16:00 Continue writing a review audit/paper on the treatment and investigation of anaphylaxis within the hospital

17:00 Home

Myth	Clinically deficient academics who never leave the lab.
Reality	Clinicians who provide a wide-ranging regional clinical service and manage an adaptable immunology laboratory informed by clinical practice.
Personality	Inquisitive, knowledgeable, and practical.
Best aspects	Time enough to ensure individual patient care is excellent, and that the service provided to the hospital by the lab is also optimized. Being able to show an interest in a research field and start practice within it.
Worst aspects	Small teams and small numbers of consultants mean that trainees and consultants may feel isolated.
Route	Internal medicine training (IMT) (p. 44), acute care common stem–acute medicine (ACCS-AM) (p. 37), or paediatric level 1 training (p. 49), then specialty training in immunology (ST3+). Exams: MRCP or MRCPCH; FRCPath (Immunology).
Numbers	90 consultants, of whom 40% are women.
Locations	Teaching hospitals with an immunology laboratory.

Life — Work

Quiet On-call — Busy On-call

Boredom — Burnout

Uncompetitive — Competitive

Low salary — High salary

Infectious diseases

Infectious diseases (ID) is a growing and dynamic specialty. Since microbes are not picky as their hosts and do not neatly confine themselves to a single organ system, ID physicians are trained as generalists adept at managing patients of all ages presenting with a broad array of clinical problems. ID doctors diagnose and treat the weird and wonderful, but also bring expertise in managing common infections in patients with complicated medical problems. ID is a continually evolving specialty where recent research has yielded significant successes. HIV management, for example, is unrecognizable, compared to 20 years ago. But as new pathogens emerge and old ones adapt to outpace treatments, many challenges await that will ensure a career in ID remains exciting and varied.

The patients

Everyone—young and old, from all walks of life and every corner of the globe. ID physicians see patients with home-grown, common or garden ID, and also travellers returning from far-flung climes who may harbour more exotic bugs. They see patients whose immune systems are impaired due to any number of insults (e.g. HIV, chemotherapy, organ transplantation) who may present with unusual infections or unusual manifestations of common infections or something else entirely.

The work

Every day is gratifyingly different. Patients are seen in all departments of the hospital: the student in the emergency department (ED) with meningococcal meningitis; the visitor from Nigeria on the intensive care unit (ICU) with complicated falciparum malaria; the man on the ward with undiagnosed fevers despite weeks of investigation; the elderly woman on the isolation ward with a further recurrence of *Clostridioides difficile* diarrhoea; or the man in clinic with recently diagnosed HIV, making a rapid recovery from *Pneumocystis jirovecii* pneumonia. ID training and practice are increasingly integrated with the traditional laboratory specialties of microbiology and virology, enabling ID physicians to facilitate optimal use of laboratory diagnostic technologies.

The job

Often based on dedicated ID units that typically include isolation facilities for airborne infections. Outpatient clinics may be general, including patients with an array of conditions, or specialized (e.g. HIV, hepatitis C) where ID physicians often work alongside specialist nurses. Some units operate a consult model where ID physicians advise other teams on the management of infections that are complicated, e.g. as a result of multidrug-resistant pathogens or concurrent medical problems. ID physicians accredited in microbiology or virology will spend time in the laboratory, managing the smooth running of tests and interpreting results (see Medical microbiology, p. 216; Virology, p. 316).

Extras

Training in ID opens doors to a world of possibilities. ID doctors often choose to participate in research and there are opportunities to balance a clinical and academic career. There are excellent opportunities for work overseas in many varied roles. ID lends itself well to work alongside clinicians from other disciplines to develop innovative services, both within the hospital (e.g. specialist neurological infection clinic) and the wider community (e.g. prison health services).

For further information

British Infection Association (BIA). Tel: 01772 681 333. Web: http://www.britishinfection. org Email: bia@hartleytaylor.co.uk Twitter: @biainfection

09:00   Board-round of current inpatients with the ward multidisciplinary team (MDT)

09:30   Teaching ward round on the ID unit

12:00   Consult of patient on the ICU with suspected encephalitis

12:30   Review of patient receiving intravenous antibiotics in community for infective endocarditis

13:00   Tuberculosis multidisciplinary meeting

14:00   HIV clinic

16:30   Back to the ward to troubleshoot any problems and review new admissions

17:00   Teleconference to discuss research proposal

18:00   Cycle home in Lycra, eat vegan food, and play the board game Pandemic

03:30   Call from the ED—'Do you think that this man with fever and cough who has just arrived from Saudi Arabia has Middle East respiratory syndrome (MERS)?'

Myth	Super smart nerds suggesting long lists of tests for obscure unpronounceable bugs you've never heard of.
Reality	An incredibly varied and dynamic specialty with something for everyone.
Personality	Open-minded dynamic thinkers with an eye for detail, coupled with a broad outlook.
Best aspects	Immense satisfaction of watching many patients with infections making full recovery with treatment; a world of career opportunities to explore.
Worst aspects	Failing to clinch the diagnosis as a patient with a weird array of symptoms deteriorates.
Route	Internal medicine training (IMT) (p. 44) or acute care common stem (ACCS-AM) (p. 37), followed by combined infection training (CIT) (p. 53), then specialty training in ID (ST5+). Can be combined with general internal medicine (GIM) (p. 44), microbiology (p. 52), or virology (p. 52). Exams: MRCP; FRCPath.
Numbers	400 consultants in ID and tropical medicine, of whom 35% are women.
Locations	Teaching hospitals.

Life					Work
Quiet On-call					Busy On-call
Boredom					Burnout
Uncompetitive					Competitive
Low salary					High salary

▌ Intensive care medicine

Intensive care medicine (ICM) is a rapidly evolving area of healthcare, combining some of the most scientific aspects of healthcare with some of the most human. The specialty has been at the forefront of the battle against the recent COVID-19 pandemic and the work done in intensive care units (ICUs) has been well documented. The demand for ICM is dramatically increasing due to multiple factors, including an ageing population, increasing complexity of cases, comorbidities, and others e.g. polypharmacy, obesity, drug resistance, and substance misuse. ICM remains closely related to the acute specialties of internal medicine (p. 114), anaesthesia (p. 118), and emergency medicine (EM) (p. 154). Those wishing to train in ICM must complete the core components of one of these specialties before accrediting solely in ICM or obtaining a dual CCT with their parent specialty.

The patients

Intensivists care for the sickest patients in the hospital, including those admitted with unplanned life-threatening emergencies, major trauma, and elective high-risk surgical patients. Patients admitted to the ICU are those requiring invasive monitoring and support for single or multiple organ failure. Patients may be young, fit, and usually well, or more commonly elderly with multiple comorbidities. Turnaround on the ICU is normally quick, but some patients require prolonged stays. All patients require a high level of care and support, but despite expertise and advanced treatment, mortality remains high at 10–20%. For this reason, the specialty has an important role in providing end-of-life care and leading discussions on the difficult, but important issue of organ donation.

The work

ICM provides a challenging, exciting, stressful, and unpredictable workload. The focus of care is early, goal-directed therapy by optimizing initial resuscitation and providing treatments offered only in intensive care. Patients may require invasive ventilation, cardiovascular support, and renal replacement therapy, as well as regimented review of nutrition, microbiology, endocrinology, and psychological aspects of care. ICM is a very practical specialty, with specialists frequently performing skills, including placing central lines, intubation, and inserting percutaneous tracheostomies, to name a few, as well as using bedside echocardiography and bronchoscopy. A working knowledge of physiology, pharmacology, and technology is required, and good communication, often at times of crisis, is paramount.

The job

The job of the intensivist is expanding, and it extends throughout the hospital as part of cardiac arrest and trauma teams, managing deteriorating ward patients, as well as a commitment to intensive care follow-up clinics. ICU beds are a limited and expensive commodity and intensivists have an increasing role in managing admission and transfer of patients. It is a specialty dependent on the MDT—physiotherapists, dieticians, pharmacists, microbiologists, and technicians, as well as a highly skilled and experienced nursing staff who spend the most time with the patients. Close working relationships are essential.

Extras

There is some limited scope for private practice. Some intensivists choose to undertake research, and subspecialization is possible with separate neurosurgical, paediatric, cardiac, and liver ICUs in regional centres. When not in ICM, intensivists who are dual-accredited return to their base specialty, allowing for a varied and interesting job plan. Many are often found teaching, particularly where high-fidelity simulation and practical skills are involved.

For further information

The Faculty of Intensive Care Medicine (FICM). Tel: 020 7092 1653. Web: https://www.FICM.ac.uk Email: contact@ficm.ac.uk Twitter: @FICMNews

Intensive Care Society (ICS). Tel: 020 7280 4350. Web: https://www.ics.ac.uk Email: info@ics.ac.uk Twitter: @ICS_updates

A day in the life ...

07:45	Change out of normal clothes into battle pyjamas (scrubs)
07:50	Review bed availability and booking diary for elective surgical cases and transfers—yay or nay to go ahead with surgical cases—prepare for surgeon tantrums
08:00	Handover—sit down (coffee if lucky)
09:00	Daily reviews of all patients; review of acute treatments and progress, set goals for the day, ventilation-weaning strategy, further investigations, etc.
13:00	Journal club and morbidity and mortality meeting with trainees and consultants
14:00	Microbiology ward round—review all antibiotics and rationalize with micro results
15:00	Critical care outreach ward round to review patients of concern on the general wards
16:00	Major surgical cases begin to arrive to ICU from theatre
17:00 -20:00	On the unit: anything can happen—misplaced tubes, crashing patients, electrolyte abnormalities, ventilator tweaking, etc.

Myth	Pyjama wearing, laryngoscope-wielding superheroes, using scary drugs to save every sick patient.
Reality	Fast-paced and dynamic clinicians working in an ever-changing environment. Demanding-medically, physically and psychologically. Making tough decisions that will occasionally upset people.
Personality	Adaptive, calm under pressure, team player, mental toughness with element of obsessiveness and stickler for detail, but ability to see the bigger picture. Loves an arterial blood gas.
Best aspects	Practical skills, applied physiology, teamwork, lots of gadgets and toys, and the chance to ensure patients and families are supported in life-threatening or life-ending illnesses.
Worst aspects	Tiring, high psychological impact, being the person to say 'enough is enough', management of beds, high mortality rates. Chronic patients, with limited progress. The hours can be long.
Route	Core training in anaesthetics (p. 39), EM (p. 37), acute care common stem—acute medicine (ACCS-AM) (p. 37), or internal medicine training (IMT) (p. 44), then specialty training in ICM (ST3+) as a single or dual specialty. Exams: exam relevant to core training; FFICM.
Numbers	Number of ICM consultants variable between reports. Over 80% dual CCT in anaesthesia, and around 20% are women.
Locations	Regional/district hospitals and also subspecialist centres.

Life						Work
Quiet On-call						Busy On-call
Boredom						Burnout
Uncompetitive						Competitive
Low salary						High salary

Locuming full-time

Locum work is temporary work to fill a gap on a clinical rota (e.g. due to training, maternity leave, sickness, etc.). Most doctors will do some locum shifts to supplement pay or gain additional experience alongside—or between—clinical or research jobs. Being a full-time locum is not a medical subspecialty, rather it is a career pathway that can apply to any area of medicine. It requires having a high degree of flexibility with your working hours, places of work, and even monthly income. The locum life means hospitals and colleagues change on a daily basis—for better or worse. It does, however, allow full control over working hours and commitments, making it easier to maintain whatever work/life balance is best suited to you as an individual.

The patients

The patients can come from whichever area of medicine in which you find yourself working. The only thing they are likely to have in common is this: scepticism of you as a locum. Whether in a vibrant A&E department or a silent medical ward, patients are likely to assume that, as a locum, you are nothing but a 'soldier of fortune', selling your wares to the highest bidder, and who might offer them inferior care compared to your full-time colleagues.

The work

Locums exist to plug the holes left in certain departments by either absent colleagues or unfilled posts. The shifts might become available months in advance or on a few desperate hours' notice. Hence compulsive email-checking is where the locum will rise or fall. You will need to belong to either a locum agency or a hospital's Staff Bank to have access to these shifts—both of which require a bounteous amount of paperwork. Which of these two is the superior option is a debate that has raged among locums for time immemorial, with no definitive answer in sight.

The job

The work will obviously vary, depending on which area of medicine you are locuming in. What it will entail is frequently arriving at new hospitals and having to prove yourself to your generally dubious colleagues. It requires both good clinical and interpersonal skills to allow yourself to be accepted into the herd sooner rather than later. You are usually excluded from formal teaching, so it requires high levels of self-discipline to maintain your own ongoing medical education. It is also particularly well suited for those who seek that most forbidden of medical fruits: the social life.

Extras

Locum pay is usually higher than equivalent full-time posts, but without the benefits of paid leave and, in some cases, indemnity or pension. Locuming isn't usually a life-long decision. It's very common for doctors to choose this route for a short period of time—either just to take a break from a particularly gruelling year or to earn money to go travelling, or to spend more time with a young family. It is as lucrative or as relaxed as you want it to be. That is its single greatest draw card.

For further information

NHS Professionals (NHS locum agency). Tel: 0333 014 3652. Web: https://www.nhsprofessionals.nhs.uk Twitter: @NHSPbank

12:30	Arrive for shift at new hospital 30 minutes early to try and find way around
12:40	Already lost, you console yourself with a coffee
12:50	Find correct department, introduce self to all the staff, attempt to charm nurse in charge. Usually fail
13:00	Quick orientation of department
13:15	Attempt to tackle unfamiliar IT system. Phone IT department about faulty IT system
13:30	Begin seeing your patients for the day
14:00	Impress sceptical colleagues with clinical knowledge—gain acceptance into the herd
17:00	Dinner with newly impressed colleagues in canteen
17:30	Continue seeing patients, but with renewed confidence
22:45	Handover of patients
23:00	Departure, with fresh promises of returning for more shifts soon

Myth	Unambitious, greedy slackers who leech off the NHS instead of doing 'real' work.
Reality	Adaptable, personable doctors who are an indispensable part of the NHS.
Personality	Sociable people who seek a greater work/life balance.
Best aspects	Working in various hospitals with various staff means the working environment never gets boring. Full control over own working hours.
Worst aspects	Pervasive negative perceptions about locums.
Route	Any and all fields need locums, often of all levels of experience from F1 to consultant/GP.
Numbers	10 200 GP locums, 3500 hospital locums at consultant level; 9000 locums neither on the specialist/GP register nor in training.
Locations	Everywhere.

Life					Work
Quiet On-call					Busy On-call
Boredom					Burnout
Uncompetitive					Competitive
Low salary					High salary

Media medicine

'Media medicine' is a unique area of work that has been relatively under-recognized. Traditionally, it took the form of the 'couch doctor' offering advice on television shows or a health column in a newspaper or magazine. Nowadays there are doctors from a range of different backgrounds and specialties doing everything, from TV presenting to writing for the national press. With the increasing part that modern, and particularly social, media play in our day-to-day lives, media medicine really has started to gain strength as a powerful form of health promotion and education, as well as entertainment. Media medics are not just doctors—they are writers, advisers, producers, broadcasters, presenters, and entertainers. Media medicine is not one format but encompasses a whole range of platforms, including television, radio, online, and print. Because of these factors, the role can be entirely unique to each professional.

The patients

Since media medicine is not technically a clinical specialty, there are no 'patients' as such. However, depending on the particular role (e.g. on screen, on radio), media medics are likely to be communicating with the general public quite a lot. Therefore, it is very much a public health role and effective public engagement is a core aspect.

The work

The exact job very much depends on each individual. Some media medics offer advice or information on daytime TV. Some do radio phone-ins on general or specific medical issues. Some write for magazines or websites on health topics. Some have developed presenter roles on popular shows (e.g. Channel 4's *Embarrassing Bodies*) or children's TV! As easy as it may seem and as much as some people may *want* to work in the media, not everyone is suited to it and in many respects, the industry chooses the person. As well as having the right set of skills and being desirable to the industry, they must also be popular with the public. Furthermore, it is not a stable career and there are never any guarantees—a thick skin is definitely necessary. It's not an easy path, and knock-backs and rejection are commonplace!

The job

Media medics work all over the country in various environments, depending on the project in which they are involved. This could be on a studio set, at a radio station, or even on location in a remote part of the world. It also means being prepared to travel, and sometimes at relatively short notice. Because it requires a significant amount of flexibility, it doesn't always work for those who have full-time clinical or personal commitments as it must fit in around other activities. Also, media medics have to constantly keep up-to-date on both their specific area or niche and medicine as a whole. That means doing *a lot* of reading and research!

Extras

Media medicine is a bespoke profession—it can offer many varied opportunities if the individual is prepared to work hard for them. If successful, it gives the ability to carve out a unique role (provided the work is there!). There are some perks too: being invited to glitzy events and parties is always fun (although not that frequent)!

For further information

Medical Protection Society. Press support for members. Available at: https://www.medi-calprotection.org/uk/about-mps/media-centre/a-guide-for-doctors-on-handling-the-media
Medics in the Media (2011) by Neil Chanchlani. *BMJ* 2011;342:d1461. Available at: http://careers.bmj.com/careers/advice/Medics_in_the_media

06:30 Alarm goes off!

07:30 Travel from home to TV studio—do some research/reading en route

08:30 Into hair and make-up to get ready, grab a cup of tea/coffee

09:00 Briefing for on-screen item with production team ± rehearsal

09:30 Reading and research to check all information is up-to-date, get relevant statistics/facts, plan for questions

10:45 Live on-screen item (lasting 5–7 minutes)

11:00 Tidy up loose ends from on-screen item

11:15 Travel from studio to hospital for clinical shift

12:00 Clinical shift in hospital

20:00 Leave hospital and travel home

21:00 Catch up on emails from the day (work and media)

22:00 Write health piece for magazine

23:00 Write journal club presentation for work, update e-portfolio, catch up on social media

24:00 Bedtime!

Myth	Fluffy media darlings with poor clinical skills.
Reality	Passionate individuals in a cut-throat industry that demands hard work, drive, creativity, and up-to-date medical knowledge, as well as physical stamina and mental resilience.
Personality	Proficient communicators with a skill for getting information across to the public, engaging, go-getters, able to handle negative reviews/rejection.
Best aspects	Working in a dynamic and exciting industry alongside a variety of interesting people, being recognized and valued by the public, opportunity to support or represent charities.
Worst aspects	Early starts, travel, balancing with other family or work commitments, giving up 'days off' at the last minute, negative reviews from press or public, poor job stability.
Route	Opportunistic, usually requires a concurrent clinical role which can theoretically be in any specialty, but often at a certain level (e.g. GP, ST4+) so that you are relevant/credible.
Locations	Anywhere in mixture of settings/roles, but most major media organizations are based in/near big cities.

Life					Work
Quiet On-call					Busy On-call
Boredom					Burnout
Uncompetitive					Competitive
Low salary					High salary

Medical education

The word 'doctor' comes from the Latin '*docere*', meaning 'to teach'. Fortunately, gone are the days where an all-knowing consultant could humiliate their minions in a game of 'guess what I'm thinking' on ward rounds and call it teaching. Gone too is the cliché that 'those who can, do; those who can't, teach'. In the last two decades, there has been growing appreciation of the specific skills required by educators, the need for integration of educational theory and evidence with practical teaching, and a developing interest in medical education as a specialty in its own right. The GMC now requires medical educators to have appropriate qualifications to teach. A multitude of PGCert, PGDip, and Masters programmes in medical, clinical, and health professions education are available to prospective educators—offered via face-to-face, blended, or online options.

The patients

Medical educators may work with real or simulated patients in their education role(s), depending on the setting. Teaching in hospital or general practice often involves working with patients; clinical skills and clinical communication teaching may make use of actors as simulated patients; some teaching involves manikins, high-fidelity simulators, or even virtual reality. Learners may be undergraduate students, postgraduate trainees, or those undertaking continuing professional development. They might be in uni-professional or multi-professional groups. A vital aspect of teaching is considering *who* the learners are, in order to meet their learning needs. This will help to determine the content and structure of teaching.

The work

There is something for everyone—teaching in a classroom, clinical, or online setting; explaining, facilitating, supervising, mentoring, and pastoral roles; working with individuals, pairs, small groups, or large groups; creating resources; running assessments; evaluating programmes; designing curricula. One can dip a toe in the waters of medical education or become fully immersed.

The job

Some educators separate clinical and educational work, e.g. combining part-time clinical work with a faculty role in a medical school, whereas others have roles that blend the two— consultant posts usually have teaching in their job description, and many, particularly GPs, become clinical or educational supervisors (p. 97) for trainees. The majority of educators also work clinically, but it is possible to transition completely to become a full-time educator. The job is generally flexible and works well in combination with other commitments such as family, hobbies, and other work roles. It is hugely rewarding and lots of fun!

Extras

Medical education opens up a host of opportunities—as well as face-to-face teaching, one can get involved in research, course design, assessment, writing, and many other projects. The community of medical educators is a friendly, supportive, collaborative one, with a pretty flat hierarchy—especially on Twitter and at conferences which are recommended as a good way to network, share your work, and find out what's 'hot' in medical education.

For further information

Academy of Medical Educators (AoME). Tel: 029 2068 7206. Web: https://www.medic aleducators.org Email: info@medicaleducators.org Twitter: @MedicalEducator

Association for the Study of Medical Education (ASME). Tel: 0131 225 9111. Web: https://www.asme.org.uk Email: info@asme.org.uk Twitter: @asmeofficial

---

09:00	Check emails, review teaching notes for the day
10:00	Team meeting: collaboration, research ideas, planning teaching, staff development, curriculum development, evaluation and quality assurance/improvement, budgets
12:00	Lunch with colleagues
12:30	Check room setup for teaching session
13:00	Teaching session
16:00	Marking/session planning/online feedback/emails
17:00	Head home for dinner and time with the family
19:00	Evening webinar/review teaching materials for the next day

Myth	Clinical expert = expert teacher.
Reality	Sometimes the hardest thing is not giving your knowledge, but helping people to find theirs.
Personality	Outgoing, organized, enthusiastic.
Best aspects	Teamwork, innovation, making a difference to future generations of healthcare professionals.
Worst aspects	Balancing teaching and clinical commitments—two part-time roles always equal more than one full-time!
Route	There are numerous formal and informal ways in. Increasingly, postgraduate education qualifications are needed.
Locations	Hospitals, community, universities around the UK and abroad.

Life						Work
Quiet On-call						Busy On-call
Boredom						Burnout
Uncompetitive						Competitive
Low salary						High salary

Medical entrepreneur

Entrepreneurship involves the development of a successful business that addresses an unmet demand or radically improves existing performance. Medical entrepreneurs focus on improving patient outcomes and improving efficiency in the delivery of care. There is no established training programme and no qualification that defines expertise-individuals make their own path aided by the guidance of mentors. Glorious failure should be worn as a badge of honour so that mistakes are not repeated, yet the attainment of success can be both elusive and difficult to define. There is growing recognition of the role entrepreneurs can play to cope with increasing demand in the face of diminishing resources. In a conservative financial climate, they are uniquely placed to drive meaningful change through the acceptance of personal risk. Entrepreneurs will not be discouraged or diverted by 'experts' with a vested interest in the status quo but strive to build a better world and a positive balance sheet.

The patients

Whilst patients must be the ultimate focus, a medical entrepreneur is unlikely to be involved in direct delivery of clinical care. Instead, the 'patients' are individuals or organizations who are responsible for funding the nascent idea and subsequent purchasing of the finished product or service. Selling to the NHS presents its own unique challenges due to budgetary constraints, differing strategic priorities among organizations, and often opaque procurement pathways. Clinicians often see the value of innovation early, but ultimately it is managers who decide on implementation. The greatest responsibility for every entrepreneur is to secure sufficient liquidity to give the business every chance of success-building relationships with individual and institutional investors must begin early.

The work

The work of a medical entrepreneur varies greatly, depending on both the business plan and stage of development. Those embarking on a new project should be focused on generating data that can influence purchasing decisions and building a final product or service through an iterative process. Meeting prospective clients and/or investors is key to moving forward, and perfecting an inspirational 'elevator pitch' is vital. Successful entrepreneurs need to develop a skill set that is quite distinct from those nurtured in clinical practice where treatment options are rarely presented as 'time-limited offers' and signing of legal documents has little personal implication. Business administration is a constant chore.

The job

Working as an entrepreneur does not provide the job security or peer support of a conventional medical career, with outcomes primarily resting on few shoulders. The development of a core team helps share this burden and sensible recruitment enhances the chances of success. On-call commitments must be considered with any project involving a service agreement.

Extras

Mentoring is the foundation of the entrepreneur community and is not dissimilar to supervising junior doctors. International travel may be required to access investment or to explore new markets. For those who remain in clinical practice, the development of a broader perspective and non-clinical skills should enhance future career option.

For further information

NHS Accelerated Access Collaborative. Clinical entrepreneur training programme. Web: https://www.england.nhs.uk/aac/what-we-do/how-can-the-aac-help-me/clinical-entrepreneur-training-programme/ Twitter: @AACinnovation

Doctorpreneurs (non-profit organization for doctors and medical students interested in healthcare innovation and entrepreneurship). Web: https://doctorpreneurs.com Email: info@doctorpreneurs.com Twitter: @Doctorpreneurs

A day in the life ...

07:30   Respond to emails during commute to work

08:30   Start day job (medical registrar)

13:30   Telephone calls and urgent emails over lunch

17:30   Finish day job and respond to day's emails during commute home

18:30   Home for dinner and family time

20:00   Telephone call with co-founder to review status of current projects

20:30   Review latest software build from development team

21:00   Work on specification document for a new client

22:00   Business administration

22:30   Produce jobs list for tomorrow

Myth	A member of the flat white drinking, hipster elite with a jet set lifestyle and a bank balance to match.
Reality	We walk among you and have a non-prejudiced attitude to all caffeinated beverages. Success can be measured in many ways, but few ventures result in £1 billion companies.
Personality	Unquestionable self-belief backed by single-minded dedication and a desire to disrupt the status quo. Require leadership skills to inspire and managerial skills to deliver.
Best aspects	Taking an idea and transforming it into something tangible that can have a positive impact on patient outcomes.
Worst aspects	Designing an innovate solution to a problem no one wants to solve. Never having enough time.
Route	There is no established route, although clinical seniority is advantageous for generating traction. The decision of whether to continue clinical medicine in parallel is very difficult.
Locations	No restrictions, providing ability to travel to meet clients. Anywhere with Wi-Fi and caffeine is usually sufficient.

Life					Work
Quiet On-call					Busy On-call
Boredom					Burnout
Uncompetitive					Competitive
Low salary					High salary

Medical ethics

Medical ethics is a branch of philosophy that studies questions of morality specific to medical practice and research. Whilst not a medical specialty per se, ethics has always been recognized as an important part of medicine. The formal requirement for explicit teaching in medical ethics emerged partly in response to the Nuremberg Trials after the Second World War, when it became clear that doctors had participated in some of the worst horrors in Nazi Germany. Later in the twentieth century, new developments in medical technology posed additional ethical challenges for doctors, particularly in the fields of organ transplantation, assisted reproduction, and end-of-life care. At the same time, the doctor–patient relationship was undergoing a shift away from the kindly paternalism of the past to a more autonomy focused ethos. This placed new emphasis on doctors' abilities to communicate effectively to ensure that patients could make informed decisions, rather than simply obeying the doctor's orders.

The patients

All doctor–patient encounters engage some degree of ethical consideration. Often this is just routine: gaining informed consent; maintaining confidentiality. The most challenging situations are those that involve a clash between ethical values, e.g. a patient who wants to refuse lifesaving treatment or a risk that keeping the patient's condition confidential may harm others. For this reason, a medical ethicist's work is unlikely to be confined to one group or one category of patients. Equally, a medical ethicist's role involves doctors and other healthcare professionals as much as patients. Most professional medical ethicists in the UK work in medical schools, and the bulk of their work will involve training medical students.

The work

Medical ethics usually involves a number of different activities. An ethicist may spend much of their time teaching medical students and is likely to be closely involved with one or more teaching hospitals. In addition to teaching work, medical ethicists often participate in clinical ethics committees and contribute to local and national policies and guidelines. In common with other academic medical school staff, medical ethicists will have administrative and advisory roles, as well as their teaching and assessment obligations. Medical ethicists often have a specific field of expertise within the discipline: public health ethics, reproductive ethics, or research ethics, for example. They will be expected to conduct research in their field and to publish their work.

The job

Medical ethicists will spend much of their time in the lecture theatre or seminar room on a university or medical school campus. They may also spend time in hospitals, participating in grand rounds or (less commonly in the UK) at the bedside. Ethicists may not be part of a team per se but will often work closely with clinical colleagues. Medical ethicists are often invited to contribute to education and training days for medical specialties.

Extras

The job of a medical ethicist can be quite diverse, and many opportunities exist for outreach activities, media work, and research. Perhaps the most exciting aspect of medical ethics is the fact that it is such a dynamic field; it responds to every new development in medical technology and evolves alongside changes in legislation and regulation.

For further information

Institute of Medical Ethics (IME). Tel: 01925 299 733. Web: www.instituteofmedicalethics.org/website/ Twitter: @IMEweb

UK Clinical Ethics Network (UKCEN). Web: http://www.ukcen.net Email: info@ukcen.net Twitter: @UKCEN

08:30 Catch up with emails

09:30 Lecture to 180 students on the ethics of organ transplantation

10:00 Supervision meeting with a student doing a project on direct-to-consumer genetic testing

11:30 Meeting with colleagues about a research project involving people who lack capacity

13:00 OMG! A major breakthrough in a highly controversial area of medicine has erupted, and you are asked to give a comment on the news ...

13:45 Snatch a quick sandwich, then a training session with junior doctors on advance directives

15:30 Review a paper submitted to an ethics journal of which you're on the editorial board. Ask for substantial revisions and chuckle nastily

16:30 Meeting of the local clinical ethics committee: the dilemma is whether to initiate gastrostomy feeding for an elderly post-stroke patient whose prognosis is poor, but whose family want 'everything done'

19:00 Revise a paper you've submitted for publication that has come back from the reviewer, requiring a lot of irritating and unnecessary changes

22:15 Watch the news, spot an item on patients above a certain BMI being denied treatment that neatly illustrates an issue in tomorrow's seminar

Myth	It's all a matter of common sense.
Reality	As medicine has become more complex, so have the ethical dilemmas.
Personality	Analytical, open-minded, meticulous, articulate.
Best aspects	Grappling with some fascinating and gripping dilemmas; helping and supporting doctors and patients.
Worst aspects	Doctors who deny they ever encounter ethical challenges.
Route	First degree in medicine, law, philosophy, or sociology; masters or PhD in medical ethics.
Numbers	No centralized data recording, but an estimated 75 people teaching ethics at undergraduate and postgraduate level.
Locations	Universities, teaching hospitals.

Life					Work
Quiet On-call					Busy On-call
Boredom					Burnout
Uncompetitive					Competitive
Low salary					High salary

▍ Medical management consultancy

Medical management consultancy is at the interface between business and medicine. As we move further into the digital age, it is likely to be an ever expanding field. Medical data sets are sensitive, personal, and often unfathomable without a clinical degree. Additionally, the Data Protection Act strictly protects such identifiable data. However, despite the well-publicized difficulties with some national programmes, more and more hospital data are being made electronically accessible. The ability to extract trends and unexpected findings from large data sets means we're about to enter a whole new area of development. Very few doctors make the leap into management consulting, so they are often the only medically qualified person on a team that could be researching the background of multimillion-pound projects, assessing problem figures, interpreting findings, proposing strategies, planning the steps of transformational projects, or guiding delivery in clinical care.

The patients

No patients, but lots of 'clients'. The clients can be doctors and staff working wherever a change project is needed. Inevitably, the more clinicians involved, the more differing opinions there are, and it can feel rather like the proverbial herding of cats. The opinions, frustrations and concerns of local staff must be translated into the language of business. It often falls to the doctor on the consultancy team to explain back to the clinicians why all of their requests cannot be met and delivered as the project progresses.

The work

Management is all about data and clinical interpretation of the outcomes is essential. A medical management consultant acts as this necessary bridge between data relevance and technicians, data analysts, hospital managers, policymakers, fund holders, etc. With this clinical oversight, when the inevitable data transformation in healthcare does occur, it's easy to see the immense opportunities both in terms of individual patients and for large-scale research. The work, however, requires intense problem-solving and interpersonal skills.

The job

A variable work environment consisting of meetings, interviews, presentations, and report writing. This can range from on site at local hospitals to the consulting firm offices or NHS and Department of Health buildings. Projects generally require both clinical interpretation and business acumen, and working to meet demanding deadlines. By listening and supporting change, regardless of whether projects are enormous, transformational overhauls, or simply delivering small local improvements, the job can be very rewarding.

Extras

Initially, do not expect to be paid more because of your medical degree—you're learning from scratch again. A first-year consultant earns approximately £32 000, increasing to around £74 786 after 5 years. After 20 years, employees earn an average of £97 601. However, a partner at a top firm would bring home considerably more, but this will be when the competitive aspect of the job can really ramp up. International travel can be a perk and the travel allowances are often very generous.

For further information

Contact any of the big firms.
Management Consulting Association (MCA). Tel: 020 7645 7950. Web: https://www.mca.org.uk/ Email: info@mca.org.uk Twitter: @TheMCA_UK

08:00   Travel to client site

09:00   Run workshop to review specific treatment options with relevant clinical personnel; identify areas for improvement and associated difficulties

12:30   Working lunch chatting to workshop attendees

14:00   Back to the office: plan suitable solutions and materials for the client in an internal team meeting

15:00   Liaise with client to problem-solve issues that have arisen

17:00   Manage the ever-growing email stream

18:00   Head home with (nearly) no chance of being disturbed

Myth	Forsaking your clinical brethren to seek your fortune in the evil world of management.
Reality	Using clinical knowledge to be the necessary bridge between busy practising clinicians and non-clinicians to ensure both clinical oversight and realistic targets are present in big-change projects.
Personality	Ability to jump quickly between the big picture and the relevant minutiae. A good listener. Amiable, but iron-willed when it really matters.
Best aspects	Impacting hundreds (or thousands) of patients at a time when you manage to steer the juggernaut of change in clinically appropriate ways.
Worst aspects	Watching unrealistic or irrelevant ideas harnessing resources you know would be better used elsewhere.
Route	No fixed route. A broad sampling of junior doctor clinical experience, with the realities of working in healthcare and its daily inefficiencies, will provide the unique perspective you will bring to change projects. Other management or business training could be useful.
Locations	Any clinical environment. Travel is a big part of the job. If it's a big project, teams will be based at the project site for a couple of years or more.

Life					Work
Quiet On-call					Busy On-call
Boredom					Burnout
Uncompetitive					Competitive
Low salary					High salary

Medical management

Medical leadership is now widely recognized as an important non-clinical skill. All doctors are required to lead their colleagues at times, to improve the quality and effectiveness of services, and to speak up when things go wrong. Some doctors take up formal medical management roles. Many future medical managers get involved in medical school societies. Junior doctors are essential in creating change since they are at the heart of clinical teams working with patients and can identify what works and what doesn't by rotating between jobs. Later, some consultants and GPs do formal medical manager jobs, and most continue clinical work alongside these roles. At any level, formal qualifications or training can be undertaken. Many learn leadership skills on the job supported by coaching and learning sets. It's a privilege at any level to be involved in creating a compelling vision for the future of health and care and to play a part in making it happen.

The patients

Medical managers get to work with the other clinical professions, professional managers, accountants, patients, politicians, and the public, all of whom will have strong views about how things should be done. Leading other doctors can be hard. Colleagues will often say that medical managers have 'gone to the dark side' when, in fact, they are simply trying to develop services which deliver the best quality and are value for money.

The work

Every day is different. Medical managers oversee improvements in the quality and safety of services, develop vision, strategy, and plans for their organizations, and help decide how best to spend public money. Most get involved in investigating when things go wrong. Increasingly, medical managers are at the forefront of explaining change in the way services are delivered to the public.

The job

Many medical managers split their time between clinical duties and their medical manager roles, which can be based in separate places. It's essential to read and assimilate large amounts of verbal and numerical information quickly since there are a lot of meeting papers and reports to deal with daily. Managers need to be able to communicate at different levels, speaking to large groups and one to one. Difficult conversations with patients or with colleagues aren't uncommon. Progress can be slow. Most overestimate what they can achieve in a month and underestimate what they can achieve in a year.

Extras

The Faculty of Medical Leadership and Management (FMLM) and the NHS Leadership Academy offer personal development in relevant skills and opportunities for electives and fellowships. These offer great opportunities to learn from others and in settings not usually encountered by clinicians.

For further information

Faculty of Medical Leadership and Management (FMLM). Tel: 020 8051 2060. Web: https://www.fmlm.ac.uk Email: enquiries@fmlm.ac.uk Twitter: @FMLM_UK

08:00 Breakfast meeting with general managers going through waiting lists and finance

09:00 Chair Quality and Patient Safety Committee

12:00 1-2-1 meetings with senior nurse managers

12:30 Working lunch with other doctors to discuss ideas for improving quality and reducing costs

13:00 Attend a meeting on a new strategy and delivery plan

14:00 Weekly afternoon clinic or surgery

18:00 Phone calls to colleagues on the way home

19:00 Home to help the kids with homework and collapse on the sofa

Myth	Mediocre docs trying to escape medicine to 'go to the dark side'.
Reality	Committed colleagues trying to improve the lives of patients, the public, and staff.
Personality	Confidence, conviction, ability to listen, ability to weigh up evidence and opinion, organized, excellent time management.
Best aspects	The opportunity to make a real difference and inspire others.
Worst aspects	Those with opinions unsubstantiated by facts; dull and seemingly endless meetings.
Route	No fixed route. Occurs alongside medical training/work; initial involvement in local leadership roles, gradually working up to local, regional, and national ones.
Numbers	Several thousands at some level.
Locations	All hospitals and Trusts (acute, mental health, and primary care); meeting-based, with frequent travel.

Life					Work
Quiet On-call					Busy On-call
Boredom					Burnout
Uncompetitive					Competitive
Low salary					High salary

Medical microbiology

Medical microbiology deals with the diagnosis, management, and prevention of infectious diseases, linking the delivery of laboratory services with clinical assessment and care. Medical microbiologists work closely with laboratory scientists and may share overlapping clinical roles with infectious diseases (ID) physicians. They provide a diagnostic and clinical service to all hospital specialties and have close links with pharmacy, infection control, primary care, and public health. Alongside diverse clinical and laboratory-based practice, this specialty offers a multitude of interesting opportunities for travel, teaching, and research.

The patients

Microbiology consultations cover a huge range of patients, from obstetrics and paediatrics to elderly care. They may also be in a variety of settings, including medical or surgical wards, intensive care, or the community, in the UK or abroad. Inpatient consultations are based on results from the microbiology laboratory, arise as a result of ward rounds or MDT meetings, and can be generated by calls for advice from other specialties. Investigation and care of immunocompromised patients are an increasingly important part of the workload. There may be opportunities to contribute to specialist clinics, e.g. HIV, TB, viral hepatitis, or patients receiving outpatient intravenous antibiotic therapy.

The work

This varies between settings, ranging from management and delivery of a predominantly laboratory-based service to clinical practice involving direct patient contact. Teams usually comprise consultants and specialist registrars; sometimes with more junior trainees. Medical microbiologists are represented on hospital infection control teams, in the delivery of antimicrobial guidelines and stewardship, in daily contribution to critical care environments, and in clinical care across hospital specialties. Developing patient-based and public health strategies for the management of emerging pathogens and multidrug-resistant organisms is a current and increasing challenge.

The job

Microbiologists feel equally at home in the laboratory as when providing a peripatetic clinical service. Training can be combined with clinical ID and there may be time to pursue research interests. There are opportunities to subspecialize in sepsis management to musculoskeletal infection, clinical virology, molecular diagnostics or infection prevention or control. There is a spectrum of On-call duties range from answering occasional phone calls to full 'hospital-at-night' general medicine; the reality is usually somewhere in between.

Extras

Research opportunities, both at home and abroad, range from molecular diagnostics, immunology, and genetics to clinical trials, field epidemiology, and public health. Tackling the global problem of increasing antimicrobial resistance is currently a headline concern, and the COVID-19 pandemic highlights the crucial role of infection specialists in a public health crisis. Microbiology is unlikely to be a route to your first million; this is not a specialty for anyone with a strong interest in private practice.

For further information

The Royal College of Pathologists (RCPath). Tel: 020 7451 6700. Web: https://www.rcpath.org Email: info@rcpath.org Twitter: @RCPath

Healthcare Infection Society (HIS). Tel: 020 7713 0273. Web: https://www.his.org.uk Email: admin@his.org.uk Twitter: @HIS_infection

---

A day in the life ...

08:30   Review lab results generated overnight; discuss new cases with on-call team

09:00   Meet with pharmacy and infection control teams to discuss patients needing anti-microbial review

10:00   Visit wards to review patients—cases are often flagged up by new lab results

11:00   Attend MDT meeting with another team (e.g. transplant, haematology, neurosurgery)

13:00   Grab a sandwich, signing clinic letters, or catching up with emails

14:00   Intensive care ward round and review other general ward inpatients

16:00   Run a teaching seminar for medical students

17:00   Call clinical teams with important culture results.

18:00   Home time, possibly dealing with further phone queries during the evening

21:00   Try to fit in an hour or two of academic work at home

01:00   Answer a phone call from the emergency department about a septic patient. Liaise with the lab to ensure appropriate handling of relevant samples

Myth	Goggle-wearing geek in a dirty white coat; likes to hide in a secluded lab and sniff agar plates.
Reality	Sociable, interdisciplinary expert caring for complex patients; roles in travel medicine and global health; research; management of high-consequence pathogens, epidemics, and pandemics.
Personality	Collaborative teamworker, with an interest in molecular and diagnostic medicine; clinical and holistic skills underpin high-quality clinical care.
Best aspects	Key player in MDT: diverse patient mix: wide opportunities for audit, research, teaching, travel, and varied leadership roles.
Worst aspects	Being the bearer of bad news: advising the removal of a long line or the need for (another) operation.
Route	Internal medicine training (IMT) (p. 44) or acute care common stem–acute medicine (ACCS-AM) (p. 37), followed by combined infection training (CIT) (p. 52), then medical microbiology training (ST5+). Can be combined with general internal medicine (p. 44), infectious diseases (p. 52), or virology (p. 52). Exams: MRCP; FRCPath.
Numbers	Approximately 450 consultants in England.
Locations	The laboratory, the wards or the wider world!

Life						Work

Quiet On-call						Busy On-call

Boredom						Burnout

Uncompetitive						Competitive

Low salary						High salary

Medical oncology

Medical oncologists lead treatment of patients with cancer using systemic anticancer therapy (SACT) such as chemotherapy. The specialty originated in academic centres where medical oncologists led research into cancer biology and the development of new drugs to treat cancer. It is a fascinating and rewarding specialty combining cutting-edge science with holistic patient care, supported by enormous advances in treatment made in recent years.

The patients

By definition all patients will have cancer, and in many cases, this will be a potentially terminal illness. Patients may be having SACT to increase the chance of cure or else ease symptoms and prolong life. They will likely be going through some of the most challenging times in their lives. Although most are in the older age group, patients may present at any age from late teens. Paediatric oncology is a separate paediatric subspecialty. The majority of patients will have been diagnosed by other clinicians although diagnostic skills are still required to identify complications of the cancer or its treatment.

The work

Medical oncologists need to have an interest in the science and research underpinning the specialty and are often involved in research and clinical trials. The field is fast-moving, and treatments can involve chemotherapy, therapies targeting specific genetic mutations, and, more recently, immunotherapy. As well as an academic aptitude, oncologists need an interest in people and empathy, so they can support patients through potentially complex decisions and sometimes arduous treatments. Supportive and palliative care is also an essential part of the role, as the aim is not just to prolong life, but to assist patients and their families to make decisions appropriate to them, maintain quality of life, and receive excellent planned end-of-life care. Oncologists are also involved in leadership of the cancer care pathways to constantly improve standards of care.

The job

Most patients are seen as outpatients; the majority of patients on treatment for cancer are outside hospital, continuing with their lives. There are some inpatients who may be admitted with complications of cancer or its treatment. Some oncologists may supervise laboratory research or clinical trials, whilst others have roles in providing acute oncology services to optimize the management of cancer patients in general hospitals. Oncologists subspecialize in specific cancer types and will work with MDTs and specialist nurses to manage patients. With ever-increasing knowledge, it is challenging to stay up-to-date across the field. Oncologists can build ongoing relationships with patients, which can increase job satisfaction but prove emotionally challenging when patients deteriorate. This ongoing responsibility can lead to a significant workload outside planned sessions, such as clinics and ward rounds, with a constant flow of queries from patients, their families, plus clinical colleagues.

Extras

Oncologists are usually involved in teaching trainees. To stay up-to-date, present data, and network with colleagues, most attend conferences, some international, which also provide motivation and peer support. There is some private practice, which varies according to subspecialty and location of work.

For further information

Association of Cancer Physicians (ACP). Web: https://www.theacp.org.uk Twitter: @ACPUK

A day in the life ...

08:00 Catch up on emails, letters, and other work such as prescribing

09:00 Subspecialty multidisciplinary team meeting with other clinicians and nurses to discuss patient management. May discuss 15–60 patients

10:30 Ward round with junior doctor and nurse to see inpatients and their families

12:00 Telephone calls to patients or GPs to answer queries or provide information

12:30 Meet clinical trials team to review new trials and complete paperwork for existing trials

13:00 Appraisal session with registrar

13:30 Lunch at desk

14:00 Cancer clinic—see new and follow-up patients, dictate letters, prescribe treatment

17:30 Check for urgent emails and then head home

20:00 Prepare slides for talk at regional meeting on new cancer treatments

Myth	Boffins who don't know when to stop giving dying patients chemotherapy.
Reality	Caring and empathetic doctors, with an interest in the science of medicine, who strive to improve cancer care and provide patients with longer, good-quality lives.
Personality	Diligent, caring, fairly academic, team players who are interested in people.
Best aspects	Opportunity to help patients with serious illnesses at a critical time in their lives. Underpinning of fascinating science and rapid advances. Strong teamworking ethos, with connections locally and nationally.
Worst aspects	Ever-increasing workload with more patients and more treatments. Ongoing patient responsibility that does not fit with a sessional job plan. Repeated emotionally charged consultations and breaking bad news.
Route	Internal medicine training (IMT) (p. 44) or acute care common stem–acute medicine (ACCS-AM) (p. 37), followed by specialty training in medical oncology (ST3+). Exams: MRCP; SCE in Medical Oncology.
Numbers	575 consultants, of whom 48% are women.
Locations	Teaching and local hospitals, usually in specialist departments. Many have sessions in academic research or trials units, or with universities.

Life						Work
Quiet On-call						Busy On-call
Boredom						Burnout
Uncompetitive						Competitive
Low salary						High salary

Medical politics

Politics is all about changing things, not Westminster's party-political back and forth. What is deemed 'quality improvement' in the clinical setting is called medical politics in professional life. It can be local, regional, national or international, by medical students, juniors or seniors. Democratic structures allow people's views to be heard. The British Medical Association (BMA) is the most obvious route for national medical politics, but other routes exist (Royal Colleges, GMC, specialist societies etc).

The patients

While medical politics can effect change to benefit patients, it also helps your colleagues. Though they can be hard to please, helping colleagues is what gets most people involved for the first time in medical politics. Most medics think of medical politics as something done by someone else, but it isn't just what is done in BMA House or government buildings – it happens at every level.

The work

Locally, your colleagues need a voice on various committees and boards that make decisions affecting their studies, work, and medical lives. Nationally, government policy needs input from ordinary doctors and students, as does the work of many non-governmental organizations affecting medical care, including Royal Colleges, the GMC, and others.

The job

Medical politics involves meetings (some fun), reading (some interesting) and many conversations. More change happens through informal, individual chats than (rare!) formal negotiations. Committees bring with them endless emails (8000 in one year for one committee for this author!). Chairing a committee needs a command of the brief, finessing of interpersonal relations with committee members and external stakeholders, and providing the committee's public face, including on social media.

Extras

Bringing about positive change (or averting negative change) can be hugely rewarding. Team work on intense, difficult issues can forge long-lasting friendships. Work on national issues can involve media appearances, for which training is provided. International travel opportunities abound, though teleconferencing is increasingly common. Opportunities such as the National Medical Director's Fellowship can broaden management experience.

For further information

British Medical Association (BMA). Tel: 0300 123 1233. Web: https://www.bma.org.uk Twitter: @TheBMA

Faculty of Medical Leadership and Management (FMLM). Tel: 020 8051 2060. Web: https://www.fmlm.ac.uk Email: enquiries@fmlm.ac.uk Twitter: @FMLM_UK

A day in the life ...

BMA National Committee Chair

06:00	Train to London for the day's meetings (emails and meeting papers en route)
08:30	Early meeting with Postgraduate Dean to discuss shared agenda for next week's GMC meeting
10:00	Chairing national committee meeting
13:00	Lunchtime meeting with specialist association and patient representatives
14:00	Off to Whitehall to hear about medical workforce planning
16:30	Opportunistic discussion with senior civil servant to try to prevent an awkward issue escalating
18:30	Dinner with deputy chairs to plan actions from today's meetings
22:00	Emails on the late train back, before 'early' bedtime—back on the wards tomorrow!

Myth	Self-interested CV-padders hoping for knighthoods in due course; weird policy drones who have forgotten what a hospital looks like inside.
Reality	Working doctors and full-time students cramming in meetings on their days off, working hard for the benefit of their colleagues and patients.
Personality	Wide variety. Some people are detail-focused; others are personably brilliant at persuading people to do the right thing. A few are wholly driven by a single issue they pursue to the end.
Best aspects	The opportunity to effect change at a national level, which can deeply and positively affect the lives of many.
Worst aspects	So. Many. Emails. Numerous papers to read for meetings. Clinical colleagues can offer opinions without offering to help.
Route	Involvement often starts as student or junior doctor, from local to national levels. Almost always alongside study/clinical work; Rare positions are full-time.
Numbers	Thousands of doctors and students at all levels, but fewer than 100 people as their main role.
Locations	National meetings happen in London, or else in the devolved capitals. Bigger roles require travel, though teleconferencing is on the increase.

Life					Work
Quiet On-call					Busy On-call
Boredom					Burnout
Uncompetitive					Competitive
Low salary					High salary

Médecins Sans Frontières

Médecins Sans Frontières/Doctors Without Borders (MSF) is an international humanitarian organization delivering emergency medical aid. Funded by donations, MSF can operate independently and observe neutrality and impartiality. MSF's greatest asset is its workforce: dedicated volunteers who undertake potential personal risk to deliver the best possible care, in an ethical fashion, while observing the MSF founding principles. The organization is exemplary in its response to crises often overlooked by the international community, including MSF's persistent presence during the 1994 Rwandan genocide, and their early response to the 2014 West African Ebola outbreak. A hard-earned MSF T-shirt is a true badge of honour.

The patients

Patients are those of all ages affected by armed conflict, epidemics, and natural and man-made disasters, and those who are excluded from healthcare. They are people in the very greatest of need from populations in distress, who have been abandoned and are economically disadvantaged. A patient may be a victim of sexual violence in Democratic Republic of Congo, a child refugee with a complex medical condition in Bangladesh, a woman requiring assistance during labour in Afghanistan, a migrant in Libya with a war wound, or a displaced person with COVID-19 in Yemen. Care is delivered irrespective of gender, race, religion, creed, or political convictions. MSF's message to its patients is simple: you are not forgotten.

The work

Despite sometimes needing to make near-impossible compromises, the work couldn't be more rewarding. Initiative and resourcefulness are essential. There is great camaraderie with a truly international workforce, and total immersion in a culture is possible. Medicine is often the least challenging aspect: volunteers receive training, may have relatively few therapeutic options and may see a very high case volume. Beyond patient care, doctors may find themselves setting up new care programmes, solving an epidemiological mystery, or negotiating MSF's presence with local authority figures.

The job

A medic might take a full year out of training, while a surgical consultant might do annual, 6-week deployments. A minority opt for `career MSF'. `Missions' depend on what the crisis demands, from a well-supplied hospital through to a basic rural clinic. Working hours vary widely. Placement intensity will dictate duration: acute/high-stress missions mandate shorter postings or more frequent R&R breaks.

Extras

MSF doctors are frequently expected to train national MSF and Ministry of Health (MoH) staff. Research opportunities abound, and can be presented at the annual MSF scientific day.

For further information

MSF UK. Tel: 020 7404 6600. Web: https://msf.org.uk Email: office-ldn@london.msf.org
Twitter: @MSF_uk

A day in the life ...

Multidrug-resistant tuberculosis (MDR-TB) programme, Uzbekistan

07:30 Drive with translator/assistant to designated district, via the laboratory to collect latest sputum results

09:00 With MoH counterpart, see emergency TB cases

10:00 Review MDR-TB cases at a 'DOT corner'

12:00 Visit non-ambulatory MDR-TB patients in their own homes

14:00 Discuss new hospital x-ray machine with MoH Chief Medical Officer

15:00 Visit new confirmed cases of TB and consent them to commencing treatment

17:30 Travel to MSF office in the capital to update medical team leader and project co-ordinator and liaise with infection control nurse, epidemiologist, and logisticians

19:00 Play volleyball with other staff before supper in front of a box set

Myth	Arrogant adrenaline junkies who think they are here to save the world.
Reality	Deplorers of injustice with an itch not quite scratched by their medical elective.
Personality	Earnest, resilient, and dynamic; adaptable and able to leap outside their comfort zone. An understanding family is helpful.
Best aspects	Nothing is comparable with sensing that you have saved the life of a grateful patient who had otherwise thought they had been completely abandoned and forgotten.
Worst aspects	Psychological impact; not being unable to 'unsee' the worst atrocities; the guilt felt on leaving patients and peers when the mission is over; reverse culture shock on returning home.
Route	Depends on specialty, e.g. ST2+ for medical doctors, ST3+ for paediatricians: Diploma in Tropical Medicine/Infectious Diseases required for both; ST5+ for O&G; 'proven experience' for anaesthetists; post-CCT/FRCS for surgeons. Minimum 3 months' travel/work experience in developing countries. French or Arabic desirable.
Numbers	More than 2500 international staff join 30 000 locally hired staff annually.
Locations	Ranging from safe, but impoverished countries to war zones.

Life					Work
Quiet On-call					Busy On-call
Boredom					Burnout
Uncompetitive					Competitive
Low salary					High salary

Medico-legal adviser

Medico-legal advisers are employed by one of three medical defence organizations (MDOs). They are medically qualified and also usually hold at least membership of a Royal College. Some advisers are also dual-qualified as lawyers. Advisers give advice and assistance on medico-legal matters to members of the defence organization for which they work. Most doctors choose to be a member of one of the MDOs and a variety of other healthcare professionals may also be members. Consultants who practise privately are required to have their own indemnity as they are not covered by NHS indemnity. Dental members are advised and assisted separately by specialist dentally qualified advisers. This specialty has received increased recognition over the past few years, with the formation of the Faculty of Forensic and Legal Medicine (FFLM) within the Royal College of Physicians (RCP).

The patients

There is no direct patient contact and no responsibility for patient care as such. Medico-legal advisers advise members of the relevant MDO directly. They do not give clinical advice but need to have a good understanding of the clinical framework in which a problem has arisen. Part of the role of an adviser is to support a doctor through what can be very stressful events, and so excellent communication skills are required. Some cases can go on for a considerable amount of time and so an adviser can form close relationships with members they advise and assist.

The work

Medico-legal advisers provide advice and assistance on ethical matters, complaints, coroner's inquests, fatal accident inquiries, GMC cases, and disciplinary investigations. They advise on cases from all four major jurisdictions in the UK, as well as others such as Isle of Man and Channel Islands, even worldwide, depending on the organization. The work itself is varied, as every case is different. An adviser will deal with doctors from all specialties and is not confined only to cases of their own original medical specialty. Advice can be given on the telephone, including on the 24-hour advice line and in writing for ongoing case work. Advisers may accompany members to meetings or hearings. There are also opportunities to lecture, teach, and contribute to publications by the MDO.

The job

Medico-legal advisers are either office-based or home-based. Some initial training is required, and most advisers have a previous medico-legal qualification such as an LLM (Master of Law) or MA in Medical Ethics and Law. Advisers can work towards Membership of the FFLM (MFFLM) of the RCP. The job itself is varied, challenging, interesting, and rewarding. Most advisers will have on-call commitment to a 24-hour telephone advice line. The role is demanding and requires good written and verbal communication skills. Advisers need to be able to prioritize tasks and be organized, as they have an ongoing and varied case load.

Extras

Some advisers may agree with their employing MDO to retain a small clinical commitment, although most no longer practise clinically. However, all advisers remain fully registered with the GMC, and the MDO is usually the adviser's designated body. There is no opportunity for private practice as such, although there may be scope, with the employing MDO's agreement, for part-time work as part of a portfolio career.

For further information

The Faculty of Forensic and Legal Medicine (of the Royal College of Physicians), London.
Web: https://fflm.ac.uk Email: forensic.medicine@fflm.ac.uk Twitter: @FFLMUK

08:00	Providing telephone advice on the 24-hour advice line
09:00	Reading emails and incoming messages or documents for ongoing cases
09:30	Multidisciplinary team (MDT) meeting, to discuss general administrative matters and any ongoing difficult cases
11:00	Preparing a lecture to be given to trainee GPs
12:00	Telephone discussion with a doctor regarding an ongoing disciplinary investigation
13:00	Lunch break, including travel to next meeting
14:00	Meeting with a doctor, solicitor, and a barrister regarding a forthcoming GMC hearing
16:00	Travel back to the office
16:00	Reading emails or incoming documents, further provision of written advice, including on new matters
18:00	On-call overnight, providing urgent telephone advice only

Myth	An easy job far removed from clinical practice.
Reality	A varied and demanding role, requiring a thorough understanding of both clinical and legal medicine, and ongoing revalidation with the GMC.
Personality	Excellent communication skills; team players. Advisers should be able to multitask and prioritize, and have good writing and public-speaking skills.
Best aspects	Intellectually stimulating and challenging, a varied case load, and opportunities to do other tasks such as articles and press summaries.
Worst aspects	Workload can be unpredictable as cases can evolve or become more demanding over time.
Route	Medical training in a specialty to membership level, postgraduate legal or medico-legal qualification, on-job training; MFFLM exams.
Numbers	Approximately 100 UK-wide throughout the three MDOs.
Locations	Either office-based or home-based throughout the UK, depending on the MDO. Some travel required for case work and/or lecturing.

Life					Work
Quiet On-call					Busy On-call
Boredom					Burnout
Uncompetitive					Competitive
Low salary					High salary

Metabolic medicine

Metabolic medicine is a subspecialty of chemical pathology (p. 136) or general internal medicine, that typically recruits trainees following completion of stage 1 internal medicine training (IMT) (p. 44). Metabolic medicine specialists diagnose and manage patients with deranged biochemistry including those with conditions that are genetic (e.g. with inborn errors of metabolism), acquired (diabetes) or iatrogenic (parenteral nutrition). Most UK trainees train jointly in chemical pathology and metabolic medicine so, as a specialist, time is split between reviewing patients in clinics or wards and providing clinical support to the laboratory.

The patients

Metabolic medicine is primarily an adult specialty that includes the transition from adolescent to adult clinics. Patients are referred by GPs and other hospital specialists and will reflect the specialist nature of metabolic medicine. In addition, there are requests for advice about patients in the care of other specialists or in the community.

The work

There are five main areas of metabolic medicine and typically a specialist will only use one or two of these skills in depth. These include nutrition (e.g. obesity and bariatric surgery patients), diabetes, cardiovascular assessment and treatment (primarily lipid management but also hypertension), metabolic bone disease and inherited metabolic diseases. The work is diverse and flexible. Large hospitals may require subspecialization whilst a smaller hospital may require a generalist. Clinical overlap with the chemical pathology laboratory service is common with involvement in the organisation of the diagnostic laboratory service. Rarely, consultants may have responsibilities to the general medical on-call rota.

The job

Depending on the hospital, there is usually an equal split between outpatient clinics and laboratory-based work; there may be ward rounds (e.g. parenteral nutrition in intensive care). Laboratory duties vary but can include advice on test requests and interpretation, and oversight of general laboratory work, rather than providing results or performing bench work. On-call periods may be frequent, but calls vary, dependent on the specialist service offered and most out-of-hours work will be from home.

Extras

It is easy to become involved with any and every department in the hospital as well as the community and you have freedom to choose projects that suit your abilities. Work can be arranged to maintain areas of interest including teaching, research and management activities. Training is flexible and out-of-program experience is easily achieved. Academic work is supported, and the work life balance can be adjusted to suit most requirements. There is some private practice, with involvement in local private laboratories or specialist outpatient review.

For further information

The Royal College of Pathologists (RCPath). Tel: 020 7451 6700. Web: https://www.rcpath.org Email: info@rcpath.org Twitter: @RCPath

A day in the life ...

08:00 Review of abnormal specimen results on the laboratory IT system

09:00 Outpatient lipid clinic: five new patients and 15 familiar faces, with a range of conditions

13:00 Review of equipment tenders with laboratory managers over lunch

14:00 External quality assurance review of tests, checking comparability and reviewing problems with analyte measurement

15:00 Clinic notes, dictating letters, and literature research where required

16:00 Medical student teaching

17:30 Review laboratory work schedule for evening, depart for home

Myth	Test tubes, pipettes, large glasses, and bow ties.
Reality	Busy specialty with emphasis on patient contact, but time to pursue interesting cases and own research interests.
Personality	Good communication skills, enjoys teamwork, sense of humour, academic, systematic, numerate.
Best aspects	Good variety, ability to reassure patients, good overview of all hospital practice.
Worst aspects	Blood sciences laboratories are highly automated, and an appreciation of technical aspects are important to make the case for instrument improvement and staff retention.
Route	Chemical pathology (ST1+) (p. 52), IMT (p. 44), or acute care common stem–acute medicine (ACCS-AM) (p. 37), followed by specialty training in metabolic medicine (ST3+). Exams: MRCP; FRCPath.
Numbers	30 consultants, of whom 14% are women.
Locations	Mostly teaching hospitals and larger district general hospitals.

Life						Work
Quiet On-call						Busy On-call
Boredom						Burnout
Uncompetitive						Competitive
Low salary						High salary

National healthcare policy and leadership

Moving from clinical practice to work in the Department of Health (DH), NHS England (NHSE), NHS Improvement (NHSI), Care Quality Commission (CQC), or any other national government-funded healthcare organization is often perceived as having crossed an important divide, or even going over 'to the dark side'. In reality, delivering healthcare for whole populations needs policy development and strategic planning informed by medical professionals with real clinical experience. There is no formal career structure or typical route of entry, meaning it is open to any hospital, community, or public health doctor, but typically those with significant managerial experience at clinical, divisional, or medical director level. Managerial roles are enormously rewarding and allow doctors to use a wide range of both broad and specialist, clinical and non-clinical skills to represent their specialty—they can influence healthcare in a wider setting than that of an individual's clinical practice.

The patients

Most managerial roles cannot be fulfilled without negotiating time formally set aside from clinical work. The vast majority of doctors, however, continue to practise to some degree to maintain their skills and interest. It is also true that clinical practice can provide a 'safety net', should the national role not be as expected or the clinician not deliver as anticipated.

The work

This involves being on committees and contributing to publications and presentations. Building teams and involving key stakeholders from the delivery end of healthcare services are vital components. Leadership skills and an ability to manage complicated political situations are essential. The work requires effective communication with medical colleagues, government and departmental officials, politicians, the press, and the public. Doctors need to be an ambassador for their employing or seconding organizations. At times, this requires delicate diplomatic skills to represent the organization without jeopardizing clinical reputation and judgement.

The job

Jobs vary in their time commitment, with some being permanent and others being secondments from NHS work. Secondment contracts protect NHS terms and conditions, and under employment law, the 'host' Trust for such doctors has to provide a full-time contract for secondees when a secondment ends. This specialty of medicine was previously the preserve of senior medical professionals, but there are now schemes for junior doctors, such as the National Medical Director's Clinical Fellow scheme, which annually recruits around 25 junior doctors to work within a national healthcare organization, such as National Institute for Health and Care Excellence (NICE), NHSI, or NHSE, for 1 year. Formal local and regional management and leadership schemes for junior doctors also exist.

Extras

National healthcare management and leadership roles provide plentiful opportunities for travelling around the UK and further afield. The job involves working with a wide variety of other professionals, which can be both challenging and very interesting. This kind of lifestyle can limit private practice and also tilt the work–life balance firmly in favour of work.

For further information

Faculty of Medical Leadership and Management (FMLM). Tel: 020 8051 2060. Web: https://fmlm.ac.uk Email: enquiries@fmlm.ac.uk Twitter: @FMLM_UK

06:00   Travel to London, processing emails en route
09:00   Meeting to discuss clinical strategy at NHSE
10:00   Chairing a national committee for medical managers
13:00   Meeting with other clinical leads
14:00   Strategy planning meeting with team
16:00   Travel home
20:00   Emails, reading and editing documents

Myth	Doctors who are no good at medicine playing at being politicians and medical managers.
Reality	Doctors wishing to extend their interest, and impact, in medicine beyond their own field by using managerial and communication skills.
Personality	Communication and public-speaking skills are essential; pragmatic, good time management, thick-skinned.
Best aspects	Variety of working environments and colleagues; ability to influence strategic planning of healthcare and national policy.
Worst aspects	Usually working in an advisory role which can be ignored; job can fill every waking (and sleeping) hour.
Route	Training in any clinical specialty, with managerial experience before or after CCT.
Locations	Work often involves travelling; for example, NHSE is based in London and Leeds, NHS Scotland in Edinburgh, etc.

Life					Work
Quiet On-call					Busy On-call
Boredom					Burnout
Uncompetitive					Competitive
Low salary					High salary

Neonatal medicine

Neonatal medicine deals with babies born too early or too sick to be cared for on postnatal wards or at home. It is now the largest paediatric subspecialty (p. 49) but was only born in the 1960s. The range of problems is wide. It requires excellent hand–eye co-ordination, compassion, stamina, and attention to detail. Neonatal networks comprise 'neonatal intensive care' (NICUs), 'local neonatal', or 'special care' units. In 2009, the Department of Health published standards mandating access to 24-hour transport services to ensure babies can be 'uplifted' and 'repatriated' as required. The British Association of Perinatal Medicine (BAPM) publishes regular guidance on optimal service configuration.

The patients

Like policemen, premature infants seem ever younger and smaller. Babies of 23–24 weeks' gestation weighing below 600 g are not unusual and typically require prolonged intensive care. Outcomes have improved dramatically, but some will have long-term problems and some don't make it home. In neighbouring cots, there could be a 5kg infant of a diabetic with hypoglycaemia, a term baby with hypoxic–ischaemic encephalopathy receiving therapeutic hypothermia, and a baby with a complex dysmorphic syndrome, Unfortunately, there remains an over-representation of babies from families with major social problems.

The work

Whatever GPs and geriatricians say, neonatologists are actually the last truly general medics. They do endless ward rounds to fine-tune ventilators, inotropes, fluids, and electrolytes. They attend deliveries to resuscitate babies and counsel families during inpatient stays, and after discharge or death. Some are expert ultrasonographers; all can cannulate invisible veins and impalpable arteries. Most follow up babies post discharge up to age 2 - 3 years. They work closely with obstetricians, midwives, surgeons, and cardiologists, and may seek advice from geneticists, nephrologists, endocrinologists, and even orthopaedic surgeons! They depend on excellent neonatal nurses, specialist pharmacists, radiographers and radiologists, speech and language therapists, dieticians, and physiotherapists. Input into child protection conferences is sometimes required. There are also lots of twins and, in the IVF-age, some higher multiples, which can be exciting but stressful.

The job

NICUs are invariably in teaching/large hospitals. Opportunities for travel sometimes arise, typically to retrieve a sick infant from a neighbouring hospital at 3 a.m.! As trainees, all paediatricians do a year or more of neonatology and maintain these skills, knowing they will often be the ones left 'holding the baby' until the transport team arrives.

Extras

There are opportunities for clinical and laboratory research, and for presentation overseas. Many trainees are 'flexible'. There is essentially no private neonatal practice in the UK.

For further information

British Association of Perinatal Medicine (BAPM). Tel: 020 7092 6085. Web: https://www.bapm.org/ Email: bapm@rcpch.ac.uk Twitter: @BAPM_Official

The Neonatal Society. Web: https://www.neonatalsociety.ac.uk Twitter: @NeonatalSociety

---

08:31   Handover from night consultant, neonatal Grid ST7, and nurse practitioner

09:13   Meet neonatal pharmacist; prescribe IV nutrition for babies not yet on milk

09:42   Ward round of intensive care patients with day ST5 paediatric trainee and F2 doctor

12:27   Combined coffee and lunch break

12:46   Meet with parents of ventilated 24-week gestation baby to update them on progress

13:11   Discussion with ward sister and obstetrician about the 26-week twins who need to be delivered because their mother is dangerously hypertensive

13:26   Supervise the ST4 doing cranial ultrasounds on two babies and do a cardiac echo on one to see if the arterial duct needs referral for surgical ligation

15:49   Cup of tea and piece of cake with the juniors and nurses before handover to night consultant

16:35   Go to office, check emails, sign clinic letters, and arrange a supervision meeting with the ST1 about to rotate to paediatric oncology

17:45   Go home. Not on-call tonight, so sleep like a baby (i.e. wake every 3 hours)

Myth	Miracle worker.
Reality	It's hard work—physically, intellectually, and emotionally—but very rewarding.
Personality	Slightly obsessive/compulsive, lots of stamina, good at relating to and working (sometimes very closely) with all types of people.
Best aspects	Waving off home a baby plus elated, nervous parents whom you've supported for several weeks. Supportive multidisciplinary environment despite very challenging and demanding work.
Worst aspects	Seeing a normally formed term baby dying from overwhelming infection. Heavy and unpredictable out-of-hours on-call commitments.
Route	Specialty training in paediatrics (ST1+) (p. 49), then neonatal Grid Training (ST6+). Exams: MRCPCH.
Numbers	470 consultants; further 190 general paediatricians with a special interest in neonatal medicine.
Locations	In 42 hospitals, all with large maternity/fetal medicine departments.

Life					Work
Quiet On-call					Busy On-call
Boredom					Burnout
Uncompetitive					Competitive
Low salary					High salary

Neurology

Neurology involves disorders of the brain and nervous system. Having been established as an independent discipline during the time of Charcot in the mid-1800s, it is a fairly old specialty. However, with newer treatments for chronic diseases e.g. multiple sclerosis (MS), epilepsy, and Parkinson's, neurology has disproven its reputation of being an intellectual pursuit without treatments. And with one of the biggest research budgets globally, this trend towards more sophisticated and effective treatments in neurology will continue. In addition, neurologists are increasingly involved in acute stroke and areas that were previously ignored e.g. head injury and dementias. This has brought different working patterns, new models of care, and stronger links with other specialties such as psychiatry (p. 55; pp. 268–278) and stroke medicine (p. 300).

The patients

Adults with any disorder of the central and peripheral nervous system. The most common problems referred to neurology are headache, dizziness, weakness, and paraesthesia. Many patients have conditions needing long-term treatment. There are more rare disorders in neurology than in any other specialty; but, increasingly, new treatments are becoming available. The variety and challenge keep neurologists interested and up-to-date as constant learning is a necessity.

The work

Around 20% of acute medical patients have a neurological condition, so referrals from acute medical and surgical specialties form the bulk of the work. Only the most complex patients are admitted to a neurology inpatient bed; most remain under medical teams, with neurologists advising on investigations and plans. Most patients, particularly those with long-term conditions, are managed in outpatient clinics. On-call work is dominated by stroke, with more and more neurologists being involved in thrombolysis and thrombectomy. The specialty workload is an interesting mix of thorough history and examination, with lots of time spent thinking, and fast-paced assessment and decision-making.

The job

Neurology is mostly based in secondary care, with most areas operating a 'hub-and-spoke model'—most neurologists are mainly based in a large neuroscience centre with stroke and neurology inpatient units, which provides remote support to surrounding district general hospitals (DGHs). Consultants also spend a few days a week visiting DGHs for outpatient clinics and reviewing referrals; this can involve some travelling, but getting to know different colleagues and hospitals adds variety and interest.

Extras

Most neurologists develop a subspecialty interest; these can include the fields outlined earlier, as well as others e.g. movement disorders, peripheral nerve disorders, muscle disorders, functional neurological disorders, and neuro-ophthalmology. Being a traditionally academic specialty, many neurologists complete a research degree (MD or PhD) before or during registrar training. Many consultants are involved in research and teaching alongside their clinical work, and some may spend most of their week in an academic research post, working at a university.

For further information

The Association of British Neurologists. Tel: 020 7405 4060. Web: https://www.theabn. org Email: info@abn.org.uk Twitter: @theABN_Info

---

08:30	Board round on the inpatient ward with nurses, junior doctors, and therapists
09:00	Ward round of the 20 inpatients and the two neuro-intensive therapy unit (ITU) patients; scans and electrophysiology reviewed, and treatment plans put in place
11:00	Reviewing referrals across the hospital—good walking shoes required
12:00	Journal club or grand round, followed by lunch and catching up with colleagues
13:20	General neurology clinic: migraine, neuropathy, optic neuritis, functional neurological disorder; a good mix of new and follow-up patients
16:50	Final catch-up with the ward
17:30	Heading home—need to search the literature for a challenging case on the ward and new journal issues waiting to be read!

Myth	Spend lots of time making a clever diagnosis for which we can do nothing.
Reality	Managing a wide range of conditions with complex therapeutics; good mixture of fast-paced acute neurology and stroke work, with slower-paced outpatient clinics.
Personality	Thorough, inquisitive, methodical, team player, good communicator.
Best aspects	Never being bored; from the acutely unwell stroke patient to complex MS therapeutics, managing epilepsy, and communicating a new diagnosis of motor neurone disease, neurologists see and treat all!
Worst aspects	Few neurologists (less than 50% of average in other European countries) lead to long waiting lists and delays, as well as heavy workload.
Route	Either internal medicine training (IMT) (p. 44) or acute care common stem–acute medicine (ACCS-AM) (p. 37), then specialty training in neurology (ST3+). Exams: MRCP; SCE in Neurology.
Numbers	1000 consultants, of whom 30% are women.
Locations	Hub-and-spoke model, mostly in tertiary centres/teaching hospitals, with some time in DGHs.

Life					Work
Quiet On-call					Busy On-call
Boredom					Burnout
Uncompetitive					Competitive
Low salary					High salary

Neurosurgery

Neurosurgery has a reputation as an exciting 'high-octane' specialty staffed by classic 'type A' surgical personalities. This is only partly true. In fact, the surgical neurologist is a meticulous and considerate being who carefully weighs up the evidence and the wishes of the patient before deciding whether to proceed with surgery. The complications of any surgery can be life-changing, but in neurosurgery, the stakes are particularly high. A patient going blind from a tumour knows they must have surgery to preserve their remaining vision, but also that surgery carries the risk of blindness. It is an enormous privilege to be part of that decision.

The patients

Neurosurgeons manage a wide range of pathologies in patients of all ages, although most large centres have dedicated paediatric neurosurgeons. Consultants can be divided broadly into cranial and spinal neurosurgeons. Cranial surgeons cover pathology within the skull, e.g. aneurysms, brain tumours, and functional neurosurgery, e.g. epilepsy, movement disorders, and pain. Most neurosurgeons do some degenerative spine work, e.g. discectomies and laminectomies, whilst complex spine surgeons (p. 296) perform surgery which requires the insertion of metalwork. The risks of surgery are not insignificant. It is very rewarding to 'fix' patients, but devastating to damage them. And you will do both.

The work

The focus of the week is the operating list, which may range from tumour resection to implantation of deep brain stimulation. Outpatients is the 'shop front' where surgeons meet their patients and discuss the risks and rationale for surgery (or why it would be futile). It is important to have a deep understanding of the condition and its imaging, and to be able to explain this to the patient. Due to the complexity of elective cases, neurosurgeons often only have a handful of patients under their care when not on-call.

The job

Most operating is consultant-led. For trainees, the tight collaboration with senior colleagues may be intensely rewarding. Others may feel frustrated they are not 'running the show' by the end of training. Senior trainees can handle most decisions (often for patients in different hospitals) and out-of-hours emergency surgery. On-calls are busy during training, but consultants rarely have to operate overnight. The specialty relies heavily on the MDT, and close working with other specialists aids complex decision making.

Extras

As some highly complex operations are carried out infrequently, there are opportunities to develop surgical training programmes with cadaveric labs, virtual platforms, and simulation training. All trainees are encouraged to present research at national and international conferences. Neurosurgery is a small specialty, and this leads to strong ties (and rivalries) across the UK and internationally. There are opportunities for private practice, but the high-risk nature of the work makes indemnity premiums high and postoperative care often cannot be delegated.

For further information

The Society of British Neurological Surgeons (SBNS). Tel: 020 7869 6892. Web: https://www.sbns.org.uk Email: admin@sbns.org.uk Twitter: @The_SBNS

The British Neurosurgical Trainees' Association (BNTA). Web: http://e1v1m1.co.uk Twitter: @e1v1m1

07:50   Arrive at work, grab a coffee, go to handover

08:15   Team brief for theatre—two trans-sphenoidal resections of pituitary tumours or a vestibular schwannoma resection (all day case)

08:30   Quick ward round whilst the team get the patient ready

12:00   Grab lunch during skull base MDT

14:00   MDT clinic with clinical nurse specialists, oncologists, and neuro-, ENT, and max-facs surgeons

18:00   Home if the tumour is all out and the on-call is under control

02:00   Contacted by the on-call registrar to discuss an acute haemorrhage with hydro-cephalus in a young woman who needs urgent intervention

Myth	Brusque 'Type A' colleagues.
Reality	Delicate operations, thoughtful individuals.
Personality	Suited to a wide spectrum of personalities. Common traits include meticulous attention to detail and considered decision-making.
Best aspects	Intricate surgery, privilege to be involved in critical decision-making.
Worst aspects	Busy on-call. Difficult decision-making, including end-of-life cases. Surgery carries high risks, even if benign disease.
Route	Run-through training (p. 61) in neurosurgery (ST1+) or entry at ST3 with completed Neurosurgery Alternative Certificate of Core Competence. Post-CCT fellowship training usually required. Exams: MRCS; FRCS (Surgical Neurology).
Numbers	300 consultants in England across approximately 20 units.
Locations	Large regional units or centres in teaching hospitals. Training rotations in London include three or four units, but elsewhere training is usually in one or two hospitals.

Life					Work
Quiet On-call					Busy On-call
Boredom					Burnout
Uncompetitive					Competitive
Low salary					High salary

Nuclear medicine

Nuclear medicine (NM) is the use of radioactive drugs to diagnose and treat disease. It may sound unreal—radioactive nuclei are injected into, and decay inside, patients, release gamma rays, cause scintillations in crystals, are detected by tubes in arrays, and ultimately produce images of physiology—but it is all true. Not only is it true, it is also often essential to provide diagnostic information not available via any other modality and effective treatment for benign and malignant conditions.

The patients

Some of the most wide-ranging of any medical specialty—although you may not necessarily have direct contact with many of them! Patients' ages range from 0 to 100+ years and the conditions they have may be acute or chronic, benign or malignant, uni- or multisystem, and simple or complex. NM can have an important role to play in patients with a wide range of malignancies, cardiovascular diseases, complex orthopaedic conditions, dementias, urological conditions, thyroid and parathyroid disorders, and hepatobiliary disorders. Most patients only visit the NM department for diagnostic purposes, but some are also treated there.

The work

NM classically images organ function, requiring a good understanding of physiology, as well as physics and pathophysiology. With the increasing use of hybrid imaging, good anatomical knowledge is also required. The majority of clinical work in NM consists of reporting images—with many similarities to diagnostic radiology (p. 282): sitting in a dark room, staring at a computer screen, and trying not to overdose on coffee! However, patient contact is still maintainted—to a greater or lesser degree, depending on subspecialty interests—via treating patients with NM therapies (a growing field) or assisting with cardiac stress test lists. Other important roles include attending MDT meetings, helping the rest of the NM team, audit, research, and teaching.

The job

NM is quite a niche specialty—if it is your dream to work in a small district general hospital in a fairly rural area, then don't choose NM! Consultants working in bigger NM departments can have NM-only jobs, but in smaller hospitals, NM work is usually combined with radiology. There is very little NM-specific on-call (in general, it is 9–5 only), but in the future, NM consultants will be dual-trained in radiology and participate in radiology on-call. NM is also truly multidisciplinary, requiring close work with technologists, physicists, nursing staff, and the admin team.

Extras

NM is a fast-evolving specialty, with development in novel radiotracers, technological advances in cameras, and increasing focus on treating malignant conditions with the emergence of targeted treatments (referred to as theranostics) as a major field of investment and research. NM is very accommodating for flexible and part-time work due to its predominantly non-acute nature. As NM is quite a small specialty, there are good opportunities for research and involvement in national committees and societies. Overall a very scintillating career!

For further information

British Nuclear Medicine Society (BNMS). Tel: 0738 529 7906. Web: https://www.bnms. org.uk Twitter: @BNMSnews

European Association of Nuclear Medicine. Tel: +43 1 890 44 27. Web: https://www. eanm.org Email: office@eanm.org Twitter: @officialEANM

A day in the life ...

08:30 Attend MDT meeting: help contribute to patient management decisions

09:30 Reporting: usually a wide variety of systems and pathologies

11:30 Review a patient on the cardiac stress list about whom the team have concerns (it's nice to have a change from reporting and talk with a patient)

11:45 More reporting (fuelled by tea or coffee)

13:00 Lunch: either with colleagues, in a meeting, or whilst catching up on emails

13:45 Departmental meeting to discuss protocol changes, scan waiting times, updates on staff changes, etc.

14:45 Thyroid clinic: review patients referred for radioactive iodine treatment

16:00 Reporting: usually urgent cancer or inpatient scans in the afternoon

17:05 Go home: it's rarer to leave late in NM than in many other specialties!

Myth	'Unclear medicine' interpreting uninterpretable blobs on a screen.
Reality	Using increasingly accurate imaging modalities (particularly positron emission tomography computed tomography (PET-CT)) as the problem-solver or decision-maker for a patient's treatment.
Personality	A bit geeky—NM specialists have chosen to think about physics, physiology, and pathology, use language other doctors don't understand, and spend less time with patients.
Best aspects	Deals with multisystem pathology which is often more interesting than reporting the same system over and over again. Can provide information that will really change a patient's management. Lower stress than in many other specialties.
Worst aspects	Can feel relatively distanced from the rest of the hospital and other colleagues, and disconnected from patients and their clinical management.
Route	Core training in medicine (p. 44), then specialty training in NM (ST3+)—alternative routes from core surgical training (p. 61) or paediatric level 1 training (p. 49). Also possible to train as a radionuclide radiologist (slightly different to a specific NM-trained consultant) via radiology (p. 59). Exams: exams relevant to core specialty; FRCR and Diploma in Nuclear Medicine.
Numbers	90 consultants, of whom 35% are women.
Locations	Most acute hospitals have an NM department; major NM departments are concentrated in larger tertiary hospitals in large cities.

Life					Work
Quiet On-call					Busy On-call
Boredom					Burnout
Uncompetitive					Competitive
Low salary					High salary

Obstetric medicine

Obstetric medicine is a medical subspecialty that deals with the management of medical problems in pregnancy and the puerperium. Medical problems arising in pregnancy are becoming more common as more women are entering pregnancy with pre-existing medical conditions and previous pregnancy problems. Acute medical problems in pregnancy are also on the rise; thus, obstetric physicians are valued members of the multidisciplinary team (MDT), working alongside obstetricians, obstetric anaesthetists, midwives, and specialist physicians to deliver holistic care to women and their families in what can be an emotional and vulnerable time.

The patients

Some patients are referred prior to pregnancy for pre-pregnancy counselling (PPC) to ensure their medical problems and medication are optimized for pregnancy. Most women will be seen antenatally either in specialist clinics or as inpatients. Increasingly, women present to emergency medicine and ambulatory care, as opposed to directly to maternity, so obstetric physicians are key to reviewing women in these areas, as well as developing local protocols and care pathways within their hospitals. Obstetric physicians must have a strong general medical background, as well as a good understanding of obstetrics. Obstetric training is not necessary, but training within the maternity team and shadowing obstetricians on the labour ward and in antenatal clinics will help gain an understanding of obstetrics.

The work

Understanding pregnancy and pregnancy physiology is key, and understanding how diseases manifest in pregnancy is also important. Early recognition of problems and prompt and appropriate management are essential. Knowing what tests are suitable in pregnancy, and what are normal ranges or findings, is vital. Some women have very complex conditions and have multiple people looking after different problems; in these cases, it is the role of the obstetric physician to act as a 'project manager'. This means supporting obstetricians with the medical aspects of care, and specialist physicians with the obstetric aspects of care, whilst ensuring that the woman and her family understand the care plan. Most obstetric physicians still do general internal medicine on-call; not only does this ensure that good clinical skills and general medicine knowledge are maintained, but it also ensures links outside of maternity are fostered.

The job

Obstetric medicine is hospital-based in centres that have maternity, fetal medicine, and usually neonatal expertise. Teamwork is essential and a close working relationship with obstetricians and midwives is key. Increasingly, close liaison with general practice, emergency medicine, and acute medicine occurs, as women frequently present to these areas and specialist input is required. The diversity of work and the people with whom one works makes the job challenging, exciting, and deeply rewarding.

Extras

There are opportunities for research, lecturing, and teaching, including simulation-based teaching. Multidisciplinary education, including education outside of maternity on external courses, is possible. Private practice is also possible.

For further information

MacDonald Obstetric Medicine Society (MOMS). Web: https://www.obstetricmedic.org.uk/ Email: macdonaldobstetricmedicine@gmail.com Twitter: @MOMSuk

---

08:00	Journal club
09:00	Obstetric medicine ward round
11:00	High-risk pregnancy multidisciplinary team meeting
12:00	Educational supervision of obstetric and medical trainees
13:00	PPC
14:00	Obstetric medicine clinic
17:00	Travel to meeting
18:00	Deliver lecture at educational meeting/dinner
20:00	Home
17:00-21:00	General internal medicine on-call (approximately 1 in 16)

Myth	Obstetrically trained; therefore, can deliver babies.
Reality	Physicians who cannot, and certainly should not, deliver babies.
Personality	Caring, driven, holistic, able to handle raw emotion and tears. Ability to think clearly and be decisive when required.
Best aspects	Teamwork, sheer gratitude from women and their families. Postnatal reviews/baby cuddles when women bring in their babies.
Worst aspects	Occasionally battling against myths regarding medication and investigations—frequently re-requesting tests or explaining that medication is safe.
Route	Post-CCT or out of programme for experience (OOPE) (p. 101) fellowships for medical trainees (ST3+). Soon subspecialty training may be available for those undertaking general internal medicine. Watch this space. Maternal and fetal medicine is a separate subspecialty of obstetrics and gynaecology (p. 240).
Numbers	Currently, fewer than 12 practising obstetric physicians in the UK, of whom most are women.
Locations	Mixture of hospitals with co-located maternity and neonatal services. Most obstetric physicians are based in London, but hopefully as more are trained, this will change.

Life					Work
Quiet On-call					Busy On-call
Boredom					Burnout
Uncompetitive					Competitive
Low salary					High salary

Obstetrics and gynaecology

Ask the general public what an obstetrician does and, surprisingly, many will not have a clue. Add to this mention of your being a gynaecologist, or both, and then it is usually a complete conversation stopper. The word obstetrician comes from the Latin *'obstare'*—to stand by or in front of. If only. The actual job is more akin to running around a battlefield populated solely by pregnant mothers. A gynaecologist, on the other hand, deals with medical or surgical management of benign or malignant problems of the female genital tract. Obstetrics is very diverse, involving the creation of embryos, nurturing the fetus and mother after conception, and helping mother and baby throughout the pregnancy, delivery, and postnatal periods. However, when things go wrong, they can do so horrendously. Whilst delivering a mother of a much-wanted child is truly magical, witnessing the loss of a baby can be devastating. The ability to cope with triumphs and disasters, and to 'treat those two impostors just the same' is essential. Meanwhile, whenever problems occur somewhere along the female genital tract, a gynaecologist may be useful.

The patients

For obstetrics, all female and of reproductive age. If you want to look after blokes, children, or old people, this job is a non-starter. Managing the fetus is challenging, not least because one relies on indirect examination and investigations. So whilst there are plenty of opportunities to talk to mother and partner, conversations with the baby are somewhat one-sided. The challenge is looking after at least two people at the same time—mother and baby, especially when their interests conflict. For gynae, again all female patient population but can be of all ages. Areas of interest include fertility medicine (p. 164), early pregnancy, urogynaecology (p. 310), and gynae oncology (p. 188).

The work

The joy of obstetrics is that one is both physician and surgeon to the pregnant mother. Some obstetricians prefer to be known as Mr/Miss, whilst others as Dr—reflecting their place on this surgery/medicine spectrum. Generally, all issues occuring in pregnancy come within an obstetrician's remit and this makes for great variety. Whilst there is a steady stream of clinics to attend, the core of every obstetrician's job is on the delivery suite where almost anything can happen. Blood loss can be monumental and enough to make even the most stoical quiver in their wellies. Gynaecology is like any branch of surgery—except it happens to be all to do with female bits. Gynae surgeons divide into open, laparoscopic, vaginal, and, more recently, robotic surgeons. In addition, the specialty has pioneered the development of day-surgery and office-based minor procedures.

The job

A typical job plan includes clinics, ward rounds, scanning sessions (if a fetal medicine specialist), delivery suite sessions, and on-call. The specialty of obstetrics and gynaecology (O&G) is increasingly becoming divided. So although all trainees come out qualified in both specialties, many consultant jobs are either one or the other. As a gynaecologist, the job plan mainly consists of theatre sessions and gynae outpatients.

Extras

O&G provides great opportunities for research and teaching. Gynaecology has a reasonable component of private practice. Many specialists travel to the developing world to help improve obstetric services.

For further information

Royal College of Obstetricians and Gynaecologists (RCOG). Tel: 020 7772 6200. Web: https://www.rcog.org.uk Twitter: @RCObsGyn

08:00 Handover on delivery suite

08:30 Scrub up and perform two elective Caesarean sections

10:00 Attend the ward to manage various complications in labour/pregnancy, including a mother who presents with mildly raised blood pressure

10:45 Emergency call to attend a mother carrying twins who is bleeding at 32 weeks

12:00 Training meeting on diabetes in pregnancy interrupted by a call to attend a mother whose fetal heartbeat has suddenly slowed down

13:30 Elective gynae surgical list—a case of endometriosis, followed by vaginal prolapse requiring laparoscopic or vaginal surgical skills

17:00 Check in on the ward team

18:00 Prepare a lecture for a surgical skills training course

Myth	A jolly happy job delivering healthy, happy babies.
Reality	This is not midwifery. Obstetricians deal with death, disaster, and risk. Adrenaline junkies need only apply—with a spare pair of pants.
Personality	It helps to be cool, calm, and collected, and never to be seen to panic. Good communication skills are essential—mothers are often under extreme stress and a display of human kindness can transform the situation.
Best aspects	Rescuing a baby from near death or saving a mother from life-threatening haemorrhage.
Worst aspects	Managing unrealistic expectations about having a waterbirth to the sound of Balinese wind-chimes when, in fact, an emergency Caesarean is required.
Route	Run-through training in O&G (ST1+) (p. 47). Exams: MRCOG.
Numbers	2700 consultants; 60% do both O&G; 80% of trainees are women.
Location	Mainly district general or teaching hospitals.

Life					Work
Quiet On-call					Busy On-call
Boredom					Burnout
Uncompetitive					Competitive
Low salary					High salary

Occupational medicine

Occupational medicine is concerned with the multifaceted interaction between health and work. There are many, often complex or hidden, factors that determine how people function, perform, and behave at work, and whether and when they attend. The diversity of people and their jobs offer enormous variety of clinical experience. As well as individual patients, occupational physicians also liaise with their employers, managers, employee representatives, and colleagues in other specialties and disciplines. Occupational health is not part of the NHS that is funded through taxation; responsibility for its provision lies with employers rather than with the state. So although some occupational physicians work in the NHS, many work for large employers with in-house occupational health services or for independent occupational health providers serving a number of different employers.

The patients

Are usually employees of an organization for whom the occupational physician provides a service. Patients are usually referred by their managers, or self-referred, rather than referred by other clinicians. However, in 2015, the UK government launched the 'Fit for Work' service, enabling GPs to refer patients on long-term sick leave for return to work advice. Patients' expectations may differ from those in other specialties, and this can affect the doctor–patient relationship. Patients may not have chosen to be referred, so the challenge is to build rapport and trust.

The work

Occupational physicians apply a functional, as well as a medical, model in assessing interactions between health and work. Relevant questions include: what can the patient do? What are their limitations? What barriers or obstacles are preventing them from functioning effectively at work? What is likely to help them stay at work or return to work? Occupational physicians need good negotiating and influencing skills in order to achieve positive outcomes for employees and employers. A clear understanding of consent and confidentiality issues and relevant employment law is essential.

The job

Occupational physicians usually work as part of multidisciplinary occupational health teams, which may include specialist occupational health nurses, psychologists, counsellors, welfare advisers, administrators, physiotherapists, ergonomists, occupational therapists, occupational hygienists, and safety professionals. Occupational physicians may be asked to advise about environmental issues, including the impact of organizational activities on the natural environment. On-call requirements vary; often there are none. Part-time work is possible and work–life balance is usually good (if you practise what you preach).

Extras

Occupational physicians may work in teaching hospitals or academic centres. There may be opportunities to participate in research and/or to teach undergraduates and train postgraduate doctors specializing in occupational medicine. National-level work and media exposure may also be possible if you seek out the opportunities. Travel and overseas placements are available with multinational companies.

For further information

Faculty of Occupational Medicine (FOM). Tel: 020 7242 8698. Web: https://www.fom.ac.uk Email: fom@fom.ac.uk Twitter: @FOMNews

Society of Occupational Medicine. Tel: 0203 910 4531. Web: https://www.som.org.uk Email: admin@som.org.uk Twitter: @SOMNews

08:00 Drop off the kids at school and travel to work

09:00 Clinic: six patients referred by their managers because of sickness absence or concerns about their health at work

12:00 Media interview with a journalist writing an article about work-related stress

13:00 Lunchtime meeting with Chief Executive Officer (CEO) and director of human resources, interrupted by a call to review an employee with acute psychosis

14:00 Health and well-being at work meeting or in environmental working group

15:00 Case conference to discuss absence and/or performance management with managers and human resources advisors

15:30 Meeting with senior nurse/service manager to discuss operational issues

16:00 Meeting with occupational medicine trainees

17:00 Head home on the train, checking emails or agenda items for tomorrow's meeting, or sleeping/listening to Spotify, or reading the newspaper

Myth	Agents of uncaring employers forcing the sick to work.
Reality	Using specialist expertise and experience to find workable solutions where health and work interact.
Personality	Listening skills, team player, innovative problem-solver, flexible, able to manage uncertainty, able to understand and assimilate different perspectives, non-judgemental.
Best aspects	Making a positive difference to people's working lives.
Worst aspects	Incorrect assumptions and misunderstandings about your role.
Route	Specialty training in occupational medicine (ST3+) from almost any core training pathway, e.g. medicine (p. 44), anaesthetics (p. 39), general practice (p. 42), paediatrics (p. 49), psychiatry (p. 55), public health (p. 57), radiology (p. 59), and surgery (p. 61). Exams: exams relevant to core/initial specialty; MFOM; research-based dissertation.
Numbers	Approximately 575 doctors working at consultant level.
Locations	NHS premises are just one of many. Often office-based. May be on-site, off-site, in a variety of workplaces. May involve travel and assessments in workplaces.

Life					Work
Quiet On-call					Busy On-call
Boredom					Burnout
Uncompetitive					Competitive
Low salary					High salary

Oncoplastic breast surgery

Oncoplastic breast surgery is a relatively new, exciting, and constantly evolving specialty open to surgeons who have trained in either plastic and reconstructive or general surgery. It combines the principles of surgical oncology with plastic and aesthetic surgical techniques to improve the outcomes of patients undergoing treatment for breast cancer. It includes breast reconstruction using implants or patients' own tissue (often from the abdomen or back), as well as breast conservation techniques to minimize the risk of deformity and asymmetry, and the enormous psychological impact this can have after a cancer has been removed.

The patients

Most patients have a diagnosis of breast cancer, although some have risk-reducing surgery due to high-risk family history or genetic mutations. Breast cancer is unfortunately common, but most patients can expect to be cured with treatment. Although this is incredibly rewarding, it is an emotive topic, and a large responsibility is looking after patients' psychological well-being, which is often related to their cancer experience and treatment. Many patients are young women with young families. This is challenging emotionally to the surgeon and the patient.

The work

The majority of interactions with patients are on an outpatient basis. There may be multiple visits to clinic preoperatively to obtain a diagnosis, attend for further imaging, biopsies, and results, and ultimately plan surgery. Most operations are performed as day cases, with few requiring inpatient admission, except in larger reconstruction cases. Clinics include 'one-stops' where patients are triple-assessed with clinical examination, radiology, and biopsy. Review clinics monitor patients following completion of cancer treatment to detect signs of recurrent disease and oversee endocrine therapies. Oncoplastic clinics are combined oncoplastic breast and plastic surgery consultant clinics where complex or revisional cases can be assessed, ensuring patients have access to a full range of techniques and skills that may be appropriate in their care.

The job

Oncoplastic breast surgery is performed in general and central hospitals, often linked to a breast screening centre. A team approach to care is fundamental. You depend upon, and work closely with, many pan-specialty colleagues, particularly radiology, pathology, and oncology, and specialist nurses in breast cancer and breast reconstruction. Often you will operate with another consultant, particularly in reconstruction or bilateral cases.

Extras

Breast cancer treatment is a fast-moving practice, with an enormous evidence base facilitating its progress. Surgeons are expected to participate in audit and publish figures against national standards, e.g. mastectomy, complication rates etc. Research and recruitment to trials are routine for most patients, so staying abreast of current evidence through personal reading and regular attendance at conferences—both surgical and oncological—is mandatory. This does, however, encourage opportunities to travel. Many breast surgeons complete a higher research degree during training. They are also expected to contribute to surgical training, and most larger centres will have an oncoplastic fellow, as well as registrars.

For further information

Association of Breast Surgery (ABS). Web: https://associationofbreastsurgery.org.uk/ Twitter: @ABSGBI

British Association of Plastic Reconstructive and Aesthetic Surgeons (BAPRAS). Tel: 020 7831 5161. Web: https://www.bapras.org.uk Email: secretariat@bapras.org.uk Twitter: @BAPRASvoice

---

07:30   Grab a coffee, then head to the surgical day unit to mark patients for theatre

08:30   Morning theatre list (2–3 lists per week); skin and nipple sparing mastectomy with implant reconstruction and sentinel node biopsy, then total duct excision

13:55   Grab a sandwich on the way to clinic

14:05   Outpatient clinic: one-stop breast clinic—assess 12 new patients with breast lumps or other symptoms, who each have clinical examination; radiology (mammogram ± ultrasound) and core biopsy/fine-needle aspiration in one streamlined clinic

17:30   Admin, review cases/results of patients to present in tomorrow's multidisciplinary team

18:30   Swing by day unit to check on postoperative patients, then home

Myth	The 'easy' option for trainees who don't like doing on-call.
Reality	Demanding specialty involving comprehensive training in two specialties. Team approach is key. Evidence-based practice +++.
Personality	Team player, caring, methodical, able to apply principles of both oncology and aesthetics in planning surgery.
Best aspects	Genuine relief and gratitude from patients postoperatively. Rarely involves antisocial hours working.
Worst aspects	Breaking bad news, dealing with operative complications.
Route	Core surgical training (p. 61), then specialty training in general (p. 184) or plastic (p. 266) surgery. Last 2–3 years purely breast surgery, often with peri-CCT Oncoplastic Fellowship. Exams: MRCS; FRCS.
Numbers	Approximately 600 consultants.
Locations	Central and district hospitals; breast screening centres.

Life					Work
Quiet On-call					Busy On-call
Boredom					Burnout
Uncompetitive					Competitive
Low salary					High salary

Ophthalmology

Ophthalmology deals with the diagnosis, treatment, and prevention of conditions that affect the eye and visual system. Ophthalmology is indeed spelt with a superfluous 'h'—blame the ancient Greeks. Thankfully, much has changed since then, with innovative techniques, including stem cells, gene therapy, and increasingly complex intraocular devices, working their way into daily practice. As one of the few truly combined medical and surgical specialties, it offers a wide range of opportunities to its practitioners. It includes, but is not limited to, prevention and (where possible) restoration of sight loss. Although the eye may appear an isolated organ, it does have a profound relationship with other body systems.

The patients

Eye disease accounts for around 8% of outpatient, and 3% of emergency attendances in the NHS. Patients are of all ages (from premature infants to centenarians) and backgrounds, and come with an enormous range of conditions. Some may be discharged on their first visit or after surgery; some may stay with you for their (and your) lifetime, e.g. glaucoma, macular degeneration. Some may be at risk of sight loss, death, or life-changing morbidity and it is the ophthalmologist's mission to identify and manage these different groups appropriately.

The work

Ophthalmology has a very high patient throughput. Outpatient clinics tend to be large, and operating lists busy. However, taking an appropriate history and tailored examination is just as important as any other specialty (though usually involves patients taking off fewer clothes). Most ophthalmologists are surgeons, increasingly working in a specialized patient group or anatomical area of the eye. Most also perform cataract surgery, which is the most common operation performed worldwide. It is also one of the most successful operations, with a resultant glow of satisfaction for the doctor. Surgical exposure for trainees is generally excellent from day 1 and they can expect 2–3 theatre sessions per week. The remainder of time is split between clinics and eye casualty. For those less interested in operating, medical ophthalmology is an expanding subspecialty, as is emergency ophthalmology.

The job

A hospital specialty with increasing community involvement, the vast majority of the workload occurs during 'office' hours, with little ward work. Ophthalmologists work closely with a number of specialized allied healthcare professionals, including hospital optometrists, orthoptists, photographers, and nursing staff. Ophthalmologists often liaise with other medical specialties (e.g. neurology, rheumatology, oncology). As eye emergencies are relatively common and approached with fear by non-ophthalmologists, most departments have an eye emergency system. These emergencies do not go away at night and all units have an on-call rota. However, the chances of having a night's sleep are relatively high when on-call.

Extras

There are a number of centres producing high-quality research in ophthalmology and it is possible to have a satisfying academic career—full- or part-time. As ophthalmology is a mystery to most other doctors, the opportunities for teaching, lecturing, and writing are easily satisfied. Private practice can be lucrative, and there are plenty of opportunities for clinical experience or voluntary work abroad.

> ### For further information
>
> **The Royal College of Ophthalmologists (RCOphth).** Web: https://www.rcophth.ac.uk
> Twitter: @RCOphth

08:00 Morning consultant-led teaching session

09:00 General clinic. Some new and follow-ups: 25–30 patients between the consultant and registrar

12:45 Lunchtime teaching

13:15 Preoperative ward round. Patient examination, consent, and lens selection

13:45 Cataract theatre list. Trainees completes two cases as per preoperative discussion. Consultant completes more complex cases

17:00 On-call today, so head down to emergency department. Fairly steady patient traffic, including one admission with a corneal ulcer

20:45 Head home. Several late evening calls and one overnight from A&E and walk-in centres, but no overnight reviews needed

Myth	Glorified opticians who also perform cataract surgery. Speak and write in code that only they understand.
Reality	Highly variable, high-volume clinical and surgical workload. Focuses on prevention or management of morbidity rather than mortality.
Personality	Meticulous, with good organizational and interpersonal skills. Thrives under pressure. Empathy is essential, as many patients are fearful of going blind. Manual skills and courage are required.
Best aspects	Many patients are very pleased with outcomes, which are often rapidly achieved. Use of evolving technologies (and associated gadgets to play with). Early surgical exposure. Little ward and night work.
Worst aspects	Patients and other medical colleagues don't really understand what you do. Daytime can be very busy. The eye can be an unforgiving organ and errors may not heal in the way that the skin or bone might.
Route	Run-through training in ophthalmology (ST1+). Exams: FRCOphth; Refraction Certificate. Specialty training in medical ophthalmology (ST3+) is separate and follows internal medicine training (IMT) (p. 44) or acute care common stem–acute medicine (ACCS-AM) (p. 37).
Numbers	1500 consultants, of whom 30% are women.
Locations	Secondary care: mixture of hospitals, with certain subspecialties only in larger units. Increasing peripheral/community-based clinics.

Life					Work
Quiet On-call					Busy On-call
Boredom					Burnout
Uncompetitive					Competitive
Low salary					High salary

Oral and maxillofacial surgery

Oral and maxillofacial surgery (OMFS) is the specialty responsible for treating pathology of the face and neck. It is one of the youngest surgical specialties and continues to grow in scope. It is now responsible for managing many conditions that other specialties used to in decades past, which, on occasion, is a surprise to patients and colleagues alike. It is the only discipline in which specialist trainees and subsequently consultants are dual-degreed in both medicine and surgery. There is a common misconception that OMFS training takes longer than other comparable disciplines and may thereby put off those wishing to have a family; however, with shortened degree courses and many other specialties requiring higher degrees to secure a consultant job, there are now equal numbers of female and male trainees and the average age of OMFS consultants being appointed is little different to others.

The patients

OMFS is the only specialty in which referrals come from both dentists and doctors, providing significant diversity in presenting conditions. A referral could be for possible oral cancer from a dentist, a salivary gland tumour from a general practitioner, craniofacial and cleft referrals from paediatrics, orthognathic surgery from an orthodontist, or facial trauma from the emergency department. All ages of patients are encountered, with operating based upon a mixture of theatre-based general anaesthesia and clinic-based local anaesthesia.

The work

Few specialties can boast the breadth of patient encounters that are managed by oral and maxillofacial (OMF) surgeons, ranging from draining an orofacial abscess almost occluding the airway to resecting half of a mandible and reconstructing it with a fibula free flap. Although 'generalists' within the specialty occasionally still exist, most modern OMF surgeons are subspecialized to some degree, with the core based around facial trauma and oral pathology. The largest subspecialism is head and neck cancer, the majority of which originates from the oral cavity; these lesions often require large facial resections in combination with neck dissections, and free tissue transfer. Skin cancer and orthognathic surgery, by which the positions of the facial bones are moved, represent the next largest workloads of the specialty. Tertiary referral centres include OMF surgeons practising cleft or craniofacial surgery, managing vascular anomalies, and temporomandibular joint surgery.

The job

OMFS is a predominantly hospital-based specialty, with most consultants spending approximately one-third of their time operating and two-thirds in clinic. Clinics are often multidisciplinary, reflecting the range of other specialties and healthcare disciplines that they work with. These include, in particular, radiologists, ENT, orthodontists, speech and language therapists, and orthoptists. True emergencies are rare out of hours, but those that do occur can be highly challenging, generally due to the close proximity (and importance) of the airway.

Extras

OMFS is the only specialty that is responsible for teaching both medical and dental students, and in whom the majority of core trainees are primarily dentally qualified. There is the opportunity for private practice in a wide range of disciplines, including facial aesthetics, implantology, and oral medicine.

For further information

British Association of Oral and Maxillofacial Surgeons (BAOMS). Tel: 020 7405 8074. Web: https://www.baoms.org.uk Email: office@baoms.org.uk Twitter: @BAOMSOfficial

Saving Faces: The Facial Surgery Research Foundation. Tel: 020 8223 8049. Web: https://savingfaces.co.uk Email: info@savingfaces.co.uk Twitter: @Saving_Faces

---

07:45 Ward round incorporating a twice-weekly journal club

09:00 Clinic starts: ten patients, most new with a variety of problems

13:00 Lunch on the hop, consolidating new admissions and discussing challenging cases with colleagues

13:30 Multidisciplinary team meeting to determine best care for current oncology patients

14:30 Clinic-based procedures list

16:30 Research meeting with a strong coffee

17:15 Postoperative ward round

18:15 Home time

Myth	Glorified dentists.
Reality	A busy and demanding surgical specialty, managing a broad range of conditions and undertaking complex surgery in a multidisciplinary environment.
Personality	Since originating as dentists decades ago, the specialty remains widely recognized for humility and helpfulness, as most emergency department nurses will attest to.
Best aspects	The sheer diversity of clinical practice, even in those who have subspecialized to some degree.
Worst aspects	Misconceptions about the role remain, hampered by the name of the specialty, which only partially describes practice.
Route	Equal numbers of trainees now undertake medicine first, as those who are initially dentists. Core surgical training (CST) (p. 61), then specialist training in OMFS (ST3+). Run-through training also available (ST1+). Exams: MRCS; FRCS ± MFDS.
Numbers	Approximately 340 consultants in England, of whom 11% are women.
Locations	Secondary and tertiary care, in both district general hospitals, teaching hospitals, and highly specialized units.

Life — Work

Quiet On-call — Busy On-call

Boredom — Burnout

Uncompetitive — Competitive

Low salary — High salary

Orthopaedic surgery

Orthopaedics is the pinnacle of all clinical specialties. It deals with the management of fractures, tendon and ligament injuries, and problems with joints such as arthritis. Despite the stereotype of orthopods being knuckle-dragging gorillas banging things with hammers, orthopaedics is actually the perfect harmony of basic biological science, anatomy, pathology, biomechanics, sports sciences, psychology, communication skills, teamworking, and surgery (including microscopes, arthroscopes, lots of shiny high-tech kit, and yes, also with hammers too). Orthopaedics accomplishes something that most other specialties fail to achieve, which is to *fix* things (which means mobility, function, and lifestyle, not just bones!).

The patients

Orthopaedic patients cover the entire range of ages: from children with hip, foot, or spine problems, to young adults with sports injuries, and all the way up to older people needing joint replacements. The case-mix depends on location and subspecialty focus. Most jobs in orthopaedics are so busy that you meet many patients, although the length of time you spend with each individual might not be as long as in some of the more 'chronic' specialties.

The work

The workload may be big, but the work itself is very varied. Nowadays, surgeons tend to subspecialize, e.g. hip, knee, foot and ankle, upper limb, hand, spine (p. 296), paediatrics, trauma (p. 308), or oncology. The key to the job lies in diagnosis and formulating the right management plan, with many patients not actually needing surgery. Despite this, there is still a lot of operating, ranging from tiny delicate hand and spinal surgery to major physically demanding surgery such as hip and knee replacements.

The job

Patient contact is in outpatient clinics (which are normally extremely busy), on ward rounds (which are normally fairly fast), and in theatre (where the patients are mostly asleep!). Your actual job as an orthopaedic surgeon can vary enormously, depending on whether you might be a trauma surgeon in a major trauma centre, more of a generalist in perhaps a small town in a more rural setting, or a top-level full-time elite private knee surgeon in the middle of London!

Extras

There are great opportunities for academic work, including teaching and research. Orthopaedics can also be a financially, as well as personally, rewarding job—more so than most other specialties. However, this very much depends on geography and subspecialty (i.e. there's more private work in knees, but very little in paediatrics). Only a small minority make it to the dizzy heights of the 'top' of their specialty where the rewards can be high; however, this comes at a price, as this requires almost obsessive focus, dedication, and determination. Importantly, however, if money's your motivation, then frankly you're in the wrong profession!

For further information

British Orthopaedic Association (BOA). Tel: 020 7405 6507. Web: https://www.boa.ac.uk
Twitter: @BritOrthopaedic

British Orthopaedic Trainees Association (BOTA). Web: https://www.bota.org.uk Twitter:
@bota_uk

07:30	Trauma meeting to discuss the previous night's emergency admissions
08:00	Preoperative ward round to see patients due for theatre that day and any postoperative patients who are still inpatients from previous theatre lists
08:30	Theatre (maybe four minor cases, or two minors and one major, or two majors)
12:30	Postoperative ward round to see day-case patients from the morning before they're discharged
13:00	Meetings/admin catch-up/rushed bite to eat, if you're lucky!
14:00	Outpatient clinic (20+ patients for elective clinics, 50+ patients for fracture clinics)
17:30	Ward round to see post-op patients from major cases
18:30	Private clinic in the nearby private hospital
20:30	Head home
21:00	Family time/dinner then admin catch-up at home
00:00	Bed

Myth	Thick, brash, arrogant, type A personalities who can't read an ECG.
Reality	Technically minded, highly intelligent, Type A personalities who **can** read an ECG... but who simply pretend that they can't and who are more than happy to let the medics do all the boring bits!
Personality	Hard-working, determined, confident, able to make big decisions fast and have the courage to perform under pressure.
Best aspects	Interesting varied work, with the emotional reward of fixing people's problems; good mix of young and older patients. Not too many nasty smells and not too much death or long-term suffering to deal with. Good propensity for private work.
Worst aspects	Very hard work and very long hours. Highly competitive. Constant interference from politicians/managers/insurance companies who all want things 'cheap' (as opposed to 'best').
Route	Core surgical training (CST) (p. 61), followed by specialty training in trauma and orthopaedic (T&O) surgery (ST3+); run-through training from ST1 available in Scotland. Exams: MRCS; FRCS (T&O).
Numbers	2550 consultants in England (combined with trauma surgery), of whom 6% are women.
Locations	Hospitals.

Life						Work
Quiet On-call						Busy On-call
Boredom						Burnout
Uncompetitive						Competitive
Low salary						High salary

Paediatric cardiology

Paediatric cardiologists deal with children with both congenital and acquired heart disease. For obscure historical reasons, training is overseen by the adult Royal College of Physicians (RCP) and is not part of paediatric Grid Training (p. 50). Most consultants have a specialist interest, in addition to general paediatric cardiology, such as fetal cardiology, intervention, advanced imaging, electrophysiology, or adult congenital heart disease (ACHD). This means that the specialty attracts (and suits) a wide range of personality types and skills.

The patients

Patients range from those seen in early fetal life to older children who may also be followed into adulthood. Paediatric cardiology offers the opportunity to lead the acute management of heart disease at first presentation, then to follow the same child for many years, forming a close relationship with the patient and their family. Being able to effectively communicate with children of all ages, as well as their families, is a key part of this specialty.

The work

The majority of patients are born with congenital cardiac lesions, although acquired heart diseases such as cardiomyopathies also form part of the workload. Experience in neonatology is useful, as neonates form a large part of the inpatient group. Consultants spend their time on the ward and intensive care units, as well as in frequent general outpatient and specialist clinics. The care of children following cardiac surgery and intervention forms the majority of inpatient work. Experience in the catheter laboratory is an important part of training, and previously all consultants were expected to be able to perform basic interventional techniques. Nowadays, in most centres, the vast majority of invasive cardiology is undertaken by consultants with a specialist interest in cardiac intervention.

The job

Paediatric cardiology in the UK is practised in a limited number of tertiary centres, located in major cities. Most consultants have a commitment to undertake outreach clinics in smaller hospitals in the local region. There is an exceptionally strong emphasis on teamwork and shared decision-making, meaning that almost all-important decisions on patient management and surgery are made during multidisciplinary team meetings. Close co-operation with other specialties, especially cardiac surgery, intensive care, and neonatology, is essential. All trainees and consultants in paediatric cardiology are expected to be competent in echocardiography, and this skill is often utilized by other specialties in the management of critically ill children with and without heart disease.

Extras

Research is encouraged, and some trainees undertake a higher research degree during their training. Many trainees also undertake a period out of programme (p. 101) outside the UK as the specialty is dynamic and the international community is surprisingly close-knit. Less-than-full-time training is still uncommon but is becoming more accessible. Some private practice is available, but far less than in adult cardiology.

For further information

British Congenital Cardiac Association (BCCA). Tel: 020 7380 1918. Web: https://www.bcca-uk.org Email: bcca@bcs.com Twitter: @bcca_uk

Association for European Paediatric and Congenital Cardiology (AEPC). Tel: +41 229 080483. Web: https://www.aepc.org Email: office@aepc.org

08:00 Attend handover of cardiology patients on paediatric intensive care unit (PICU), mostly perioperative

08:30 Teaching session on echocardiography by advanced imaging consultant

09:00 Ward round of cardiology ward, PICU, and neonatal intensive care unit (NICU) with cardiology multidisciplinary team

12:00 Lunch

12:30 Urgent MDT meeting discussing a new baby born with an antenatal diagnosis of hypoplastic left heart

13:30 General cardiology clinic. Mostly follow-up patients, with some new patients with possible heart disease referred by local paediatricians

17:00 Evening handover with junior medical team

18:00 On-call. Visit theatre to perform a transoesophageal echocardiogram on a post-op patient. All's well—patient transferred to PICU

23:00 Answer telephone call from on-call cardiology registrar, to give advice about the postoperative patient on PICU who is stable but with an abnormal heart rhythm

Myth	Aggressive egomaniacs that paediatricians dread phoning to ask for ECG advice.
Reality	A varied and rapidly developing specialty that attracts many types of doctor, with the opportunity to make a bedside diagnosis, e.g. with echocardiography, then to follow the child long term.
Personality	Depends on specialist interest; excellent communication skills and ability to comprehend complex haemodynamic and imaging data.
Best aspects	A rare example of a specialty that combines acute work with providing ongoing care throughout and even beyond childhood. Extremely varied; can be tailored to suit individual skills and personalities.
Worst aspects	Poor outcomes or severely impaired quality of life in some can be challenging. Strong media attention on outcomes can increase pressure.
Route	Either internal medicine training (IMT) (p. 44) or acute care common stem–acute medicine (ACCS-AM) (p. 37) and/or paediatrics level 1 training, then specialty training in paediatric cardiology (ST4+). Exams: MRCP or MRCPCH.
Numbers	Around 150 consultant paediatric cardiologists in the UK (30% women), with a larger number of paediatricians with expertise in cardiology (PECs).
Locations	Small number of tertiary centres located in major cities across the UK, with outreach clinics in smaller district hospitals.

Life					Work
Quiet On-call					Busy On-call
Boredom					Burnout
Uncompetitive					Competitive
Low salary					High salary

Paediatric surgery

Paediatric surgeons specialize in surgery on babies and children, ranging from extremely premature neonates weighing a few hundred grams to 17-year-old teenagers weighing a hundred kilograms. Paediatric surgery is a niche surgical subspecialty working closely alongside paediatricians, neonatologists, and paediatric intensivists in children's hospitals. Surgeons manage a wide variety of congenital anomalies, as well as common emergency surgical conditions of infancy and childhood e.g. pyloric stenosis and appendicitis. Common day-case elective procedures include inguinal and umbilical hernia repair, cyst excisions, and circumcisions. Opportunities to specialize, e.g. in neonatal, oncology, and trauma surgery, exist, and some become super-subspecialized in rare conditions, including biliary atresia and separation of conjoined twins.

The patients

The patients are sick babies and children, almost always accompanied by their anxious parents. When children are well, they run around the ward playing with their toys and are delightful. When they are unwell, they can be quiet and withdrawn, or screaming their heads off! Babies and infants are unable to tell you what is wrong, so it's up to the paediatric surgeon to figure out what is causing their green vomit or abdominal distension. Their parents need detailed explanation, reassurance, and close involvement in every step of their child's care.

The work

Paediatric surgery is one of the last bastions of general surgery. Dissection in an extremely premature neonate must be delicate and precise. Much operating is performed using loupes (with magnification ranging from 2.0 to 4.0 times). Skin incisions will grow with the child and their closure should therefore meet the exacting standards of a plastic surgeon. Close cooperation with paediatricians and the wider MDT, including radiologists, dieticians, psychologists, and play therapists, is essential. A high proportion of the work is urological, and trainees spend at least a year in paediatric urology performing procedures, including cystoscopies and reconstructive urological surgery.

The job

A paediatric surgeon's working week will usually involve 2–3 operating sessions, 2–3 outpatient sessions, a 24-hour period on-call for emergencies, and 2–3 sessions set aside for audit, clinical governance, teaching, management, and/or research. Although the surgeon is usually based in a tertiary centre with access to the neonatal intensive care unit (NICU) and paediatric intensive care unit (PICU), many also provide outreach services to network hospitals in the form of outpatient clinics and day-case lists on a weekly or monthly basis.

Extras

Most consultant paediatric surgeons develop an academic, managerial, and/or educational role, in addition to their clinical commitments, with senior lecturers and professors travelling widely to speak at international conferences. Audit and research collaborations are common both nationally and internationally. Minimally invasive surgery is becoming standard for many conditions, and this field is rapidly evolving with miniaturization of robotic equipment. Opportunities for private and international practice do exist, but the volume is not comparable to that seen in adult surgical subspecialties. A significant number of trainees are less than full time, and paediatric surgery attracts many female trainees.

For further information

British Association of Paediatric Surgeons (BAPS). Tel: 020 7430 2573. Web: https://www.baps.org.uk Email: info@baps.org.uk Twitter: @BAPS1953

07:30 Arrive at work (either at base hospital or at a network district general hospital (DGH) as part of outreach work). Consent parents

08:15 Theatre team briefing

08:30 Morning operating list, including two herniotomies and a long case, e.g. a tumour resection

12:30 Outpatient clinic: 22 patients between consultant and registrar

16:00 Multidisciplinary team meeting with radiology, histopathology, and intensive care

18:00 Postoperative ward round reviewing the patients from this morning's list

18:30 Dictate letters, check correspondence

20:00 On-call overnight, covering neonatal and paediatric surgical emergencies, e.g. necrotizing enterocolitis, intussusception, and acute appendicitis

Myth	Egomaniac perfectionists who spend their time straightening 'wonky willies'.
Reality	True general surgeons of childhood, equally comfortable with neck, vascular, thoracic, abdominal, pelvic, and groin dissections. Work within MDTs to provide holistic care to children and their families.
Personality	Patient, gentle, meticulous, fastidious, dedicated, delicate surgeons. Excellent communication and teamworking skills.
Best aspects	Nothing in life is more rewarding than curing a child of illness. Endless variety in pathology and surgeries performed. Opportunities for research into rare diseases and new techniques e.g. tissue engineering, fetal surgery.
Worst aspects	Emotional challenges of dealing with non-accidental injury and life-limiting conditions such as incurable cancers. Long hours. Training consortia spread over large geographical areas.
Route	Core surgical training (CST) (p. 61), followed by specialty training in paediatric surgery (ST3+). Exams: MRCS; FRCS (Paediatric Surgery).
Numbers	200 consultants in England, of whom 25% are women.
Locations	Hospital-based in large tertiary hospitals and a few DGHs.

Life					Work
Quiet On-call					Busy On-call
Boredom					Burnout
Uncompetitive					Competitive
Low salary					High salary

Paediatrics

General paediatrics involves providing specialist medical care to children of all ages and supporting their families. It requires a wide range of multisystem clinical knowledge and excellent communication skills, flexibility, and adaptability. In a single week, a paediatrician might intubate a premature baby, treat a miserable toddler with severe eczema, and resuscitate a teenager with meningitis. It is a busy, demanding, varied, and hugely rewarding specialty, with a great team culture.

The patients

General paediatricians care for all children, from premature infants to adolescents. The majority of the case load is under 5 years of age. In smaller centres, paediatrics includes managing neonates, but in larger hospitals, this is a separate specialty (p. 230). Patients can present with a huge range of problems, from life-threatening emergencies to long-term conditions, and with single-organ to complex multisystem disorders. Children are usually referred by their GP or from the emergency department, but may also be referred by their school, social worker, or even the police. Children don't exist in isolation, and a key part of the job of a paediatrician involves the skilful and sensitive communication with children's parents, siblings, and wider family. Families are often followed up for many years.

The work

Paediatrics is a busy, interactive specialty. Clinical work varies from seeing urgent, life-threatening cases in the emergency department and acutely unwell children to cases that can be seen and managed as outpatients. Much of the acute workload involves infectious diseases, such as gastroenteritis and viral respiratory illnesses, from which most children make a rapid and full recovery. At the other end of the spectrum, there is a growing cohort of children with long-term conditions and complex medical needs requiring a skilled team to manage their care. There is a strong social care element and paediatricians frequently liaise with colleagues in primary care, education, and social services to deliver optimal outcomes for children.

The job

Paediatricians mainly work in hospital settings and are usually based in children's wards, the emergency department, and outpatient clinics. There are close links with other specialists in the hospital, including obstetrics, psychiatry, radiology, haematology, and microbiology. The job can be quite active and can require chasing children round the ward and getting down on your hands and knees—and you may have to be a good sport—joining in a game of 'Where's Wally' or 'I Spy'. Most paediatricians will do some work at night and at weekends throughout their careers, as children can become sick at any time.

Extras

Paediatrics is a broad specialty, with lots of options to shape your career path as you gain experience. There is plenty of capacity to develop subspecialist interests and skills. The specialty offers extensive teaching and research opportunities and the chance to go to international conferences, to work abroad—including in developing countries—and also to develop private practice if desired. Flexible training and working are well established.

For further information

Royal College of Paediatrics and Child Health (RCPCH). Tel: 020 7092 6000. Web: https://www.rcpch.ac.uk Email: enquiries@rcpch.ac.uk Twitter: @RCPCHtweets

---

A day in the life ...

08:30 Paediatrics team teaching

09:00 Night team handover of new admissions and inpatients

09:30 Consultant-led ward round reviewing inpatients and doing urgent jobs

12:00 Multidisciplinary team meeting discussing complex cases and safeguarding issues

13:00 Teach fourth-year medical students at the bedside

13:30 Team lunch—opportunity to catch up with colleagues and prioritize work for the rest of the day

14:00 Acute paediatrics clinic seeing urgent GP referrals: one patient with a fever and a rash needs admission

16:00 Afternoon handover round

17:00 Evening on-call in the emergency department seeing acutely unwell children

20:30 Handover to night team

21:30 Home for a large glass of wine

Myth	Mickey Mouse ties and tiny stethoscopes.
Reality	Demanding, varied, intense, but rewarding multidisciplinary specialty, managing all manner of conditions.
Personality	Dynamic, enthusiastic, flexible, creative, resilient, soft-on-the-inside but tough-on-the-outside, team player.
Best aspects	Huge range of pathology, physiology, and psychology from premature babies to late adolescents; being a specialized generalist in a committed team.
Worst aspects	Seeing children suffer, communicating with distressed parents, exposure to challenging safeguarding cases, emotionally draining.
Route	Run-through training in paediatrics (ST1+) (p. 49), with the option to work in a paediatric subspecialty via the National Training Number (NTN) Grid Scheme (p. 50). Exams: MRCPCH and START assessment.
Numbers	4300 consultants, of whom 55% are women.
Locations	Mixture of general and specialist hospitals and community settings.

Life					Work
Quiet On-call					Busy On-call
Boredom					Burnout
Uncompetitive					Competitive
Low salary					High salary

Paediatrics: community

Community paediatrics is a diverse and rewarding specialty involving the care of children in their own environment rather than in hospital. Community paediatricians work with children with complex needs, vulnerable children, and families in need. It can be a clinically demanding specialty which involves the collation of multiple investigations and assessments over a period of time. The role involves multidisciplinary working with tertiary specialists and allied health professionals, and multiagency working with social care or education. It is a truly holistic specialty involving varied skills.

The patients

Generally, children aged 0–18, although some areas also include young adults up to the age of 25. Family members often have similar difficulties to their children or social needs, and this increases the challenges of assessments. Patients can be from all walks of life, but many children are from disadvantaged backgrounds. Referral criteria vary between different areas and are becoming stricter as the patient population increases.

The work

Varied caseload includes work with vulnerable children through adoption medicals or looked-after children assessments, safeguarding including child protection medicals, and management of children with neurodisability, educational needs, behavioural issues, or developmental difficulties.There is a big difference from hospital paediatrics in that many patients cannot be 'cured' but their lives can be improved by good paediatric management. Some roles include joint clinics with child and adolescent mental health services (p. 268), neurologists or geneticists. There are opportunities to work in palliative care (p. 262), or in public health (p. 280). There is also the possibility of being involved in the rapid response team for sudden unexpected deaths in childhood. The ability to take a thorough and detailed clinical history is vital and good communication skills with both children and families are necessary.

The job

Community paediatrics is based in community healthcare settings e.g. clinics, schools, and sometimes in the patient's home. The specialty offers a fantastic opportunity to see families in the real world and to provide follow-up for some children with complex needs over many years. Appointments are longer than in acute paediatrics, allowing in-depth assessment of needs. Posts have different mixes of the various strands of community paediatrics and job plans can be adapted according to personal interests. There is no on-call with purely community-based posts, although many consultants find that admin pressures mean they work long hours.

Extras

Some areas combine community work with part of the week as an acute paediatrician for those who want the best of both worlds. There are opportunities to get involved in creating patient care pathways and develop diagnostic services and an increased emphasis on improving the amount and quality of research. There is scope to be involved with improving the health of children countrywide through public health initiatives. Flexible working can be accommodated. Private practice is possible, but not substantial.

For further information

British Association for Community Child Health (BACCH). Web: https://www.bacch.org.uk Email: bacch@rcpch.ac.uk Twitter: @CommChildHealth

Royal College of Paediatrics and Child Health (RCPCH). Tel: 020 7092 6000. Web: https://www.rcpch.ac.uk Email: enquiries@rcpch.ac.uk Twitter: @RCPCHtweets

08:30 Arrive at locality clinic to review notes prior to development clinic

09:00 First patient is a 10-year old with cerebral palsy whom you first saw as a 1-year old and who is making excellent progress in the mainstream school which you supported her to attend

09:30 Development clinic

12:00 Phone call from a colleague with a child protection dilemma

12:15 Review a looked-after child medical report whilst grabbing lunch

13:00 Multidisciplinary meeting with Child and Adolescent Mental Health Service (CAMHS) colleagues to assess a child with possible autistic spectrum disorder

14:00 Pre-adoption medical clinic

16:00 Sorting parent queries and email correspondence

17:00 Home time

Myth	An easy option—'nit doctors' or 'social workers'.
Reality	Improving the lives of the most vulnerable children.
Personality	Friendly, practical, and adaptable. Often good diplomacy skills are required.
Best aspects	Variety of work and getting to work with motivated and dynamic people in different disciplines. No on-call responsibilities in some posts.
Worst aspects	Increasing workload and pressure on service, coupled with decreased resources available.
Route	Run-through training in paediatrics (ST1+) (p. 49), then either Grid specialist training in community paediatrics (ST5+) or continue in a general programme and choose community posts. Exams: MRCPCH and START assessment.
Locations	Based out of hospital, often in purpose-built child development centres, community clinics, clinics in hospitals, general practice, schools, home visits.

Life						Work
Quiet On-call						Busy On-call
Boredom						Burnout
Uncompetitive						Competitive
Low salary						High salary

▌Pain management

Pain medicine encompasses the management of acute, chronic, and cancer-related pain. Most clinicians will regularly encounter patients in pain; however, despite its ubiquity, our knowledge of the biology and mechanisms which cause pain remains incomplete and therefore results in both therapeutic and academic challenges. Add to this the confounding and complex interplay with a patient's psychology and social experience that affects the nature of the pain, and its impact on the patient—this makes the difference between a successful and an unsuccessful intervention. Voltaire could have been describing pain medicine when he said 'Doctors ... prescribe medicine of which they know little, to cure diseases of which they know less, in human beings of whom they know nothing'. We are still at the frontier in making sense of 'pain'. Methods to provide effective pain management are evolving and are a specialist area in their own right.

The patients

The patients may be children or adults. They may be inpatients primarily experiencing uncontrolled acute or cancer pain, or outpatients where the pain is chronic and significantly impacting on quality of life. The interaction between doctor and patient may be short-lived and involves titration or switching of analgesia. It can also be more long term as part of a multidisciplinary team which also includes physiotherapists, specialist nurses, and psychologists who support the patient and their family/carers to reduce the magnitude of the pain and the negative impact that it has on their emotions, sleep, relationships, work, and lifestyle.

The work

This is a consultant-delivered specialty. Specialists divide their time between outpatient clinics assessing patients with chronic pain, theatre lists performing nerve blocks and even surgery in the form of therapeutic neuromodulation (electrical or chemical stimulation of the nervous system to modify pain impulses), and leading inpatient pain ward rounds assisting in the management of acute postoperative pain and other recurrent and refractory pains in medical and surgical patients. They may work closely with palliative care teams to provide interventions to manage uncontrolled cancer pain and relieve distress.

The job

Pain has a multitude of pathological causes and disabling physical and psychological consequences. Breaking the cycle of physical and psychological debility requires an analytical assessment, effective delivery of therapeutic interventions tailored to the individual, and most importantly empathy. The diversity in causes and therapeutic options allows one to take specialist interest in a particular pain type (e.g. head/facial pain, abdominal/pelvic pain, spinal pain, joint pain, palliative/cancer care) and/or a particular therapeutic approach (interventional pain medicine, including device implantation; non-interventional, more psychological approaches).

Extras

There are opportunities for education, developing professional standards, guidance, and protocols at international, national, and local levels. Research into the underlying mechanisms of pain and the evidence for all therapies is in demand. A great number of private providers offer pain management.

For further information

Faculty of Pain Medicine of the Royal College of Anaesthetists. Web: https://fpm.ac.uk/ Email: contact@fpm.ac.uk Twitter: @FacultyPainMed

---

08:00 Review clinic letters and investigation results

08:30 Outpatient clinic (ten patients, including six new referrals)

12:30 Review ward patients referred with acute-on-chronic pains or uncontrolled cancer pain

13:30 Theatre to perform injections/implantation of spinal cord stimulator

18:00 Attend multidisciplinary team meeting to discuss complex patients and agree treatment plans

19:00 Home

Myth	Management of malingerers, drug seekers, and 'heart-sink' patients.
Reality	Management of patients with genuine and disabling pain who are understandably distressed, depressed, and demanding. Requires an analytical approach to diagnosis, assessment, education, analgesia, if possible, and most essentially management of expectations.
Personality	Empathic, not sympathetic. A clear communicator. Able to manage emotional consultations and confrontation. A good teamworker who values the contribution of others and is realistic about their role in managing the biopsychosocial impact of pain.
Best aspects	Opportunity to make diagnoses and deliver definitive treatment, rather than providing a service to allow others to do the same. Being appreciated by the patients for offering support, understanding, and treatment when they felt there was nowhere else to turn.
Worst aspects	Unrealistic expectations for pain resolution and patient dissatisfaction.
Route	Core anaesthetics training (CAT) (p. 39), followed by specialty training in anaesthetics (ST3+); intermediate and higher training in pain medicine; 12 months' advanced pain training usually in ST6. Exams: FRCA; FFPMFRCA.
Numbers	Approximately 550 consultants working in chronic pain management.
Locations	Largely outpatient clinics and day-case theatres in hospitals.

Life					Work
Quiet On-call					Busy On-call
Boredom					Burnout
Uncompetitive					Competitive
Low salary					High salary

Palliative medicine

Palliative medicine involves working with anyone with a life-limiting illness. It can involve the medical, surgical, or psychological sequelae of that illness, or, more commonly, a complex interaction of several problems. It has evolved from purely hospice care for patients in the last days or weeks of life to also managing the symptoms of those receiving active treatment in acute hospitals and the community.

The patients

Nearly all patients will have an incurable illness, although they will need input at different stages in their disease trajectory. The age range is wide and contrary to perception, many patients will be young. Although paediatric palliative care is a separate specialty, teenagers and young adults (up to age 24) will be cared for by adult specialist. It can be a challenge to separate the needs of the patient from those of their family and consequently they should be thought of as your secondary patients.

The work

Although traditionally associated with cancer, palliative medicine is evolving and involved with an increasing number of non-malignant illnesses such as dementia, heart failure, respiratory illnesses, and neurological conditions, e.g. motor neuron disease. The work can be distilled down to improving symptom control and problem-solving by attention to detail, identifying what matters to the patient and their loved ones, then making often small, but hugely significant changes in pharmacological and psychosocial management. It is essential to have a solid knowledge of general medicine and oncology, with above-average communication skills and an aptitude for pharmacology and psychology—not a common combination!

The job

Palliative medicine is practised in acute general hospitals, oncology centres, the community, and the hospice setting. A job can involve working in a variety of these settings or be based in one place. There are increasing numbers of outpatient clinics, although generally less than our medical colleagues. On-call is non-resident and covers multiple sites, including on weekends and nights. There is a strong multidisciplinary ethos and recognition of our specialist colleagues' input is vital for the complex teamwork to succeed. Many posts outside of the hospice are in an 'advisory' capacity and may involve supporting colleagues in other specialties emotionally, as well as advising on symptom control or decision-making in difficult ethical scenarios. Empathy, decision-making, and diplomacy are useful skills in these environments.

Extras

Lots of opportunity for teaching on a small or large scale, as well as increasing research involvement. Due to the current shifting landscape of palliative care, there are expanding opportunities to be involved in management and policymaking. Foreign travel is increasingly an option, as the UK is often considered the worldwide leaders of palliative care. Private practice is carried out by a minority of consultants.

For further information

Association for Palliative Medicine of Great Britain and Ireland. Tel: 01489 668332. Web: https://apmonline.org Twitter: @APMPostTweets

These books may also provide further insight and inspiration: *Dear Life* **by Rachel Clarke**; *With the End in Mind* **by Kathryn Mannix.**

A day in the life …

(In a district general hospital)

09:00 Attend the acute oncology service morning meeting

09:30 Multidisciplinary meeting to discuss current inpatient list

11:00 Liaise with community team (based in local hospice) and do two home visits

13:30 Teaching medical trainees on 'breaking bad news'

14:45 Hospital ward round with trainees and specialist nurses

17:00 Admin

23:00 Phone call from on-call trainee asking for advice about a patient's terminal agitation

Myth	Appear in the last few days of life to insist on talking about dying, hold the patient's hand, and prescribe morphine.
Reality	Medically and emotionally demanding; often supporting families and colleagues, as well as patients. Hugely rewarding.
Personality	Thorough, resilient, compassionate, team player.
Best aspects	Opportunity to have a significant impact during an important time in people's lives; variety of working environment; being part of, and witness to, excellent teamwork.
Worst aspects	Can be emotionally draining, ongoing misconceptions about the nature and role of palliative care from both colleagues as well as patients and their families.
Route	Internal medicine training (IMT) (p. 44) or acute care common stem–acute medicine (ACCS-AM) (p. 37), then specialty training in palliative medicine (ST3+). Can also apply from GP. Exams: MRCP or MRCGP; SCE in Palliative Medicine.
Numbers	675 consultants, of whom 75% are women.
Locations	Balanced mix of community (home visits and clinics), hospice, district general hospitals, and larger teaching and tertiary hospitals, as well as specialist cancer centres.

Life						Work
Life	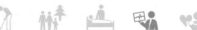					Work
Quiet On-call						Busy On-call
Boredom						Burnout
Uncompetitive						Competitive
Low salary						High salary

Pharmaceutical medicine

Pharmaceutical medicine is a diverse specialty that encompasses all aspects of drug life cycle management, be that a compound on the laboratory bench, a pharmaceutical ingredient in the development pathway, or a licensed product in use at the bedside or purchased from a pharmacy. Pharmaceutical medicine emerged during the 1970s from an increasing requirement to understand translational medicine, balance commercial and non-commercial pressures, and integrate international drug regulation, so quality, highly effective, and safe drugs are available to all. The clinical training and experience doctors bring to the many aspects of being a pharmaceutical physician can dictate the success or failure of current and future treatments in all therapeutic areas.

The patients

It is unlikely that a pharmaceutical physician directly manages patients. However, any medicine an individual receives would have been assessed in a clinical development environment and would have crossed the desk of several clinical regulatory assessors. The overarching quality, safety, and effectiveness of the therapy to a patient will have been, at some point, the pharmaceutical physicians' responsibility.

The work

Pharmaceutical physicians work in a variety of roles to drive medicine development, from early clinical pharmacology and toxicology, through clinical development, into regulatory licensure and beyond. Increasingly, development pathways vary and depend on the type of products, but scientific knowledge, medical training, and clinical experience applied through specialist areas can yield success. Pharmaceutical physicians may work as 'clinical pharmacologists' or 'clinical research physicians' to design, conduct, analyse, and interpret preclinical research studies or clinical trials in support of new products. Employment in the 'regulatory affairs' sphere ensures that companies and medicine developers adhere to regulatory authority legislation and guidance, so the safety and effectiveness to patients can be assured. The independent review of new products as a 'medical assessor' within a regulatory body, like the Medicines and Healthcare products Regulatory Agency (MHRA), enables the benefit–risk balance of authorizing or maintaining products. Physicians in a company's 'medical affairs' team work closely with sales and marketing, so that trial reports, educational information, and safety documentation are available to all.

The job

Pharmaceutical physicians work as part of multidisciplinary teams of pharmacologists, toxicologists, immunologists, pharmacists, and marketing and commercial personnel to understand and progress products into healthcare. Most work is office-based, but some may undertake trial medicals. Although there are no on-call commitments, commercial pressures may be high and require periods of extended work.

Extras

The opportunity to undertake international travel to global offices or conferences/meetings is common and salaries are often generous. Many pharmaceutical physicians migrate to work as consultant contractors or work freelance for the diversity and flexibility this brings.

For further information

Faculty of Pharmaceutical Medicine (FPM). Tel: 020 3696 9040. Web: https://www.fpm. org.uk Twitter: @FacultyPharmMed

British Association of Pharmaceutical Physicians (BRAPP). Tel: 0118 934 1943. Web: https://brapp.org/ Email: info@brapp.org Twitter: @brapp_feed

A day in the life ...

08:00 Opportunity to review emails that arrived overnight from international colleagues

09:30 Project team meeting to review status of drug development work packages, including a detailed presentation of the latest toxicology information

10:30 Update gap analysis/market assessment report to inform future project direction

11:00 Video conference with clinical trial hospital teams undertaking a large multicentre trial

12:00 Working lunch with programme manager to consider long-term approaches to paediatric regulations

13:00 Review and sign off mini-dossier for upcoming MHRA scientific advice meeting

14:00 Meet with other physicians and regulatory team to follow up serious adverse reaction data from an early phase I clinical trial

15:30 Respond to emails and finalize presentation for US meeting

16:30 Train to Heathrow for overnight flight to the USA for meeting to align clinical trials strategy for new product

Myth	Money-focused, MBA-holding doctor, with little interest in patient care.
Reality	Ability to influence, assist, and realize the clinical delivery of new and better treatments for all.
Personality	Strong communication skills, with attention to detail.
Best aspects	Well resourced to facilitate job demands.
Worst aspects	Ever-changing regulatory world.
Route	Industry entry-level jobs available after foundation years; most common to enter jobs after core training (e.g. internal medicine training) (p. 44), core surgical training (p. 61), etc. In an appropriate job, specialty training (to CCT) in pharmaceutical medicine is available. Exams: Diploma in Pharmaceutical Medicine.
Numbers	2500, of whom 40% are female; approximately 150 in CCT training.
Locations	Mostly office-based, some roles may have limited clinical and ward-based activities. UK and global sites, often with travel.

Life					Work
Quiet On-call					Busy On-call
Boredom					Burnout
Uncompetitive					Competitive
Low salary					High salary

Plastic and reconstructive surgery

Plastic and reconstructive surgery involves performing complex procedures to modify, restore, or create structures of the body—it is an umbrella under which there are many surgical disciplines, including burns, cleft lip and palate, hand surgery, breast reconstruction and microsurgery, and craniofacial surgery, to name but a few. Aesthetic surgery has become synonymous with plastic surgery. The name 'Plastic' comes from the Greek '*Plastikos*', which means to move or to shape, and has nothing at all to do with plastic as a material! Advances in surgical technique, including microsurgery, tissue engineering, and three-dimensional technology, have kept plastic surgery at the cutting edge as a specialty. Plastic surgery involves interactions with many other surgical specialties, including neurosurgery, orthopaedics, and ear, nose, and throat surgery, and this provides great opportunity for collaborative working.

The patients

There is the opportunity to treat from 'cradle to grave'. This includes children with cleft lips, young adults who have undergone trauma and burns, breast reconstruction, e.g. after mastectomies, and surgery for skin cancer. In fact, plastic surgery remains a 'general surgical specialty', in which one can take a number of surgical paths. Cosmetic surgery for aesthetic enhancement is largely funded privately by patients, but plastic surgery forms an integral part of many NHS hospitals, including for cosmetic defects where functional or psychological benefit would be gained. Many patients are 'cured' from their condition and typically make a rapid recovery.

The work

Involves many interactions with colleagues in planning and executing surgery and reconstruction. As many patients survive and do well post-procedure, it is highly satisfying and can make an enormous difference to patients' lives. Junior trainees are exposed to a variety of clinical settings and work with a number of consultant colleagues to gain experience. On-calls require management of acute emergencies, the most common of which are hand and minor injuries. Life-threatening emergencies, e.g. severe burns, are less frequent and plastic surgeons are often part of the trauma team in management of major trauma.

The job

Patients are seen in a range of clinical settings, from local hospitals to trauma centres. Procedures and techniques range from routine simple reconstruction to use of cutting-edge technology, with the ability for research into tissue engineering and innovative technology. Patients are seen largely during clinics or in theatre. Management may require the involvement of several specialists working in a multidisciplinary team in complex cases, including breast surgeons, orthopaedic surgeons, occupational therapists, and physiotherapists.

Extras

There is great opportunity to develop specialist interests in a range of clinical, research, humanitarian, and teaching roles. There is significant potential for aesthetic or cosmetic surgery, most of which occurs in the private sector, although the techniques used are often mastered during training. Many trainees are involved in teaching and there are several courses specifically set up by trainees to teach clinical and surgical skills. Through the British Association of Plastic Aesthetic and Reconstructive Surgeons (BAPRAS), there are opportunities to provide help and teaching to the developing world, and many trainees decide to obtain a higher degree if they develop research interests in specific fields.

For further information

British Association of Plastic Reconstructive and Aesthetic Surgeons (BAPRAS).
Tel: 020 7831 5161. Web: https://www.bapras.org.uk Email: secretariat@bapras.org.uk
Twitter: @BAPRASvoice
British Association of Aesthetic Plastic Surgeons (BAAPS). Tel: 020 7430 1840. Web:
https://baaps.org.uk Email: info@baaps.org.uk Twitter: @BAAPSMedia

08:00 Ward round of patients admitted as emergencies overnight and those on the morning's theatre list

08:30 Theatre briefing

09:00 Start cases. Four day surgery cases, including removal of a large skin cancer. Includes a difficult choice about what sort of music to listen to

13:00 Lunch, again a difficult choice about whose turn it is to buy coffees and lunches. The consultant inevitably loses that last battle!

13:30 Outpatient clinic: a mixture of general plastic surgical cases, then a joint case with max fax considering the technical aspects of resecting a neck tumour

17:00 See the postop patients and review the day, what has gone well, what hasn't, and a good opportunity for a debrief and team bonding

18:00 Private clinic: three follow-ups and four new patients. Two booked for surgery next week

21:30 Home

Myth	Ferrari drivers in pinstriped suits, doing nose jobs, boob jobs, and liposuction.
Reality	Surgeons who transform lives. This may be through rebuilding a nose damaged by trauma, breast reconstruction, or injecting fat cells for patients with facial deformity ... Oh OK then, maybe not just a myth ...
Personality	Knowledgeable, reliable, and dependable—what all good doctors should be; however, sociability, perfectionism, precision, and good technical ability are really important too.
Best aspects	It is the most tremendous fun, and job and patient satisfaction is very high—it's hard to beat the smile from a parent whose child's cleft lip is repaired.
Worst aspects	Long hours, repeated surgical manoeuvres, and a poor play list in theatre. In fact, there really are no 'worst' aspects.
Route	Core surgical training (CST) (p. 61), then specialty training in plastic surgery (ST3+). Exams: MRCS; FRCS (Plast).
Numbers	500 consultants in England, of whom 20% are women.
Locations	Most large teaching hospitals and smaller regional plastic surgery units.

Life					Work
Quiet On-call					Busy On-call
Boredom					Burnout
Uncompetitive					Competitive
Low salary					High salary

Psychiatry: child and adolescent

Child and adolescent psychiatrists work with children and young people from 0 to 18 years with mental health problems, although there are a growing number of 0–25 services. It is the medical component of multidisciplinary children and young people's mental health services, and is mostly practiced in the community but there are inpatient services and a range of specialist services. Problems range from neurodevelopmental disorders, through emotional disorders, to severe mental illness. Treatments are often multimodal, with social, psychological, and pharmacological components. Child and adolescent psychiatry tends to concern itself with the most complex and highest-risk children and young people.

The patients

Child and adolescent psychiatry thinks of the child in his or her system: family, friends, school, etc. The patient might be a young person who wants to be seen alone or a child seen with their whole family. Each case entails all the complexities of a child's biology, psychology, and social situation. The workload includes the diagnosis and management of emotional and behavioural problems, attention- deficit/ hyperactivity disorder (ADHD), conduct disorder, depression, and anxiety. Self- harm and eating disorders are on the rise in those aged under 18. Many cases involve physical and mental health problems, including neuropsychiatric cases, such as tics and Tourette's, and medically unexplained symptoms. Psychosis is less common than in adults, but the incidence rises during adolescence. Exciting research is finding ever-increasing treatable causes, e.g. autoimmune brain disorders.

The work

Most child and adolescent psychiatrists are based in community settings within Child and Adolescent Mental Health Services (CAMHS), also called Child and Young People's Mental Health Services (CYPMHS) in some areas. Here, there is constant collaboration among disciplines—they interact closely with paediatricians, psychologists, nurses, social workers, occupational therapists, and teachers. Consultants play significant leadership roles within multiple teams and organizations, in both inpatient and outpatient settings.

The job

Community CAMHS teams can be 'generic'or more specialized, either by age (e.g. under 11, adolescent) or by problem type (neurodevelopmental, autism, learning difficulties, forensic, children in care, early intervention in psychosis). Crisis services, community eating disorder, and forensic CAMHS have all been areas of development in recent years. Some acute trusts have specialized 'paediatric liaison' services where psychiatrists work hand- in- hand with paediatric teams. Inpatient services are divided into children's units for children under 12 and adolescent units for those aged 13 - 18. There are also medium secure adolescent units and units for children and young people with neurodevelopmental problems.

Extras

There are plenty of opportunities for multidisciplinary teaching. Some child and adolescent psychiatrists undertake expert assessments for family court proceedings. Flexible working can be supported.

For further information

The Association for Child and Adolescent Mental Health (ACAMH). Tel: 020 7403 7458. Web: https://www.acamh.org Email: membership@acamh.org Twitter: @acamh

Royal College of Psychiatrists (RCPsych). Tel: 020 7235 2351. Web: https://www.rcpsych.ac.uk Twitter: @rcpsych

---

09:00	Team meeting discussing complex patients and administrative aspects of the service
10:30	Coffee break
11:00	Assessment of a new patient with suspected ADHD
12:00	Junior doctor teaching and supervision
13:00	Journal club discussing an interesting paper on a possible new treatment for Tourette's
14:00	Consultation with social services
15:00	Follow-up clinic, with three patients with a variety of complex problems
17:00	Time to go home

Myth	Just a glorified social worker/psychologist—nothing makes a difference anyway.
Reality	The opportunity to make a real difference in children's lives with a wide range of evidence-based interventions.
Personality	Empathic, flexible, creative, a good communicator who can contain anxiety and offer hope. Good with children!
Best aspects	The complexity, the pleasure of working with children and families.
Worst aspects	Demand outstrips resources, problems with recruitment, and long-standing promises of new investment in the system only just being fulfilled.
Route	Core psychiatry training (p. 55), followed by specialty training in child and adolescent psychiatry (ST4+). Exams: MRCPsych.
Numbers	900 consultants, of whom 65% are women.
Locations	Mostly in community settings, some inpatient and some general hospital-based services.

Life					Work
Quiet On-call					Busy On-call
Boredom					Burnout
Uncompetitive					Competitive
Low salary					High salary

Psychiatry: forensic

Forensic psychiatrists assess and treat the minority of individuals with mental disorders who pose a significant risk to others. The secure hospital system that is the cornerstone of the specialty has its origins as far back as the 1860s. The central remit is also enduring—to provide humane care, rather than containment alone, to people with serious mental illnesses who have violently offended. Medical leadership of MDTs is combined with becoming expert in unravelling links between mental disorders and offending, and developing skills for a unique interface between the medical world and the criminal justice system.

The patients

Most patients are referred after a serious violent offence. Mental illness may be pre-established or come to light upon entering the police and justice system. Individuals can be diverted to psychiatric hospital at initial arrest, during court proceedings, or even when serving a prison sentence. Patients may also be referred from general psychiatric settings if there are concerns about risk. Psychotic illnesses like schizophrenia are the most common diagnoses. Many patients also have a comorbid substance misuse or personality disorder, or complex social backgrounds. Not uncommonly, a relationship with patients and their families is established over years, from initial acute admission to rehabilitation and community supervision.

The work

Core skills involve assessing diagnosis, mental state, prognosis, and risk, to guide the type of treatment and security required, and later the timing and nature of discharge. Assessments and progress are often recorded in detailed reports to feed into the various legal frameworks around care. The forensic psychiatrist has overall responsibility for the care and treatment of patients detained under the Mental Health Act. Day-to-day work involves co-ordinating multidisciplinary treatment, including ensuring physical health needs are addressed. For patients in the acute phase, optimizing pharmacotherapy is a prominent aspect, before a rehabilitative phase that involves psychological treatment and broader therapeutic activities.

The job

Posts are generally based in secure hospital units, with three tiers of security (low, medium, and high). These are healthcare, rather than prison, settings, albeit with perimeter fences and other physical modifications and procedures. Many areas also have community forensic teams who support patients following discharge. Assessing patients for transfer into forensic inpatient services involves travel to different prisons and hospitals. Prison in-reach (outpatient-style psychiatric care in prisons) can also be part, or all, of a post. MDTs include nurses, psychologists, occupational therapists, and social workers. Maintaining cohesion in the face of any challenges is an essential skill, as is effectively communicating with a range of other agencies. As a consultant on-call, commitments typically involve responding to acute needs in the inpatient forensic unit, whereas trainees may also be part of a general adult psychiatry rota.

Extras

Forensic psychiatry offers avenues for developing specific interests or expertise, e.g. in certain types of offending, adolescents, or in high security. Some forensic psychiatrists undertake postgraduate qualifications in aspects of law. Forensic psychiatrists regularly prepare court reports for patients under their care and, in some cases, give evidence in person. It is also possible to develop independent private practice as an expert witness.

For further information

Faculty of Forensic Psychiatry. Tel: 020 7235 2351. Web: https://www.rcpsych.ac.uk/members/your-faculties/forensic-psychiatry Twitter: @rcpsychForensic

---

09:00	Ward handover and community meeting on inpatient unit
09:15	Clinical team meeting (ward round) with full multidisciplinary team on inpatient unit
11:30	Liaison with Ministry of Justice about a patient's leave
12:00	Community review at supported housing site with patient, community psychiatric nurse, and housing manager
13:00	Referrals meeting on inpatient unit over lunch
14:00	Assessment of patient in local psychiatric intensive care unit for possible transfer to forensic services
15:30	Prepare assessment report
17:00	Home

Myth	Eccentrics obsessed with the psychological profiles of serial killers.
Reality	A varied specialty, sometimes challenging, but rewarding and intellectually stimulating.
Personality	Attention to detail, adaptable communicator, comfortable with leadership and expressing opinion.
Best aspects	Strong team element, diverse, continuity of patient relationships.
Worst aspects	Burden of risk, environment sometimes intense, not many Christmas cards.
Route	Core psychiatry training (p. 55), followed by specialty training in forensic psychiatry (ST4+). Exams: MRCPsych.
Numbers	560 consultants, of whom 35% are women.
Locations	Mixture of secure hospital units, community, and prison. Requires frequent travel.

Life						Work
Quiet On-call						Busy On-call
Boredom						Burnout
Uncompetitive						Competitive
Low salary						High salary

█ Psychiatry: general adult

Psychiatry is an exciting specialty with a huge range in the types of work, locations, patients, and illnesses encountered. This means psychiatrists are very rarely bored and have flexibility and variety rarely found elsewhere. The psychiatrist also holds a privileged position in society—on a daily basis, patients reveal not only their medical details, but also their most private thoughts, experiences, and (often) fascinating symptoms. Uniquely, psychiatrists hold responsibility as a doctor for their patients, but also the community in which they live, and have additional legal powers granted to exercise this.

The patients

Anyone from 18 years upwards. There is no maximum age, but patients with specific conditions may be best managed by old age psychiatry (p. 278). Patients are from all backgrounds and may present with a vast array of symptoms. These include psychosis where they may be hallucinating, be behaving in an odd or dangerous way, have delusional beliefs, or be neglecting themselves. They may have debilitating anxiety disorders, eating disorders, or severe mood symptoms, from catatonic depression to life-threatening mania, devastating extremes of personality, or addictions. Often, they have more than one diagnosis! Patients may not realize they are unwell, may have injured themselves or be suicidal, and may not want to see you. They may also come with challenging relatives and complex social or cultural circumstances.

The work

Psychiatrists frequently face tricky situations, and work can be both exciting and stressful. No two patients present in the same way, even with the same diagnosis, and there are few tests to guide diagnosis. The complexity of the work means psychiatrists spend a lot of time with their patients. There are many different risks to patient, staff, and the public to consider, so flexibility and a cool head are required. Dealing with unusual ethical questions is common. Most psychiatrists work in MDTs, comprising the psychiatrist as clinical leader, nurses, psychologists, occupational therapists, social workers, and more. The psychiatrist's work will bring them into contact with other agencies e.g. the police, local authority professionals e.g. housing and social services, legal professionals, and frequently GPs.

The job

General adult psychiatrists may lead inpatient wards or community teams, and when on-call, trainees often also see patients in the emergency departments (ED), police stations, or a patient's home. They may decide to subspecialize in roles, including liaison (based in medical hospitals, treating ED presentations and complex medical patients on the ward), addictions (alcohol, heroin, crack, sedatives, and all sorts of 'club drugs', plus associated health and social problems), and rehabilitation (supporting patients with chronic illness, e.g. schizophrenia, to independence), or may specialize in one type of illness, e.g. eating disorders or obsessive–compulsive disorder (OCD). Transcultural psychiatry is a fascinating field where medical science meets anthropology. Psychiatric treatments may be pharmacological, psychotherapy, social interventions, or specialist e.g. electroconvulsive therapy (ECT). Special qualifications are required for psychiatrists who undertake Mental Health Act (MHA) assessments to 'section' patients, if required.

Extras

There is much demand for teaching in psychiatry (undergraduates, trainees, other professionals), and there are opportunities to contribute to research. Undertaking private work is often possible and lucrative!

For further information

Royal College of Psychiatrists (RCPsych). Tel: 020 7235 2351. Web: https://www.rcps ych.ac.uk Twitter: @rcpsych

---

08:30 Emails and checking diary for the day

09:00 Multidisciplinary team meeting, clinic, or ward round begins—all possible with tea

11:00 Complex case conference with multiple agencies for a high-risk patient

12:00 Supervising trainees—helping prepare for difficult communications exam over lunch

13:00 Expected to be in a meeting to discuss new mental health initiatives in the area, but instead called away to an emergency MHA assessment—another tea on return

15:00 Asked to see a long-term patient with multiple health complaints for a medication review

16:00 Completing paperwork and reviewing a journal article for an upcoming presentation

17:00 Fielding phone call from a GP needing urgent advice

18:00 Home and on-call advising a team of juniors on night shift. Mostly clinical calls or for mental health legislation advice

Myth	Asking patients on couches about their childhood. Anything to do with *One Flew over the Cuckoo's Nest.*
Reality	Diverse, interesting medical work, making a real difference to people's quality of life.
Personality	Excellent communication skills, good teamworker, not prone to panic, able to manage complexity and ambiguity, academic.
Best aspects	Variety in both working day and career. Helping people get their lives back and seeing a real difference from your efforts. Sociable teams, fascinating work, absence of boredom.
Worst aspects	People thinking you're a psychologist—a disservice to them as much as to us! The paperwork—thank goodness for dictation!
Route	Core psychiatry training (p. 55), then specialty training in general adult psychiatry (ST4+). Dual CCT with another psychiatry specialty possible. Exams: MRCPsych.
Numbers	2550 consultants, of whom 60% are women.
Locations	Many based in community hubs, and many on the wards in mental health units. Some in primary care, medical hospitals, and clinics.

Life					Work
Quiet On-call					Busy On-call
Boredom					Burnout
Uncompetitive					Competitive
Low salary					High salary

Psychiatry: intellectual disability

Intellectual disability (ID) psychiatry sits at the intersection of health and social care. The terms ID or learning disability (LD) describe the negative effects of a range of known and unknown conditions on brain development. They cause reduced ability to learn, communicate, live independently, and participate in education and employment. People with ID have higher rates of mental and physical illness and worse health outcomes, when compared with the general population. They also have higher rates of autism, epilepsy, and sensory and motor disabilities.

The patients

Stigma and potential abuse are daily challenges for this patient group. Those with mild ID will be independent in most aspects of their lives. Those with severe or profound ID will be non-verbal and dependent on others for most of their activities of daily living. People with ID are up to three times more likely to have schizophrenia, are more likely to be on the autistic spectrum, and have higher rates of dementia. They are more sensitive to medication side effects, and cautious prescribing is essential. Additionally, they are less able to communicate their symptoms verbally and a change in behaviour is a typical reason for referral. When behaviours become disruptive for those around them, it is called 'challenging behaviour' and this is another common reason for referral.

The work

Assessments are tailored to individuals and psychiatrists will use communication styles that suit a particular patient, such as using pictures instead of words, and speak to those who know the patient best. If challenging behaviour is displayed, they will work with other members of the team to identify the reasons and appropriate treatment strategies. When required, they will use the usual range of psychotropic medication available to other psychiatrists. Additionally, ID psychiatrists are usually skilled in the management of epilepsy.

The job

ID community teams vary, and some areas will have specialist ID services for children, as well as for adults, forensic services, and inpatient units. Community teams will be made up of specialist nurses, psychologists, and occupational therapists. On-call rotas vary between areas and may be ID-specific or combined with a general adult or community Child and Adolescent Mental Health Service (CAMHS) rota.

Extras

Interest in research and clinical leadership will go far in this subspecialty. Private work is available in forensic ID and private inpatient units.

For further information

Faculty of the Psychiatry of Intellectual Disability (of the Royal College of Psychiatrists). Tel: 020 7235 2351. Web: https://www.rcpsych.ac.uk/members/your-faculties/intellectual-disability-psychiatry

Foundation for People with Learning Disabilities. Tel: 020 7803 1100. Web: https://www.mentalhealth.org.uk/learning-disabilities Email: fpld@fpld.org.uk Twitter: @FPLD_Tweets

---

09:00 Weekly team meeting at community base to discuss new referrals, complex cases, and feedback from new assessments

10:30 Home visit with nurse to assess new patient

11:45 Back to base to write up new assessment and make phone calls

12:45 Home visits. Get lunch on the go

15:30 Best interests meeting at a day centre to discuss the pros and cons of starting a patient on anti-dementia medication

16:45 Return to base, make entry in patient records, and dictate letter to GP

18:00 Home

Myth	Handing out Prozac in asylums.
Reality	Making a diagnosis is rarely straightforward and requires varying degrees of detective work.
Personality	Curious, empathetic, and compassionate.
Best aspects	Working with complex patients keeps you on your toes!
Worst aspects	Meetings, meetings, and more meetings!
Route	Core psychiatry training (p. 55), followed by specialty training in psychiatry of LD (ST4+). Exams: MRCPsych.
Numbers	390 consultants, of whom 45% are women.
Locations	Most work is community-based. There are also opportunities for ID psychiatrists in NHS and private inpatient hospitals.

Life					Work
Quiet On-call					Busy On-call
Boredom					Burnout
Uncompetitive					Competitive
Low salary					High salary

Psychiatry: medical psychotherapy

With training in medicine, psychiatry, and psychological therapies, medical psychotherapists are ideally placed to make sense of the whole patient. We all respond to people in some way—there are patients we enjoy seeing and those whom we find challenging, sometimes inspiring a feeling of 'heart-sink' or frustration. Medical psychotherapists explore why different individuals evoke these different responses, what it is about their past experiences that set up these ways of relating to others, and how these patterns are repeated in different areas of their lives, causing them problems.

The patients

Presentations are as diverse as the people we see. This is because psychotherapists tend to see people in terms of both their diagnoses *and* who they are. From a diagnostician's perspective, anxiety, depression, personality disorder, and the human sequelae of trauma are common in the consulting room. Increasingly, psychotherapists treat patients with multiple and complex difficulties e.g. complex post-traumatic stress disorder (PTSD), comorbidity, high-risk behaviours, and forensic histories. Often, these are the patients whom other services and clinicians find it hard to work with and make sense of. Medical psychotherapy can also help teams seeing these patients through case consultation or reflective practice.

The work

One of the most appealing things about this specialty is the time dedicated to getting to know and understand patients in a way that may be new for them. The focus is on the patient and their relationships—with themselves, others, and you as their doctor. Although this closeness can be rewarding, it is also the part that can be the most challenging and emotionally draining. Medical psychotherapists work with clinicians, teams, managers, and wider organizations in health and social care services to try and enable people to 'think under fire' in their various clinical or organizational situations—the objectivity and theoretical understandings gained can help others make sense of their attitudes and behaviours. Communicating complex ideas clearly is part of the challenge and fun of the job.

The job

Medical psychotherapists tend to work in office hours and sometimes do on-call work. They work across a range of settings, including outpatient psychotherapy services, inpatient specialist services, therapeutic communities, and more secure services. There is an increasing role in liaison, with primary and secondary care services, in the care and management of complex and difficult-to-manage patients. Medical psychotherapists train and specialize in a particular type of therapy, usually either psychodynamic psychotherapy or cognitive behavioural therapy. Training usually includes undergoing your own therapy, to help you understand yourself, your work, and what it's like to be a patient.

Extras

There are many teaching opportunities, plus supervision of trainees is a key component. Medical psychotherapy is an increasingly rich avenue for research and remains a good career to write and present academic papers. Private practice is possible. Medical psychotherapy is a small medical specialty, and this means that you meet, get to know, and find support from like-minded colleagues from across the UK and beyond.

For further information

Faculty of Medical Psychotherapy (of the Royal College of Psychiatrists).
Tel: 020 7235 2351. Web: https://www.rcpsych.ac.uk/members/your-faculties/medical-psychotherapy

---

08:30 Arrive at work. Catch up with secretary about appointments for the day

09:00 Meet with mentalization-based treatment team for pre-therapy group preparation

09:30 Mentalization-based treatment group for group of complex patients with borderline personality disorder

11:00 Debrief post-group, a chance to allow our own feelings to settle and to make sense of the work together

11:30 Write up the group and contact a patient's GP about an increase in their risk of self-harm

12:00 Psychotherapy journal club—a trainee presents a paper on transference and countertransference, followed by lively discussion

13:00 One-year psychodynamic psychotherapy patient and admin

14:30 New patient assessment—a man with some forensic history who has struggled to find a place with other services

16:00 Finish up admin and emails for the day. A quick cup of coffee and then home

Myth	Leather couches and an unhealthy obsession with the id, ego, and formative sexual experiences.
Reality	All medical problems involve a psychological aspect, and often our biological and pharmacological interventions fail where talking therapies can make a real difference.
Personality	Thoughtful, intelligent, resilient, empathetic.
Best aspects	Having time to spend with patients and really getting to know and thinking about them. The support and supervision of colleagues.
Worst aspects	Working with patients with the most challenging problems and those whom others find highly anxiety-provoking. This can be tiring.
Route	Core psychiatry training (p. 55), then specialty training in medical psychotherapy (ST4+). Exams: MRCPsych.
Numbers	70 consultants, of whom 80% are women.
Locations	Psychotherapy departments (outpatient) at psychiatric hospitals and clinic sites; sometimes in community outpatient settings, day hospitals, therapeutic communities, or secure services.

Life					Work
Quiet On-call					Busy On-call
Boredom					Burnout
Uncompetitive					Competitive
Low salary					High salary

Psychiatry: old age

Old age psychiatry embraces not only all the psychiatric conditions seen in general adult psychiatric practice, but also the dementias. Because the population is ageing, it is a specialty that is greatly in demand. Many patients have treatable conditions and respond well to specialist interventions—medical and psychological. Based on the principles of person-centred care, the specialty has been at the forefront of interagency and MDT working. The opportunity to make real improvements in someone's quality of life makes this an especially rewarding career.

The patients

Usually over the age of 70 (in some areas over 65) or with dementia at any age. Patients typically have coexisting physical conditions and complex social needs. They do not automatically graduate to the service on the basis of age. Although diagnosing and managing dementia is an important area of the work, the full spectrum of psychiatric disorders is encountered. Patients respond well to treatment, although they can take longer to recover. This means that we get to know them and their support networks well. The patients are often willing to participate in research.

The work

This involves clinical assessment and diagnosis in a team setting with the aim of treatment whilst maintaining a patient's autonomy and independence. History taking is commonly a fascinating process because of the length of life lived. Consultants can specialize in community, inpatient, dementia, and liaison care, although there is considerable overlap. If the psychosocial is as important to you as the biological, you will enjoy this field. If you are interested in the complexity of the ageing process, there are daily decisions to be made regarding the interaction between physical conditions, medication, and the mental health. If you enjoy thinking broadly, you will also be presented with ample opportunity to consider ethics, a variety of legislative frameworks, and family and societal systems when making formulations.

The job

Assessments are done in the patient's own home, including care home settings, as well as outpatient clinics. Memory clinics serve to provide multidisciplinary assessments for those referred with cognitive problems. Liaison work within general hospitals is at last being recognized as an important part of the holistic style of patient care that has for so long been part of old age practice and stand-alone liaison jobs are now more common. Increasingly, services are aligning to a model of crisis response, followed by treatment pathways which reflects growing demand. Teams usually comprise community psychiatric nurses, occupational therapists, psychologists, support workers, and social workers. There are often strong links with voluntary and community organizations. On-call is rarely busy and may be on a separate rota from other psychiatric specialties.

Extras

Whilst it has been a somewhat neglected specialty, there is at last a wider societal acknowledgement of the mental health needs of our ageing population and an interest in meeting them. There have been several national initiatives in recent years leading to important developments in service provision. There are plenty of research opportunities. It is a dynamic time to be an old age psychiatrist. Flexible training and working are well established.

For further information

Faculty of Old Age Psychiatry (of the Royal College of Psychiatrists). Tel: 020 7235 2351. Web: https://www.rcpsych.ac.uk/members/your-faculties/old-age-psychiatry Twitter: @rcpsychOldAge

---

A day in the life ...

09:00 Quiet night on-call ends. Check diary with secretary and speed-read emails. Meet day attachment medical student

09:30 Multidisciplinary team meeting to discuss duty work and allocation. Cases discussed

11:15 Urgent domiciliary assessment with community psychiatric nurse in the home of a severely depressed patient who has expressed suicidal thoughts to her husband

12:30 Phone GP about assessment, do some admin whilst eating lunch

13:00 Memory clinic—review seven patients, only one of whom clearly has dementia

16:00 Supervision of a trainee

17:00 Office shuts, but work done!

Myth	Have powers to make old people do what other people think is best for them.
Reality	Quietly determined individuals whose aim is to optimize and champion the mental, physical, and social well-being of some of the most vulnerable people in our society.
Personality	Curious, creative, and thoughtful. Good at big picture thinking. Enjoys team and family work. Good negotiator. And OK yes, a bit Clark Kent meets the Caped Crusader.
Best aspects	Combines the art and science of medicine. Often able to make a significant improvement in quality of life, including that of the carer. Domiciliary visits.
Worst aspects	Constant restructuring of services, chronic underfunding in social care, shortage of inpatient beds and care home places. Battling ageism.
Route	Core psychiatry training (p. 55), then specialty training in old age psychiatry (ST4+). Exams: MRCPsych.
Numbers	950 consultants, of whom 45% are women.
Locations	Community bases and inpatient units.

Life					Work
Quiet On-call					Busy On-call
Boredom					Burnout
Uncompetitive					Competitive
Low salary					High salary

Public health medicine

Public health medicine is a broad specialty focusing on improving health at a population level. Public health is a multidisciplinary specialism, with consultants coming from both medical and non-medical backgrounds. Public health has three main specialisms: health protection, health improvement, and quality improvement/healthcare public health; and although some consultants specialize in a specific domain of practice, most are generalists. Fundamentally, public health is about system changes to improve the health of the population and reduce inequalities in health outcomes, now and for future generations.

The patients

In public health, this is the population. It can be defined by place, i.e. a geographic area or workplace, by person, i.e. demographics such as ethnicity or sexual orientation, or by a community of interest/behaviour, e.g. people who smoke.

The work

Public health consultants' work is varied, ranging from 'West Wing' politics to 'Outbreak' infectious disease control. Some consultants specialize in health protection as consultants in communicable disease control. Their work is mainly about prevention and controlling outbreaks of infectious diseases like COVID-19, tuberculosis, or Escherichia coli. Others specialize in health improvement, working in local council public health teams to manage and commission programmes to address issues such as childhood obesity or physical inactivity. Some specialize in quality improvement, particularly working with the NHS on commissioning decisions and improving clinical pathways.

The job

Public health is practised in a range of settings. Some consultants work for Public Health England and its equivalents in the devolved nations; others lead teams in local councils, and some work in NHS England and NHS Trusts. Most will work as part of a small multidisciplinary team with a limited budget, making things happen through influence and use of research and evidence.

Extras

Public health is a career that involves being part diplomat, part epidemiologist, and part futurologist, and therefore lends itself to academic work, including teaching and research. There are opportunities to get involved in local and national policy development, which involves developing networks of relationships across silos and topic areas to influence change for the good of the population.

For further information

Faculty of Public Health (FPH). Web: https://www.fph.org.uk Twitter: @FPH

Royal Society for Public Health. Tel: 020 7265 7300. Web: https://www.rsph.org.uk Twitter: @R_S_P_H

08:00 Review emails and agenda for the day and touch base with team for urgent issues

09:30 Meeting with head of leisure services and Clinical Commissioning Group (CCG) well-being lead to talk about integrating physical activity into clinical care pathways

10:00 Meeting with immunization lead to review uptake

11:30 Review paperwork for child death overview panel meeting and discuss potential tensions with CCG safeguarding lead

13:30 Lunch, then meeting with local charity director to discuss their business plan and strategy

15:30 Respond to call from Public Health England health protection team about a case of TB in a local school

16:00 Review quarterly data on NHS health checks performance

16:15 Telephone call with sexual health service provider about condom distribution scheme and community HIV testing. Then more emails and paperwork

18:30 Attend council assembly meeting/health scrutiny panel

20:30 Head home

Myth	Cultural diplomats of the NHS; not quite sure what they do until disaster strikes, then it's all rubber jumpsuits and handwashing drills.
Reality	Varied, intellectually challenging, very much a career where you get to shape your future and explore your passions.
Personality	Team player, strategist, good with numbers, and great with people.
Best aspects	Opportunity to change the world and improve the outcomes for large numbers of people at once, across UK and globally. Interacting with a wide range of people across communities and organizations.
Worst aspects	Can be hard to switch off when you get attached to the issue. Some tensions around pay for those working outside the NHS.
Route	For those with a medical degree, specialty training in public health (ST1+) (p. 57) after foundation training. Typically, 10–15% of training posts go to non-medical graduates.
Numbers	Approximately 750 consultants in England.
Locations	Mix of local government, NHS, and national organizations.

Life						Work
Quiet On-call						Busy On-call
Boredom						Burnout
Uncompetitive						Competitive
Low salary						High salary

Radiology: diagnostic

The name of the game is in the title—making the diagnosis by (sometimes) irradiating the patient! Fancy, high-tech machines and increasing volumes of imaging mean that practically no patient is spared a trip to the radiology department, and that the radiologist plays a key role in the diagnosis, monitoring, and treatment of a wide variety of patients. Using a range of imaging modalities (X-ray, computed tomography (CT), magnetic resonance imaging (MRI), ultrasound, and more), a keen eye for detail, and finely tuned problem-solving skills, the radiologist works closely with other clinicians to manage patients. Despite scaremongering suggestions of being replaced by artificial intelligence, demand for general and subspecialist radiologists is, in fact, growing.

The patients

Seemingly all hospital inpatients and most outpatients get some form of diagnostic imaging. This ranges from a chest X-ray for pneumonia or an abdominal ultrasound in a wriggling child, to a postoperative CT scan or a radioisotope scan to detect cancer. Radiologists do not have overall clinical responsibility for the patient and their interactions with patients are usually a one-off. Patients can be of any age, from the preterm to the centenarian, with all manner of often as-yet-undiagnosed pathologies. If there's a patient with a rare syndrome or an interesting manifestation of a condition, they're guaranteed to have some imaging!

The work

There is a huge range of practice and radiologists are some of the few remaining 'generalists', especially in district general hospitals (DGHs), where they may see patients (and their scans) from any and all medical, surgical, and other specialties. In tertiary centres, there is usually more subspecialization in areas such as musculoskeletal, gastrointestinal, cardiothoracic, or neuroradiology, and there is often overlap with the work of interventional radiologists (p. 284)—some radiologists juggle both! Working closely with other specialty colleagues, either in MDT meetings or on an individual basis, is also an important part of the job.

The job

Generally session-based. It involves performing imaging studies (e.g. ultrasound or fluoroscopy), reporting diagnostic imaging (e.g. CT and MRI), and performing some procedures (e.g. biopsies or injections), alongside radiographers, sonographers, and imaging assistants. The demand for imaging is increasing, including out-of-hours, and on-call commitments for consultants are common—though many hospitals are moving to 'telemedicine' where scans are reported remotely by radiologists elsewhere in the UK and abroad. Trainees will have out-of-hours work.

Extras

Technological advances (better scanners as well as better digital algorithms) are revolutionizing healthcare and imaging, with radiologists at the forefront of this—if you can't beat them, join them! Research into novel techniques and future applications is encouraged, and adapting and implementing change mean that the radiologist's job is constantly evolving. As a consultant-led specialty, there are opportunities to teach trainees, students, and other clinicians. There is a generous scope for private practice, which varies depending on location and subspecialization. Less-than-full-time work is well established both in training and in consultant practice.

For further information

The Royal College of Radiologists (RCR). Tel: 020 7405 1282. Web: https://www.rcr.ac.uk
Email: enquiries@rcr.ac.uk Twitter: @RCRadiologists

08:30 Teaching with trainees

09:00 Reporting outpatient CT scans. Receive an email about an urgent scan, so report this as well

10:30 Quick coffee break to stretch the legs and refocus. Caught in corridor by clinician asking about a scan

10:45 More CT reporting. Several interruptions to discuss urgent scans requested by medics. Accept most requests and suggest better imaging modalities for the rest

12:30 Grab a quick lunch. Chat to colleagues

13:00 Lunchtime MDT—yesterday's preparation makes this run smoothly and to time

14:00 Afternoon ultrasound list—mainly outpatient, but also squeeze in an inpatient that the surgeons are worried about

17:00 Make sure urgent scans have been reported. Admin

17:30 Go home on time!

Myth	Likes hiding in the gloomy hospital basement. Doesn't like patients or being bothered.
Reality	More contact than others think with both patients and colleagues. Does also like playing medical Sherlock Holmes in dark rooms.
Personality	Academic, thorough, with a desire to figure things out. Generalist. Good communication skills. Radiology though is accommodating of all types.
Best aspects	Huge variety, interesting cases, intellectually challenging, good work–life balance.
Worst aspects	Ever increasing workload demands.
Route	Run-through training in radiology (ST1+) (p. 59). Exams: FRCR.
Numbers	4100 consultants, of whom 40% are female.
Locations	Radiology departments which can be found in all acute hospitals.

Life						Work
Quiet On-call						Busy On-call
Boredom						Burnout
Uncompetitive						Competitive
Low salary						High salary

Radiology: interventional

Interventional radiology (IR) is a subspecialty of radiology in which images are used to guide the performance of diagnostic and therapeutic procedures. Further subspecialization is possible, e.g. vascular IR, or neurointervention which deals with pathologies such as intracerebral aneurysms and stroke. With the evolution of imaging technology and rapid expansion in the development of devices, this subspecialty has grown dramatically over recent years. This has allowed specialists to carry out more complex procedures on an ever-expanding patient cohort, often where surgery is not recommended or feasible.

The patients

Patients are seen in elective, semi-elective, and emergency settings, covering a wide spectrum of pathologies, with referrals coming from nearly all surgical and medical subspecialties. Patients can range from young children to the elderly, and from elective cases, such as intravascular line insertions and embolization of liver metastases, to trauma patients requiring immediate lifesaving intervention. The patient cohort often includes the sickest patients in the hospital, many of whom are beyond the help of conventional surgery.

The work

IR utilizes imaging resources such as ultrasound, CT, MRI, and catheter laboratories with fluoroscopy to complete intricate procedures in a minimally invasive fashion. An increasing array of devices such as catheters, wires, stents, and coils, to name but a few, allow the subspecialty to treat a wide variety of conditions. Most departments now have their own IR clinics, with some having the ability to admit patients directly onto hospital wards. IR specialists may spend a small proportion of their jobs in diagnostic radiology (p. 282), giving you the best of both worlds. The varied and rapidly evolving work makes this an exciting subspecialty to be involved with.

The job

Given the increasing number and complexity of cases, close discussion and co-operation between IR and the referring medical and surgical specialties are essential. In many cases, follow-up procedures may be required and underpin the importance of joint care. Sound knowledge of multiple pathological entities and anatomy, alongside excellent hand–eye co-ordination, image interpretation, and technical proficiency, is paramount to carrying out procedures safely and effectively. In any one day, an interventional radiologist may perform multiple different procedures across different anatomical regions, e.g. lower limb angiograms and angioplasty, uterine artery embolization, biopsy of a small liver lesion. IR departments can be very busy and therefore, good teamwork with co-ordinators, nurses, and anaesthetists is essential. On-calls can become very busy in larger teaching hospitals, but there is a good balance to be found in district general hospitals, giving some degree of control to work–life balance.

Extras

With continued technological development, this is a subspecialty that is changing and expanding quickly, allowing opportunities for research and collaboration. There is plenty of scope to get involved in MDT work, in which many interventional radiologists become leaders and key contributors. Private practice is relatively limited in IR. However, with dual accreditation in diagnostic radiology, there are other options to expand your private practice.

For further information

British Society of Interventional Radiology (BSIR). Tel: 020 7406 5998. Web: https://www.bsir.org Email: office@bsir.org Twitter: @BSIR_News

The Royal College of Radiologists (RCR). Tel: 020 7405 1282. Web: https://www.rcr.ac.uk Email: enquiries@rcr.ac.uk Twitter: @RCRadiologists

---

A day in the life ...

08:00	Pre-list team meeting with whole team to plan cases and organize list
09:00	Operating list: five cases, including a biopsy of a lymph node and a nephrostomy insertion
10:23	Emergency call from the medics to insert a chest drain in a complex empyema
11:00	Continue elective list
13:00	Lunch during a gastrointestinal MDT meeting
14:00	Teaching IR trainees
15:30	Outpatient clinic: mix of new referrals and follow-ups
17:00	Clinical review of morning cases, admin
18:00	Home

Myth	Unapproachable. Mean.
Reality	A tough subspecialty requiring a vast understanding of multiple disease processes, and proficient skills to perform intricate procedures which can potentially save a life or limb.
Personality	Caring, compassionate, calm under pressure, technical, analytical, good communicator, team player.
Best aspects	Variety, making an immediate difference, excellent job prospects.
Worst aspects	Reliance on other medical and surgical specialties in referring and preparing patients. Busy on-calls. Diagnostic radiology exams whilst training.
Route	Specialty training in clinical radiology (ST1+) (p. 59), then subspecialty training in IR or neuroradiology (ST4+). Exams: FRCR.
Numbers	700 consultants, including vascular and non-vascular IR and neuroradiology.
Locations	Hospital-based, including secondary and tertiary settings.

Life		Work
Quiet On-call		Busy On-call
Boredom		Burnout
Uncompetitive		Competitive
Low salary		High salary

Rehabilitation medicine

Rehabilitation medicine (also known as physical and rehabilitation medicine (PRM)) entails improving function in patients with disabilities through diagnosis and treatment of health conditions, reducing impairments, and preventing or treating complications. The specialty predominantly deals with neurological and musculoskeletal conditions, and offers the exciting opportunity of providing both acute and long-term care. Specialists work in a balanced mixture of inpatient and outpatient settings, perform some practical procedures, and acquire a wide range of non-technical skills to provide holistic and practical care within a large multidisciplinary team (MDT).

The patients

Are mostly adults of working age but sometimes can include children (spasticity management services) and elderly individuals (trauma rehabilitation services). They have a range of medical diagnoses such as neurological conditions (including traumatic and non-traumatic brain injury, spinal cord injury, stroke, multiple sclerosis, cerebral palsy, neuropathy), musculoskeletal conditions (polytrauma, amputation, arthritis, back pain, chronic pain, soft tissue conditions), cardiovascular conditions (ischaemic heart disease, peripheral vascular disease), critical illness deconditioning, or cancer.

The work

Includes assessing the rehabilitation needs and potential of the patient and facilitating a rehabilitation programme designed specifically for that patient. The medical skills, in particular, include the diagnosis and management of medical problems in patients with disabilities such as acute/chronic pain, autonomic dysfunction, seizures, musculoskeletal problems, neurogenic bladder/bowel, osteoporosis, or nerve entrapment syndromes. Treatments include pharmacological and non-pharmacological methods and procedural interventions (by some consultants) such as botulinum toxin injection, nerve block, spinal injections, and joint or soft tissue injection. The specialist plays a vital role in educating patients and their families on medical conditions and prognoses. They are generally looked upon as the leader of the MDT; hence, teamworking and leadership skills are useful attributes for the role.

The job

Involves working as part of a team that typically includes nurses, physiotherapists, occupational therapists, speech and language therapists, psychologists, engineers, and family members. There are different levels of service based on complexity of care—acute rehabilitation units are based in tertiary care hospitals where specialists may also provide outreach input to intensive care and other acute units; intermediate rehabilitation units (e.g. for neurorehabilitation) are found in district general hospitals. Additionally, specialists may work in outpatient-based services (e.g. musculoskeletal or amputee rehabilitation services) or community-based long-term care units. On-call arrangements vary, depending on the complexity of the service, but are generally relaxed and involve providing phone advice to ward-based juniors.

Extras

There are plentiful opportunities to engage in academic activities and teaching. Research areas include basic science, technology, pharmacological agents, interventions, and health outcomes. Private practice is possible for those with special interest in musculoskeletal conditions or chronic pain. Medico-legal work is available to top up funds for those interested.

For further information

The British Society of Rehabilitation Medicine (BSRM). Tel: 01992 638 865. Web: https://www.bsrm.org.uk Email: admin@bsrm.co.uk Twitter: @BSRehabMed

---

08:30 Emails and admin

09:00 Outpatient clinic (five new referrals and two ward discharge follow-ups)

13:00 Lunch and more emails

13:30 MDT meeting to discuss ward patients' progress in their rehabilitation programmes and update goals

15:00 Medical ward round/undergraduate and postgraduate teaching

16:30 Perform a nerve block for a patient whose pain is limiting their functional recovery

17:00 Discussion with the family of an elderly patient who has progressed well since a major stroke but will still need a lot of ongoing care, support, and rehabilitation after discharge

17:30 Home

Myth	Babysitting medically fit bed-blockers awaiting social discharge.
Reality	One of the larger and more popular specialties in Europe and the USA, with reasonable opportunities for acute work, private practice, and interventional procedures, with flexibility in working pattern.
Personality	People person, team player, philosophical, patient, good sense of humour, philanthropist.
Best aspects	Working with the patient lifelong (beyond the diagnosis); restoring function and quality of life; understanding the bigger picture of life; interface of neurology and musculoskeletal medicine; MDT working.
Worst aspects	Lack of adrenaline rush in everyday job; lack of recognition and support to develop services as not a money spinner.
Route	Specialty training in rehabilitation medicine (ST3+) from one of several core training pathways, e.g. acute care common stem (ACCS) (p. 37), GP (p. 42), internal medicine training (IMT) (p. 44), psychiatry (p. 55), and surgery (p. 61). Exams: exams relevant to core/initial specialty.
Numbers	200 consultants, of whom 35% are women.
Locations	Specialist hospitals, district general hospitals, community care centres, and outpatient services.

Life					Work
Quiet On-call					Busy On-call
Boredom					Burnout
Uncompetitive					Competitive
Low salary					High salary

Renal medicine

Nephrology is an increasingly prominent specialty due to the rising prevalence of chronic kidney disease and the recognition of the impact of acute kidney injury on morbidity and mortality. Challenges in nephrology include finding practical and ethical solutions to a growing need for renal replacement therapy (dialysis and transplantation), in addition to finding effective treatments for renal disease. Nephrologists manage a diverse range of patients and pathologies, and are required to have an excellent knowledge of general internal medicine, and adopt a holistic approach to clinical problems.

The patients

Nephrologists see patients with a wide range of pathologies, and at different stages of their disease. Patients with acute kidney injury may be extremely unwell with multiple organ failure and looked after in an intensive care unit (ICU) or high dependency unit (HDU) setting. A significant proportion of outpatients may suffer chronic kidney disease due to diabetes and hypertension, and many have complex glomerulonephritides requiring immunosuppression and careful monitoring. Nephrologists also run joint clinics with, for example, HIV-specialists, hepatologists, obstetricians, rheumatologists, and haematologists. Patients on renal replacement therapy (haemo- and peritoneal dialysis and transplantation) are followed up for life, and thus develop close working relationships with their nephrology team.

The work

Inpatient work includes seeing extremely unwell patients with acute kidney injury in the ICU or HDU, managing perioperative living and deceased donor kidney transplants, dealing with access-related problems in dialysis patients, and managing complications of immunosuppression in transplant recipients. Outpatient work is similarly varied, with dialysis, transplant, chronic kidney disease, and cross-specialty clinics, and multidisciplinary meetings with radiologists and histopathologists.

The job

Nephrologists work as part of a large team that also includes transplant and vascular access surgeons, transplant co-ordinators, tissue typists, dialysis nurses, technicians, interventional radiologists, and histopathologists. Good communication skills and approachability are essential. Renal patients often have complex medical and surgical problems, and an organized, methodical approach is vital. On-calls can be very busy, and most nephrology centres have a registrar on-site 24 hours a day.

Extras

There is a strong tradition of academia in renal medicine, and clinical or basic science research and teaching is encouraged. The UK Renal Registry offers epidemiological renal research opportunities. Centres may have links to units in other countries; thus, working abroad is possible. For various reasons, private practice is minimal outside London. Flexible training and working are possible.

For further information

UK Kidney Association (previously known as The Renal Association). Tel: 0117 4148152. Web: https://ukkidney.org Email: renal@renal.org Twitter: @RenalAssoc

The UK Renal Registry. Tel: 0117 414 8150. Web: https://ukkidney.org/about-us/who-we-are/uk-renal-registry Email: renalregistry@renalregistry.nhs.uk Twitter: @UKRenalRegistry

---

A day in the life ...

08:30 Morning handover with multidisciplinary team

09:00 Ward round of inpatients on renal wards, HDU, outliers, and ICU

10:30 Procedures in theatre: one kidney biopsy and insertion of a peritoneal dialysis catheter

13:00 Lunch (may be whilst in MDT, biopsy or radiology meeting, academic presentation or journal club)

13:30 Outpatient clinic: 12 patients, four new patients with chronic kidney disease

17:00 Board round, check results, and evening handover

18:30 Home

Myth	Hypercritical sociopaths obsessed with electrolytes, anion gaps, and complex fluid regimens. Refuse to see death as a contraindication to dialysis.
Reality	Reasonably academic and extremely attentive doctors with a passion for physiology and a dedication to long-term patient care.
Personality	Attention to detail, organized, pragmatic, calm, approachable, with good communication skills.
Best aspects	Variety, blend of acute medicine and academia, long-term care of patients.
Worst aspects	Friday evenings spent inserting lines into patients who were referred by the medical team at 5 p.m., despite them not having passed urine for 48 hours.
Route	Internal medicine training (IMT) (p. 44) or acute care common stem–acute medicine (ACCS-AM) (p. 37), followed by specialty training in renal medicine (ST3+); often dual-accrediting with general internal medicine or intensive care medicine (p. 39). Exams: MRCP; SCE in Nephrology.
Numbers	750 consultants, of whom 30% are women.
Locations	Tertiary referral centre in a teaching hospital, or in a large district general hospital.

Life						Work
Quiet On-call						Busy On-call
Boredom						Burnout
Uncompetitive						Competitive
Low salary						High salary

▌ Respiratory medicine

Respiratory medicine focuses on the investigation and care of patients with lung disease, the most common being asthma, chronic obstructive pulmonary disease (COPD), respiratory infections, sleep-disordered breathing, and lung cancer. Less common conditions include tuberculosis, cystic fibrosis (CF), interstitial lung diseases (ILDs), pulmonary vascular disease, occupational lung diseases, and many more. It requires a strong foundation in general medicine with expert knowledge, alongside procedural skills.

The patients

Patients with respiratory disease are adults of all age groups, backgrounds, and ethnicities. Inpatients are often older, particularly those with COPD and respiratory failure. Patients often present with breathlessness, cough, or wheeze. They may also be referred due to abnormal thoracic imaging. The physical and social environment of the patient is highly relevant. Respiratory physicians are interested in housing, occupation, migration, substance addiction, and poverty as these all influence disease pathophysiology and treatment.

The work

Respiratory physicians work under pressure in the acute setting, particularly when caring for those with respiratory failure or severe asthma. They are experts in risk assessment: determining whether to intervene in a pneumothorax; when to thrombolyse a pulmonary embolism; when to give immunosuppression in ILD; and how to manage a pulmonary nodule. They communicate uncertainty during the diagnostic process of lung cancer, ILD, and breathlessness, whilst simultaneously providing reassurance to patients and their families. They are advocates and coaches when discussing the value of physical exercise and smoking cessation. They are adept at practical procedures, including pleural interventions and bronchoscopy. They form long-term relationships with patients, from diagnosis until death, and provide general palliative care to those with advanced disease.

The job

Most posts are hospital-based, caring for inpatients, running clinics, attending MDTs, and performing procedures. However, there are a growing number of integrated physicians who work from community hubs and general practices, as well as in patients' homes. Teamwork is key, working closely with radiologists, pathologists, oncologists, physiotherapists, psychologists, nurses, and advanced practitioners. Demand for expertise far outstrips the capacity to see every patient, so expertise in triage, running virtual clinics, and providing in-reach and education to other teams is essential.

Extras

As one of the only specialties to maintain strong general medicine expertise, respiratory physicians are well suited to take on educational roles at undergraduate and postgraduate levels. There are research opportunities spanning genomics, immunology, interventional bronchoscopy, exercise physiology, drug trials, and epidemiology. Flexible working is well established. There are opportunities for private practice for those interested. Respiratory physicians are increasingly at the centre of global issues, asked to add their expert knowledge in combatting air pollution and climate change, and to treat, control, and prevent global pandemics of respiratory viruses; working with some of the most deprived in society also often leads them to campaign on issues of climate and social justice.

For further information

British Thoracic Society (BTS). Tel: 020 7831 8778. Web: https://www.brit-thoracic.org.uk
Twitter: @BTSrespiratory

European Respiratory Society (ERS). Tel: +41 21 213 01 01. Web: https://www.ersnet.org/
Twitter: @EuroRespSoc

08:30 Triage referrals (lung cancer/sleep specialty referrals, bronchoscopy/pleural requests, GP referrals)

09:00 Board round on inpatient ward and review of new and sick patients

10:00 Bronchoscopy list with trainee

12:00 MDT with specialist nurses and colleagues from other specialties (e.g. lung cancer, CF, ILD, integrated care)

14:00 Outpatient clinic: 20 patients between consultant and trainee

17:00 Return to ward to answer queries from junior doctors and check plans for discharges

17:15 Admin, including signing off letters and answering emails. Respond to trainee queries related to ward referrals

18:00 Leave work

19:00 Prepare talk for teaching session or work on quality improvement or research project

Myth	Quite nice people with sputum obsession. Only have steroids and inhalers to offer.
Reality	Sputum-interested, kind, and committed people with a raft of interventions beyond steroids and inhalers.
Personality	Compassionate, holistic, patient, calm under pressure, skilled in managing and communicating risk and uncertainty, able to problem-solve diagnostic dilemmas, decisive, forward thinking, able to manage and lead teams.
Best aspects	Diversity of patients, pathologies and day-to-day work; mixture of acute care and long-term condition management; strong emphasis on teamwork; the intricate beauty of the chest CT.
Worst aspects	Intensity of work, particularly inpatient work over winter; emotional fatigue; feeling of powerlessness faced with diseases driven by inequality, poverty, and environment.
Route	Either internal medicine training (IMT) (p. 44) or acute care common stem–acute medicine (ACCS-AM) (p. 37), then specialty training in respiratory medicine (ST3+). Exams: MRCP; SCE in Respiratory Medicine.
Numbers	1500 consultants, of whom 30% are women.
Locations	Mostly hospitals (tertiary and district general), with increasing integrated care spanning community settings.

Life					Work
Quiet On-call					Busy On-call
Boredom					Burnout
Uncompetitive					Competitive
Low salary					High salary

▌ Rheumatology

Rheumatology deals with the investigation, diagnosis, and management of more than 200 disorders affecting joints, bones, muscles, and soft tissues. These include inflammatory arthritis and other systemic autoimmune disorders, vasculitis, soft tissue conditions, spinal pain, and metabolic bone disease. Additionally, many of these disorders affect a host of other organ systems, including the lung, kidney, skin, nervous system, and gut.

The patients

People with rheumatic conditions span all ages and backgrounds. Paediatric rheumatology is a separate paediatric subspecialty, managing patients under 16 years of age. It has been said that rheumatologists are physicians to the innocent, as in general neither lifestyle nor social class protect from autoimmune disease. Disorders such as rheumatoid arthritis are lifelong illnesses that can be treated and controlled, but not cured. Rheumatologists will develop professional relationships with patients and their families which will endure throughout their medical career.

The work

There are two major roles for the rheumatologist: the first is diagnostic; anything that presents with pain or unexplained systemic inflammation may be referred to rheumatology—one patient may have inflammatory arthritis, but the next may have cancer or a complex psychological illness. Good generalist skills are required. The second role is in management of long-term disorders, and rheumatologists must work as part of a multidisciplinary team (MDT) to deliver complex treatment programmes. Advances in immunotherapy over the last two decades have transformed the ability to control autoimmune disease beyond recognition. Rheumatologists need a detailed knowledge of immunology and therapeutics, strong interpersonal skills, and the ability to take a long-term view in collaboration with patients.

The job

There is more than one way to be a rheumatologist. About half of UK rheumatologists combine rheumatology with general or acute medicine, whilst the rest practise rheumatology as a single specialty. Rheumatology practice is predominantly based in an outpatient setting, although inpatient work remains an important component (primarily consultative and, in some cases, direct care of rheumatology beds). An increasing number of services are delivered from a community setting. Teamworking is a core part of rheumatology—specialist nurses are key colleagues, but working with therapists, GPs, and consultants in other specialties is essential. Practical skills are required in joint aspiration and injection, and many rheumatologists also have expertise in diagnostic ultrasound.

Extras

There are opportunities for subspecialization, especially in multisystem autoimmune disease or complex metabolic bone disease. These services are usually delivered from regional centres. Research and educational opportunities are excellent across the UK. Being outpatient-based, it can suit flexible working and training. Usually good opportunities to do private practice.

For further information

The British Society for Rheumatology. Tel: 020 7842 0900. Web: https://www.rheumatology.org.uk Email: bsr@rheumatology.org.uk Twitter: @RheumatologyUK

A day in the life ...

08:30 Drink coffee and triage referrals from primary care.

09:00 Ward round. Normally 1–2 inpatients (usually connective tissue disease or vasculitis) and 4–5 requests for consultation

11:00 Supervision meeting with specialty trainee

11:30 Check results from clinics, sign prescriptions.

12:30 Lunchtime team meeting. Catch up with specialist nurse and review calls to emergency helpline

13:30 Clinic: three new patients (suspected early inflammatory arthritis), seven routine follow-ups

17:00 Discuss patients seen in clinic with MDT, including specialist nurse and trainee

18:00 Make it back to office, sign extra biologics prescriptions that turned up, water office plant

19:00 Home. Check out rheumatology news on Twitter, and decide on the topic for journal club next week

Myth	Pleasant, but slow-stream clinicians prescribing steroids to elderly and disabled patients with a variety of hand deformities.
Reality	A friendly specialty. Dynamic team leaders. Transforming the lives of people of all ages with complex multisystem disease. At the cutting edge of immunological therapeutics.
Personality	Needs balance of medical and personal skills. Long-term conditions require an interest in people, as well as in diseases, and a need to take the long view. Teamworker.
Best aspects	Making a difficult diagnosis which has eluded others. Seeing treatment rapidly reduce pain and disability. Being at the cutting edge of immunological therapeutics. Teamworking. Good work–life balance.
Worst aspects	Lack of a cure for most rheumatological disorders and seeing morbidity and mortality develop over time. Understanding of specialty by colleagues (and friends and family!) often limited.
Route	Internal medicine training (IMT) (p. 44) or acute care common stem–acute medicine (ACCS-AM) (p. 37), then specialty training in rheumatology (ST3+). Exams: MRCP; SCE in Rheumatology.
Numbers	900 consultants, of whom 50% are women.
Locations	Specialist and general hospitals and increasingly in the community.

Life					Work
Quiet On-call					Busy On-call
Boredom					Burnout
Uncompetitive					Competitive
Low salary					High salary

Sexual and reproductive healthcare

Sexual and reproductive healthcare is an exciting and relatively new community-based specialty. Previously known as family planning, its name and role have evolved to encompass a wide range of contraceptive services, gynaecology, and genitourinary medicine. It involves large patient numbers and can often feel hectic, but the patients are ambulatory and usually well. Those working in the specialty find it rewarding as there is a sense of enhancing their lives in partnership with the patients, rather than making them better as in other traditional medical models.

The patients

Patients are mostly (but not exclusively) women and range from young teenagers to the elderly, and there will often be specialized work with vulnerable members of society. Hence there is no such thing as a 'typical' patient. In one day, a specialist might see a young teenager needing emergency contraception, an older woman exploring menopause treatment options, and a man with sexual problems.

The work

Services delivered include contraception, treatment of sexually transmitted infections, abortion care, gynaecological care (including procedures in outpatient settings), sexual assault (forensics), and menopause. However, mostly doctors do not end up doing *all* of these jobs at once. Most of the work is clinic-based, with much of it in community or day-case settings.

The job

The hours are reasonably sociable, with occasional evening clinics and sometimes weekends. Nevertheless, due to the breadth of areas covered, the workload can be large and you need to have excellent organizational skills to cope with the diversity of the demands and settings. It is vital to be self-motivated and determined. Much of the job involves systems leadership, so it can help if you have excellent communication skills and are a natural leader (or have the willingness to become one!). To be successful in this specialty, it is important to have the traits of a good public health doctor, i.e. to be interested in populations, as well as in individuals.

Extras

There is plenty of opportunity to get involved in teaching, as much of your clinical time will be training other doctors, nurses, and allied healthcare professionals. There are no night shifts, so the pay is lower than in some other specialties. However, the lifestyle is pleasant and offers a great work–life balance. Many work less than full time, and it is a specialty that lends itself to family life. A real plus of the specialty is that it offers such a wide variety of career opportunities. There is the possibility to create a career that is individual to you—according to your personal skill set and the local population health needs.

For further information

The Faculty of Sexual and Reproductive Healthcare (FSRH) of the Royal College of Obstetricians and Gynaecologists. Tel: 020 7724 5534. Web: https://www.fsrh.org
Twitter: @FSRH_UK

08:30 Teaching junior doctors examination skills and discussing findings from recent audit

09:00 MDT meeting and handover with other doctors, nurses, and health advisors. Allocate roles for the morning walk-in sexual health and contraception clinic

09:10 Review male patient needing treatment for rectal symptoms

10:00 Asked to review female patient with pelvic inflammatory disease

10:30 Scan female with right-sided pelvic pain; ovarian mass found. Phone referral to gynaecology on-call team

11:30 Emergency intrauterine device (IUD) insertion for post-coital contraception

13:00 Lunch break and drive to afternoon session at hospital across town

14:00 Outpatient hysteroscopy clinic in hospital. See seven patients, all with cervical blocks for endometrial biopsies and some for IUD insertions

17:10 Finish afternoon list. Catch up with emails

17:35 Leave for home

Myth	An easy option for people who don't get into O&G and prefer to live a stress-free existence.
Reality	It is highly competitive, and at times stressful. Requires the ability to 'juggle many balls'.
Personality	Proactivity, a commitment to preventative medicine, and not being afraid to raise one's head above the parapet. Highly driven and self-motivated.
Best aspects	Good work–life balance. Large variety of clinical duties keeps it interesting on a day-to-day basis. Can, to some degree, design a unique career pathway.
Worst aspects	Can be lonely (few trainees, geographically isolated, working alone in clinics). Misunderstood by other specialties.
Route	Run-through training in community sexual and reproductive healthcare (ST1+). Exams: MFSRH.
Numbers	115 consultants in England.
Locations	Mostly community-based services (i.e. integrated sexual and reproductive health departments), with some outpatient and day surgery in acute settings.

Life					Work
Quiet On-call					Busy On-call
Boredom					Burnout
Uncompetitive					Competitive
Low salary					High salary

Spine surgery

Spine surgery includes all aspects of surgical treatment of the vertebral column. There are two pathways into the career—via neurosurgical or orthopaedic specialist training. Much greater overlap has developed between these fields in recent years, with spine surgeons from both areas operating on all areas of the spine. Neurosurgeons still deal with intradural surgery, i.e. pathology inside the dural sac, such as intradural tumours, and orthopods manage spinal deformity surgery such as scoliosis. It is a hugely diverse and technically demanding branch of surgery, with the broadest range and most extensive approaches.

The patients

Are a very wide and varied group of all ages. There are an increasing number of cancer patients, as techniques have improved in this area and a lot can be done to improve quality of life with palliative procedures. There is also the chance to develop long-term working relationships with patients and their families during long-term follow-up and treatment in spinal deformity clinics. There are many patients with conditions that can be rapidly cured, such as disc prolapse with sciatica, but also those with long-term chronic pain and complex psychological issues, such as chronic back pain, who need a fully holistic approach.

The work

Breaks down into several major areas: spinal deformity, primary and secondary tumours of the spine, degenerative conditions of the cervical/lumbar spine, spinal trauma (including spinal cord injury), and infections of the spine. All of these areas try to protect or restore neurological function and treat painful instability or spinal nerve compression. Covering such a wide range often means working in large multidisciplinary groups, especially with pain anaesthetists, radiologists, oncologists, and paediatricians, as well as specialist ward and theatre nurses, physiotherapists, and neurophysiologists. A close understanding of the anatomy of the spine and the biomechanics of movement and surgical implants is required, and specialists rapidly become well versed in magnetic resonance imaging (MRI) and computed tomography (CT)!

The job

Is demanding from the point of technical ability, as well as stamina. Spine surgery, similar to vascular surgery (p. 314), has developed as a 'stand-alone' specialty, so specialization tends to be completely in the field rather than 'as an interest'. It also involves quite a bit of emergency work such as managing cauda equina syndrome or metastatic spinal cord compression. This means regularly working on a busy on-call rota, though the work is immediately rewarding. Approaching the spine may need to be done from the front and/or back in any part of the body, meaning specialists need to be able to deal with neck, abdominal, and thoracic surgery as well as the usual musculoskeletal work.

Extras

It is a relatively small surgical specialty in the UK, with a huge patient base, so you will never be bored or unemployed! There are great opportunities for international co-operation, humanitarian work, and teaching. For those who want to work privately, there is a lot of work available. The field also has many ground-breaking areas for clinical and laboratory research.

For further information

British Association of Spine Surgeons (BASS). Tel: 020 7406 1768. Web: https://www.spinesurgeons.ac.uk Email: info@spinesurgeons.ac.uk Twitter: @BASSspine

The Society of British Neurological Surgeons (SBNS). Tel: 020 7869 6892. Web: https://www.sbns.org.uk Email: admin@sbns.org.uk Twitter: @The_SBNS

08:15 Morning trauma meeting discussing overnight admissions, followed by acute ward round

09:30 Spinal clinic: 14 patients, a mixture of acute and urgent referrals

12:30 Multidisciplinary team meeting with radiology team

14:00 Operating list—a cervical total disc replacement, decompression of lumbar stenosis, and a nerve root injection block; all cases entered onto the British Spine Registry

17:30 Postoperative check with clinical nurse practitioners

18:00 Home to write teaching presentation for the Royal College of Chiropractors on 'Use of non-threatening language in back pain'

Myth	Futile surgery for the untreatable, undiagnosable, and unstable.
Reality	Technically demanding, with significant risks, but most patients get fantastic benefit.
Personality	Demands stamina, ability to concentrate for some very long operations, need to be patient and rigorous about careful workup, investigation, and preparation.
Best aspects	At best, it's life-changing surgery in areas where conservative treatment has little to offer; the most multidisciplinary of all orthopaedic specialties; huge technical developments over past decade.
Worst aspects	Ill-informed views of outcome in primary and secondary care; inappropriate referral of 'heart-sink' back pain patients due to lack of proper rehabilitation/cognitive behavioural therapy (CBT) regimes in the community; challenging complications.
Route	Core surgical training (CST) (p. 61), followed by specialty training in trauma and orthopaedics or neurosurgery. Post-CCT fellowship. Exams: MRCS; FRCS relevant to surgical specialty.
Locations	Usually teaching hospitals or large district general hospitals.

Life					Work
Quiet On-call					Busy On-call
Boredom					Burnout
Uncompetitive					Competitive
Low salary					High salary

Sport and exercise medicine

Sport and exercise medicine (SEM) is an exciting and relatively new specialty which was officially recognized in 2005. Much of the work deals with sports injuries, musculoskeletal and medical problems associated with physical activity, and advising on exercise for the inactive. The population has become increasingly sedentary and the incidence of non-communicable diseases such as cardiovascular disease and type 2 diabetes is rising. Physical activity helps to prevent the onset of such diseases and also has a role in their management. Training in SEM gives the clinician skills in the assessment and management of sports-related musculoskeletal and medical problems, and in prescribing exercise.

The patients

Patients seen in SEM clinics are not necessarily athletic or sporty (though many are); they may be young or old and experiencing symptoms due to musculoskeletal injury or dysfunction, or those related to medical problems in those who exercise. Patients in the clinic may have chronic diseases (e.g. heart or lung disease) and be attending for exercise prescription.

The work

Work is almost exclusively clinic-based and may include ultrasound and administration of diagnostic and therapeutic injections. Clinicians may become involved in the provision of cardiopulmonary exercise testing. Multidisciplinary teamworking is at the heart of the specialty, as doctors in SEM work closely with other colleagues such as orthopaedic surgeons, physiotherapists, podiatrists, and dieticians. Outside of NHS work, many SEM physicians have roles within sports teams and organizations that give them experience in caring for athletes both at elite and grass-roots level. Providing medical cover at a sport event may involve pitch side or emergency care of athletes or injured participants. Work at such events includes wound closure, assessment of acute injuries and the concussed athlete, and limb splinting or spinal immobilization in the context of more severe trauma.

The job

Patients may be seen in hospital- or community-based outpatient clinics. There are at present no on-call commitments in SEM. However, clinicians may work with sports teams and sporting events during the weekends and outside of normal working hours.

Extras

Developing an evidence base for this specialty is key and clinicians are encouraged to become involved with research. There are also opportunities to get involved with teaching at every level, including medical students, postgraduate students, and on pitch-side trauma courses. SEM is a dynamic and interesting specialty that provides a highly varied and rewarding workload. There may be opportunities to work at various sporting institutes, in the Armed Forces and in the private sector which may be as lucrative as they are exciting.

For further information

Faculty of Sport and Exercise Medicine (FSEM). Tel: 0131 527 1612. Web: https://www.fsem.ac.uk Email: enquiries@fsem.ac.uk Twitter: @FSEM_UK

British Association of Sport and Exercise Medicine (BASEM). Tel: 01302 623222. Web: https://basem.co.uk Email: enquiries@basem.co.uk Twitter: @basem_uk

08:00 Arrive at NHS sports injuries clinic. See 12 patients with musculoskeletal problems

12:00 Lunch meeting with colleagues from other specialties to talk about the benefits of physical activity promotion for their patients and how this can be delivered

14:00 Working on a grant proposal to increase the evidence base of the cost-effectiveness of delivering physical activity interventions

15:30 Journal club session with SEM registrars

16:00 Joint ultrasound for two follow-up patients

19:00 Attend sports team training session to be available to deal with any medical issues that arise

Myth	Jet-setters massaging elite athletes in exotic destinations.
Reality	Variety; the work can be taken in a number of directions, with the focus being on musculoskeletal problems, elite athletes, and/or physical activity and health promotion.
Personality	Teamworker, multitasker, innovative, able to 'sell' this specialty.
Best aspects	Getting to the bottom of why an injury has occurred rather than just fixing it; working in a team; helping to develop the specialty and its evidence base.
Worst aspects	Few NHS jobs—many consultants have had to write a business case to justify creating a new post. Constantly having to explain what you do to patients and colleagues.
Route	Specialty training in sports and exercise medicine (ST3+) is accessible from several core training pathways, e.g. acute care common stem–emergency or acute medicine (ACCS-EM) (p. 37), GP (p. 42), and internal medicine training (IMT) (p. 44). Exams: relevant membership exams of core/initial specialty; Diploma in SEM.
Numbers	30 consultants, of whom 20% are women.
Locations	Clinics are mostly in secondary or primary care; maybe travel between clinics, other institutions, and sports grounds.

Life					Work
Quiet On-call					Busy On-call
Boredom					Burnout
Uncompetitive					Competitive
Low salary					High salary

Stroke medicine

Long gone are the days of the fatalistic belief that nothing can be done for individuals with stroke. Stroke care has evolved from the observation of 'hopeless cases' on general medical wards to revolutionary acute and rehabilitation treatment by specialists in dedicated stroke units. It's incredibly rewarding to see someone walk out of hospital who previously would have been left severely disabled. Stroke medicine is a relatively new specialty, expanding rapidly in the era of hyperacute stroke treatments of thrombolysis (clot-busting injections) and thrombectomy (catheter-based clot retrieval). However, it not only deals with the management of acute strokes, but also urgent outpatient management of transient ischaemic attacks (TIAs), and post-stroke rehabilitation. As such, it combines some of the best aspects of neurology, geriatric medicine, rehabilitation medicine, cardiology, and acute medicine.

The patients

Most patients fall into one of three groups: those needing acute management, those receiving rehabilitation, and those being seen for suspected TIAs. Stroke services typically see adults of all ages, though most will be older individuals. Stroke is a heterogeneous disease, including ischaemic and haemorrhagic types, with a variety of different causes. This often means investigating for, and addressing, common treatable causes, whilst managing a range of comorbidities. Rehabilitation focuses on the spectrum of symptoms that stroke survivors may experience: physical weakness, speech disturbance, and psychological or cognitive effects.

The work

A stroke physician's day may involve moving between the emergency department, stroke unit, and outpatient clinic. Most of work is ward-based, looking after individuals who have had a recent stroke or are receiving longer-term rehabilitation. Most centres also have daily rapid access clinics for urgent reviews of individuals presenting with suspected TIAs. In clinic settings, there is a considerable proportion (sometimes up to 50%) who will be seen with acute neurological symptoms not due to stroke, so a good understanding of neurology and general medicine is essential. There is significant collaboration with a range of colleagues, including other doctors (vascular surgeons, cardiologists, radiologists, neuro-intensivists), specialist nurses, physiotherapists, occupational therapists, and speech and language therapists.

The job

Most stroke physicians split their time between acute care (responding to hyperacute stroke calls and looking after patients with recent strokes), rehabilitation, and outpatient clinics. The workload can vary considerably between these different aspects, but the variety helps keep this manageable. The shift towards becoming a more acute specialty ('time is brain') has resulted in an increasingly consultant-led service. Whilst on-calls can be busy, this often occurs in collaboration with the growing number of stroke specialist nurses trained in thrombolysis and the increasing role of telemedicine in patient assessment.

Extras

For those interested in service development, the rapid expansion and closely audited delivery of stroke services mean there are many opportunities to get involved in quality improvement and management. There are also lots of opportunities to get involved in research, which can vary from basic science to clinical and rehabilitation trials, and teaching. Private practice is relatively limited, though there are some opportunities in the outpatient setting. Flexible training is possible.

For further information

British Association of Stroke Physicians (BASP). Tel: 01506 292046. Web: https://www. basp.org Email: admin@basp.org Twitter: @british_stroke

---

A day in the life ...

08:30 Handover from night team, review imaging from new admissions

09:00 Consultant-led ward review of new admissions and hyperacute stroke unit

10:00 Registrar-led ward round of remainder of stroke unit

11:15 Thrombolysis call to emergency department—patient thrombolysed and taken back to the hyperacute stroke unit for monitoring

12:00 Multidisciplinary team meeting followed by lunch with the team

13:00 Radiology meeting to discuss cases from the week and review repeat imaging from the patient thrombolysed yesterday

14:00 TIA clinic

16:30 Thrombolysis call to the emergency department—patient appears to have had an episode of low blood sugar—re-referred to acute medicine

17:00 Meeting with a patient's family to discuss their care and prognosis

18:00 Home, put kids to bed, watch TV, plan tomorrow's medical student teaching

Myth	'Cinderella' specialty; an undesirable adjunct to the rota for reluctant neurologists, geriatricians, and generalists.
Reality	Stroke medicine will go to the ball; using skills and knowledge from neurology, geriatrics, rehabilitation, and general medicine to meaningfully improve outcomes.
Personality	Attention to detail, good team player, good communication skills, calm in emergencies.
Best aspects	Satisfaction when hyperacute treatment reduces disability; variety in clinical cases and work environment; opportunities to broaden experience in research and quality improvement.
Worst aspects	High intensity, can be emotionally draining, frequent out-of-hours commitments.
Route	Either internal medicine training (IMT) (p. 44) or acute care common stem—acute medicine (ACCS-AM) (p. 37), then specialty training (geriatrics, neurology, rehabilitation medicine, clinical pharmacology, cardiology, general internal medicine, or acute internal medicine) and subspecialty training in stroke medicine (ST4+). Exams: MRCP.
Numbers	320 consultants, of whom 25% are women.
Locations	District general and teaching hospitals. In some areas hyperacute stroke services have been centralized in a 'hub-and-spoke' model.

Life					Work
Quiet On-call					Busy On-call
Boredom			☺		Burnout
Uncompetitive	🏆				Competitive
Low salary			💰		High salary

Transfusion medicine

Transfusion medicine is a rapidly developing clinical discipline. From massive transfusion to monoclonal antibodies, practice covers all aspects of blood-based medicine and science. In the UK, it is a subspecialty of haematology, whereas in other countries, practitioners may come from a wide range of specialties. The recent developments in transfusion safety, trauma, and cellular therapy draw upon many disciplines, from genomics to behavioural science. Transfusion medicine now provides a unique opportunity to combine clinical, research, and management skills to deliver individual patient care and address public health problems.

The patients

Most patients are haematology cases of all ages receiving treatments and transplants for conditions such as leukaemia, lymphoma, and lifelong blood disorders, e.g. haemophilia. Transfusion medicine consultants also contribute to the diagnosis and management of patients in most other specialties, including trauma, obstetrics, surgery, and intensive care. Transfusion consultants may directly oversee monoclonal antibody and plasma exchange therapy. However, most patients receiving transfusions will never meet their transfusion specialist, even though the latter plays a central role in their safe and effective care.

The work

Transfusion medicine has transformed in the last 20 years from one led by laboratory-based 'blood bankers' to an independent clinical haematology subspecialty. Hospital-based practitioners are often in joint posts, working in both a teaching hospital and the blood service. Core hospital activities include close collaboration with the transfusion laboratory scientists and nurses, tailoring transfusion support for individual patients, advising high-use specialties such as surgery and stem cell transplantation, and supporting major incident planning. Blood service activities might include complex diagnostics such as identifying rare antibodies, developing new blood components, and research. The varied management work includes running regional meetings, writing policy and papers, supporting projects, encouraging audit, and delivery of education and exams.

The job

Transfusion medicine is practised in hospitals, blood services, and research units. The role may suit a wide variety of individuals. This includes those who wish to combine a clinical and academic career within the hospital setting, as well as those considering a non-patient-facing job. Posts vary considerably, with part-time options. Most include some out-of-hours on-call commitment. Recently, clinical posts have been joint appointments created between blood services and a local Trust or other organization. Others, such as donor medicine (blood, stem cells, and tissues), are confined to the national blood transfusion services. Post-holders are encouraged to hold honorary appointments with a teaching hospital and/or university.

Extras

Good opportunities exist for teaching, overseas travel, and research. UK transfusion experts are often requested to join national committees and shape international practice. Some private practice is available, and the work readily supports applications for clinical excellence awards.

For further information

British Blood Transfusion Society (BBTS). Tel: 0161 232 7999. Web: https://www.bbts.org.uk Email: bbts@bbts.org.uk Twitter: @BritishBloodTS

NHS Blood and Transplant. Tel: 0300 123 23 23. Web: https://www.nhsbt.nhs.uk Twitter: @NHSBT

A day in the life ...

08:00 Review diary for day and confirm priorities

08:30 Attend multidisciplinary trauma team meeting. Review the CODE REDs massive haemorrhage activations

10:00 Ward round with trainee and senior nurse, seeing inpatients and referrals

12:00 Review cases from transfusion laboratory. A young woman has been admitted with a rare blood disorder and is at risk of stroke, needing an emergency plasma exchange

13:00 Lunch and catch-up with research colleagues. Update clinical trial Twitter feed and plan next newsletter

14:00 Deliver training for theatre staff on non-medical 'prescribing' of blood. Provide recent evidence base and support plans for audit

17:00 Review blood results and discharge day-case patients

17:30 Home for supper. On-call remotely until tomorrow morning

02:00 Call from the acute medics—a chemotherapy patient has sepsis and no white cells. Organize an urgent transfusion of donor white cells from the lab

Myth	White-coated blood banker.
Reality	A medical magician linking the blood services to the patient bedside. A varied clinical and laboratory role in a field dominated by process and projects.
Personality	Curious, creative, well-organized communicator, capable of working as part of a multidisciplinary team within a regulatory culture.
Best aspects	Enormous variety of roles; making things happen in practice and policy; flexible and off-site working; opportunities to publish and present.
Worst aspects	Managing expectations and meetings, especially in shared posts; regulatory culture.
Route	Either internal medicine training (IMT) (p. 44) or acute care common stem–acute medicine (ACCS-AM) (p. 37), then specialty training in haematology (ST3+). Alternative routes from other pathology disciplines, paediatrics, and GP. Exams: MRCP; FRCPath.
Locations	Mixture of hospitals, blood transfusion centres and the research community.

Life						Work
Quiet On-call						Busy On-call
Boredom						Burnout
Uncompetitive						Competitive
Low salary						High salary

Transplant medicine

Solid organ transplantation is a lifesaving and life-transforming treatment option for end-stage disease of many organs. Transplant physicians manage all non-surgical aspects of a patient's care, from referral and assessment to discharge post-transplant, and often become the primary physicians for post-transplant patients. Transplant medicine is a subspecialty of any medical specialty that has a transplantable organ. Physicians train within their own medical field and general internal medicine (GIM), then subspecialize in transplant medicine, which requires in-depth knowledge of immunology, infectious diseases, post-surgical complications, pharmacology and pharmacokinetics, palliative care, rehabilitation, and radiology.

The patients

Over 6000 patients are currently waiting for a solid organ transplant. In 2019, nearly 3000 people received a transplant. All are looked after by transplant physicians to some degree. Ages range from babies to 70+ years- , and patients may be pre- transplant to waiting for their third transplant. Patients have different underlying pathologies requiring good knowledge of all organ- specific diseases and associated challenges, alongside transplant- specific knowledge. Transplant patients will turn to their transplant physicians for advice on, and treatment of, health issues, ranging from toe infection and contraception to rejection and graft failure.

The work

Reviewing all patients referred for organ transplantation, co-ordinating prospective patients' investigations, making decisions in collaboration with transplant surgeons (p. 308), and regularly reviewing those awaiting transplant. Immediately post- surgery, transplant physicians are often the primary caregivers. Post- discharge, they are responsible for transplant- related care. Empathy and clear communication skills are vital, as not all are transplantable or survive.

The job

Transplant medicine is practised in tertiary centres, but the patients are spread across the country (and sometimes beyond). Close liaison with referral centres and DGHs local to patients is key. Work is split between ward rounds, transplant assessment clinics, follow-up clinics, practical procedures, and MDTs. Research, teaching, and quality improvement are optional but provide fulfilling challenges. No two days are the same—this is an acute field, but with the challenges of immunosuppression. Transplant medicine has one of the largest and most varied MDTs, including surgeons, physicians, pathologists, pharmacists, co-ordinators, and clinical nurse specialists (CNSs). Transplant physicians often find themselves exploring the boundaries of knowledge, as transplantation is a relatively novel field with many research challenges.

Extras

Transplant medicine is the epitome of personalized patient care. You get to know your patients—you may even get invited to a wedding or two! Being in tertiary and teaching hospitals provides opportunities for ground-breaking academia and innovation. Private practice is almost non-existent. Regular international conferences provide good opportunities to share developments and transplant medicine is a close-knit community. The pool of consultants is limited, so working less-than-full-time is not well established, but colleagues are willing to help each other to provide greater flexibility. Be warned though—you are always a phone call away, even at weekends.

For further information

The International Society of Heart and Lung Transplantation (ISHLT). Tel: +1 972 490 9495. Web: https://ishlt.org Email: communications@ishlt.org Twitter: @ishlt

British Transplantation Society (BTS). Tel: 01625 664 547. Web: https://bts.org.uk Email: secretariat@bts.org.uk Twitter: @BTStransplant

---

08:00	Inpatient MDT in intensive care unit (ICU) with intensivists and transplant surgeons; quick review of any new transplants
08:30	Procedure list (e.g. bronchoscopy, cath lab, endoscopy)
12:30	Liaise with transplant co-ordinators and surgeons regarding incoming transplant referrals. Review urgent cases which may need transfer from other hospitals
13:00	Quick lunch whilst going through incoming emails/admin
13:30	Post-transplant clinic, ward round (post-transplant inpatients), or assessment (pre-transplant) clinic. See, on average, 8–10 patients in clinic or approximately 15 inpatients
17:00	Review any urgent queries, urgent procedure in ICU, or virtual MDT with a referring centre
18:00	Home, answering the phone with any queries from the junior team on site

Myth	Glorified GP. Regularly airlifted to work.
Reality	Super-specialized physician who's never airlifted to work. Working with patients through life-changing treatments, but cursed to see them die. Link between intensivists and surgeons.
Personality	Compassionate, empathic, able to deliver difficult discussions, caring, and engaging. Decisive and able to manage risk; team player, good communicator. Open to innovative treatments.
Best aspects	Witnessing life-changing treatments. Patients transition from end-stage organ failure to being well, enjoying life again and going back to work. Teamwork.
Worst aspects	Attachment to patients makes it emotionally challenging when they do badly or die waiting for a transplant. Minimal (if any) private work.
Route	Either internal medicine training (IMT) (p. 44) or acute care common stem–acute medicine (ACCS-AM) (p. 37), then specialty training in relevant specialty, e.g. respiratory, renal, gastroenterology, etc. (ST3+). During/after training, obtain experience within transplant medicine. Exams: MRCP; SCE.
Numbers	Niche field, with limited numbers of consultants in dedicated centres, e.g. <15 lung transplant physicians (30% women) in UK. Significantly more transplant nephrologists and hepatologists.
Locations	Dedicated tertiary transplantation units (seven cardiothoracic, eight liver, 24 renal).

Life					Work
Quiet On-call					Busy On-call
Boredom					Burnout
Uncompetitive					Competitive
Low salary					High salary

Transplant surgery

Transplant surgery emerged from the need to treat people with terminal organ failure who would otherwise have a very low quality of life and eventually die due to lack of a critical body function. There are nearly as many subspecialties as the number of solid organs that can be transplanted: six (heart, lung, liver, pancreas, kidney, intestine). There has been huge progress over the last 20 years in the surgical, medical, and immunological aspects of transplantation, and the number of transplants worldwide are steadily increasing.

The patients

Patients referred for a transplant either are approaching or have end-stage failure of one or more vital organs. Except for a relatively small group of pre-emptive kidney failure patients, most patients are complex with a multitude of comorbidities. Without a transplant, most patients will eventually die if left untreated, especially where the organ function cannot be substituted (e.g. liver). A transplant can provide sustainable organ function for years, or decades in some cases, and in fact 'reset the clock' for the majority of these patients. Equally important, the quality of life is hugely improved early on and most people can resume normality in their lives.

The work

Apart from elective (living donor) and urgent (deceased donor) transplants and organ retrievals, daily work also involves ward rounds, surgical assessment for activation on the transplant waiting list, and post-transplant follow-up clinics. Working across several sites is very common. Transplant surgeons interact with a range of other healthcare professionals, and have unique skill sets that cross several surgical specialties, e.g. general, vascular, and urology for kidney transplants, making them valuable team players in transplant units. Many transplant surgeons develop an area of 'special interest' within their specialty, e.g. vascular access surgery for kidney transplant surgeons. Long working hours and the intensity of the workload certainly require commitment and dedication, whilst communication, teamwork, and training in human factors are key elements. Nevertheless, transforming a patient's life with a transplant is an incredibly rewarding experience, well worth every hour of dedication and hard work.

The job

Transplant surgery is practised in tertiary referral centres, usually in busy teaching hospitals. A very small number of liver or kidney transplants from living donors are performed in private hospitals. Most transplant units are led by a joint team of transplant surgeons and physicians (p. 304) who work in close collaboration with pharmacists, transplant immunology scientists, psychologists, nutritionists, anaesthetists, perfusionists, and dedicated theatre and ward staff. Referrals for transplant assessment usually come from specialist physicians, e.g. hepatologists. Transplant surgeons also do organ retrievals, usually at a regional level, although travelling further may be required. There is no fixed schedule for either retrievals or urgent transplants, meaning surgeons spend many nights in the operating theatre.

Extras

Research and education have become integral parts of careers in transplant surgery. New technologies, better understanding of immunological mechanisms and organ preservation, novel pharmacological agents, and refinement of surgical techniques have literally transformed transplantation, with surgeons leading the way.

For further information

British Transplantation Society (BTS). Tel: 01625 664 547. Web: https://bts.org.uk Email: secretariat@bts.org.uk Twitter: @BTStransplant

Herrick Society for UK Transplant Trainees. Web: https://www.herricksociety.org.uk Email: secretary@herricksociety.org.uk Twitter: @herricksociety

08:00 Review and consent patients on theatre list

08:30 Clinic letters and admin

09:00 Post-transplant follow-up clinic: 12–15 adult patients

12:30 Lunch at one of the many multidisciplinary team (MDT) meetings

13:30 Elective transplant from a living donor

17:30 Check transplant function and immunosuppression levels from morning clinic

18:00 Write the draft of that guidance you've been working on for so long ...

Myth	Surgeons airlifted to work ... in luxury jets.
Reality	Hard-working individuals making use of suitable organs to transform people's lives, day and night, 24/7. Airlifted only in helicopters to retrieve vital organs.
Personality	Committed and ambitious, practical, analytical, 'getting things done' mindset, team player.
Best aspects	High levels of job satisfaction, challenging patients and surgery that keep your mind and body active, wide knowledge in related disciplines beyond the confines of surgery.
Worst aspects	High-frequency and intensity on-calls; most urgent transplants happen during the night, minimal private work.
Route	Core surgical training (CST) (p. 61), followed by specialty training in general surgery (ST3+), with rotation in transplant jobs (ST5+). Alternative routes through urology (p. 312) or vascular surgery (p. 314). Post-CCT fellowships are desirable. Exams: MRCS; FRCS.
Locations	Transplant units in tertiary hospitals. Outreach clinics and non-transplant operating lists in district general hospitals.

Life					Work
Quiet On-call					Busy On-call
Boredom					Burnout
Uncompetitive					Competitive
Low salary					High salary

Trauma surgery

Orthopaedic trauma surgeons treat patients of all ages who have been injured in an accident, from falling over and breaking a hip to a high-speed road traffic accident. Most orthopaedic surgeons in the UK deal with trauma, as well as another subspecialty such as joint replacement. However, with the advent of major trauma centres, trauma as a defined area of musculoskeletal medicine is becoming increasingly popular.

The patients

People of all ages get injured and orthopaedic trauma surgeons will treat injuries to bones throughout the body—the range of patients dealt with is vast. Trauma patients, particularly the elderly, have complex medical and social needs, in addition to their injuries. Efficiently preparing patients for their operation, caring for them afterwards, and ensuring they will be safe at home are important parts of the role. Not all patients will need an operation and making this decision is a key element of the job.

The work

Orthopaedic trauma is dynamic—the landscape of trauma changes over time. Equally as technology develops, new ways of treating fractures emerge. As such, learning and adaptation are key features of the specialty. Orthopaedic trauma surgery is firmly 'evidence-based'; however, not all the answers are known. How best to deal with the growing burden of 'fragility injury' as the population ages is of considerable interest currently.

The job

Orthopaedic trauma patients are seen in hospitals throughout the UK. Increasingly, however, those with the most significant injuries are sent to one of 27 major trauma centres. Serious injuries are seen in the emergency department. More minor injuries, such as broken wrists, are seen in fracture clinics. Patients who require an operation will undergo surgery as soon as it is safe to do so. This may be immediately as an emergency but often can be planned for a few days afterwards. Caring for injured patients is a team activity, of which surgeons form one part—liaising with anaesthetists, plastic surgeons, physicians, nursing staff, and therapists is essential for holistic care. Co-ordinating this multidisciplinary team to work to the benefit of the patient is an important part of the job.

Extras

Traditionally taught through an apprentice model, education and training are central to orthopaedic trauma. Abundant opportunities exist to teach junior surgeons in all clinical settings. Known for its participation in multinational trials, the orthopaedic trauma community has a strong research ethic and completion of higher degrees is encouraged. Private practice is a significant feature in orthopaedics in general and opportunities for supplementing income are available.

For further information

British Trauma Society. Web: https://www.britishtrauma.com/ Email: exec@britishtrauma.com Twitter: @britishtrauma

---

A day in the life ...

07:30 Breakfast at work, checking emails, and patient administration

08:00 Trauma meeting—junior staff and on-call consultants discuss cases admitted over the last 24 hours

09:00 On-call team splits—half do a ward round, half start the trauma theatre list

12:30 Acute fracture clinic—patients with broken bones sent from the emergency department

15:00 Take over from colleague in trauma theatre

19:30 Finish the last (planned) case of the day in theatre

20:00 Hand over to the junior team, see patients who have problems, and home for dinner!

20:30 On-call from home to cover life- and limb-threatening cases that need to go to theatre overnight and for phone advice to the on-call junior surgeons

Myth	Educationally challenged, adrenaline-charged bonesetters.
Reality	Hard-working, team-focused specialists.
Personality	Robust, driven, and uncompromising. Appreciative of high standards of patient care.
Best aspects	Teamworking and combining patient care with technical achievement and ability to interact with evolving technology.
Worst aspects	Long hours during training and the impact emergency surgery has on work–life balance.
Route	Core surgical training (CST) (p. 61), then specialty training in trauma and orthopaedic surgery (ST3+); run-through training from ST1 available in Scotland. Exams: MRCS; FRCS (T&O).
Numbers	2550 consultants in England (combined with trauma surgery), of whom 6% are women.
Locations	Most district general hospitals, but increasingly, significant trauma is being transferred to the 27 major trauma centres.

Life					Work
Quiet On-call					Busy On-call
Boredom					Burnout
Uncompetitive					Competitive
Low salary					High salary

Urogynaecology

Urogynaecologists deal with the full range of functional pelvic floor disorders, including incontinence, pelvic organ prolapse, and recurrent urinary tract infection (UTI). These are remarkably common conditions, with a huge public health impact. Although urogynaecology may seem like an unglamorous career choice, demand for services has never been higher, as awareness of pelvic floor disorders grows and the associated stigma lessens. The specialty is relatively young, having been formalized only over the last 20 years. It has evolved in parallel with female urology and shares a similar curriculum.

The patients

Pelvic floor disorders affect women of all ages, but many patients present either in the months after childbirth or at around the time of menopause, as these two life events may precipitate symptoms. For some patients, the treatment journey may be completed in a matter of months (e.g. cure of stress incontinence with a mid-urethral sling). More long-lasting doctor–patient relationships develop for women with conditions, such as urgency incontinence, that may require retreatment over many years.

The work

In most centres, the majority of patients present with urinary incontinence or prolapse; however, the remit is broader than this. It may encompass recurrent UTIs, bladder pain, bowel dysfunction, and some kinds of sexual dysfunction. Urogynaecologists typically directly manage all aspects of diagnosis and treatment for women under their care. In addition to outpatient clinics, many consultants will have one or more dedicated diagnostic sessions where they perform flexible cystoscopies, urodynamic studies of bladder function, and rectal function studies. Theatre lists include a combination of vaginal, open, and cystoscopic procedures. In some centres, many procedures can also be performed with a laparoscopic approach.

The job

The workload is similar to other benign surgical jobs, centred around outpatient clinics and predominantly day-case operating. Except in very specialist centres, most consultants will also maintain some obstetric practice, perhaps including labour ward cover or antenatal clinics. In training centres, consultants will be supported by a subspecialty trainee on a dedicated 2- or 3-year training programme who manages inpatients and co-ordinates operating lists. Outpatient clinics and diagnostics are usually supported by specialist nurses with expertise in ancillary devices such as catheters and pessaries, and by specialist physiotherapists with expertise in biofeedback and pelvic floor training.

Extras

Many urogynaecologists are very active in research, with typically several multicentre trials available UK-wide at any one time, funded through either charities or industry. There are very vibrant national (UK Continence Society, British Society of Urogynaecology) and international societies (International Continence Society, International Urogynecological Association), to which most UK urogynaecologists will make an annual pilgrimage. With the success of contemporary minimally invasive treatments, private practice can be very worthwhile in some areas.

For further information

British Society of Urogynaecology (BSUG) c/o The Royal College of Obstetricians and Gynaecologists. Tel: 0207 772 6211. Web: https://bsug.org.uk Email: bsug@rcog.org.uk

---

08:00 Preoperative ward round—clerking in patients and planning surgery

08:30 Day-case operating list, including cystoscopic injection of BOTOX® to bladder

12:00 Multidisciplinary team (MDT) meeting with urology colleagues and clinical nurse specialists

13:00 Diagnostic outpatient clinic, including video-urodynamic investigations

17:00 Postoperative ward round to discharge patients

Myth	Pacifying elderly infirm women with intractable urine leakage.
Reality	Managing women of all ages with a wide range of conditions amenable to both medical and surgical treatment.
Personality	Empathetic, team player, able to communicate about sensitive issues, keen to treat the conscious as well as the anaesthetized.
Best aspects	Delivering truly life-changing treatments to otherwise well women who have often suffered for years before coming forward for care.
Worst aspects	Inevitably some exposure to urine and faeces.
Route	Specialty training in obstetrics and gynaecology (ST1+) (p. 47), then subspecialty training or Advanced Skills Training Module in urogynaecology (ST6+). Exams: MRCOG.
Numbers	Approximately 200 consultants with either full subspecialty training or a special interest in urogynaecology.
Locations	Mixture of secondary and tertiary care, with options for practice in almost all gynaecology units.

Life					Work
Quiet On-call					Busy On-call
Boredom					Burnout
Uncompetitive					Competitive
Low salary					High salary

Urology

This job is for people with a diverse surgical interest. On offer is the possibility of major surgery, lasers, robotic operations, keyhole surgery, microscopic suturing, cutting-edge research, and more! Furthermore, there are opportunities to attend and present at meetings all around the world. All trainees start as general urologists, with limited competitive entry into fellowship programmes for those who want to be a super-specialist. With an ageing population, the urological workload is expanding.

The patients

Urology covers all ages and both sexes, but most of urology deals with the ageing male. However, it is possible to specialize in paediatric or female aspects of urology (p. 310). Generally, old men are very interesting and have many stories to tell—sometimes a problem in a busy clinic! Some of them will have lived through, or been involved in, major world events. Aside from their urological disease, they often have other medical problems that may need to be taken into account if surgical procedures are being planned.

The work

Urologists manage disease of the renal tract, including the kidney, ureters, bladder, prostate, testis, and penis. Common diseases include prostatic enlargement, renal stones, and cancer. Prostate cancer is the number one urological cancer, with an excellent prognosis in the vast majority of men. Patients requiring chemotherapy, radiotherapy, or palliation are generally managed by oncologists—medical (p. 218) and clinical (p. 142). Surgery is very variable, from transurethral resection of the prostate (TURP), to advanced endoscopic techniques, to complicated resections and reconstructions. Some of the endoscopic work requires the use of a lot of water, so you may have to invest in a pair of wellies! On-call emergencies include renal colic, testicular torsion, trauma, and urinary retention.

The job

A normal week may comprise operative surgery, diagnostic tests (keyhole examinations of the bladder, urodynamics, ultrasound-guided prostate biopsies, etc.), clinics, ward work, and administration. Whilst the days are usually busy, the nights are generally quiet, with few urgent interventions requiring a consultant urologist's expertise. Urologists work closely with radiologists, oncologists, gynaecologists, and renal physicians.

Extras

There are plenty of research opportunities in urology if you are interested. Teaching of nurses, hospital doctors, GPs, medical students, and other urologists is often an option. Most urologists will attend two or more meetings a year, including annual meetings of the British Association of Urological Surgeons (BAUS), European Association of Urology (EAU), and American Urological Association (AUA). Subspecialization is common (e.g. urological oncology, renal transplant, stone disease). Private practice is available and can pay well.

> **For further information**
>
> **The British Association of Urological Surgeons (BAUS).** Tel: 020 7869 6950. Web: https://www.baus.org.uk Twitter: @BAUSurology

08:00 Handover from junior doctors covering the previous night

08:15 Cancer multidisciplinary team meeting: discuss patient management

09:00 Clinic: 16 patients seen, good mix of new patients and follow-ups

12:30 Consent patients for theatre, then quick lunch

13:30 Operating theatre. List includes a flexible cystoscopy for a man with painless haematuria and a TURP

17:00 Postoperative ward round

18:00 On-call, but non-resident

NIGHT Calls for advice; occasionally need to go into hospital for a urological emergency

Myth	Penis doctors.
Reality	There is so much more to urology! Massively varied specialty with a good balance of operative, diagnostic, clinical, administrative, and social sessions.
Personality	Outgoing, confident, sense of humour, both feet placed firmly on the ground, good practical skills and visuospatial awareness.
Best aspects	The patients, surgery, colleagues, and no shift work.
Worst aspects	Getting called in to insert or change catheters.
Route	Core surgical training (CST) (p. 61), then specialty training in urology (ST3+). Limited number of subspecialty fellowships. Exams: MRCS; FRCS (Urology).
Numbers	1000 consultants in England, of whom 10% are women.
Locations	Hospital-based, found in most hospitals.

Life					Work
Quiet On-call					Busy On-call
Boredom					Burnout
Uncompetitive					Competitive
Low salary					High salary

Vascular surgery

Vascular (and endovascular) surgery is a challenging, technically demanding, yet rewarding surgical specialty that encompasses operations and interventions on almost every part of the body. Dealing with all things arterial or venous, they are known to the complimentary as 'Masters of the Red Sea' and to the not-so-complimentary as 'plumbers' (which also explains their affinity and success in Donkey Kong)! Excepting the upper gastrointestinal system, vascular surgeons are the first port of call for uncontrollable bleeding, and with the advent of the endovascular revolution, we are two specialties for the price of one!

The patients

Vascular surgeons meet a wide variety of patients with a multitude of conditions. These include renal failure, diabetes, ischaemic heart disease, and all the goodness that comes with being a vasculopath. This essentially means that every patient who presents to a vascular surgeon must be properly assessed from both a medical and surgical standpoint. A good vascular surgeon is one who is adept at management of acute medical issues, pre-optimization of the patient, and, of course, operating for acute and chronic vascular surgical problems. Every patient's well-being is of the utmost importance, and preserving limb and mobility is the vascular surgeon's life's work.

The work

Work as a vascular surgeon is a myriad of challenges as patients usually present with a multitude of comorbidities alongside their vascular disease. The scope of practice encompasses both open as well as endovascular work and operating on almost every body part, from the neck down to the feet. Endovascular work consists predominantly of angioplasties, stents, mechanical thrombectomies and thrombolysis, and central venous access techniques. Open surgery involves everything from thoracoabdominal aneurysms to carotids, complex bypasses, arteriovenous fistulas, and more.

The job

The job of a vascular surgeon comprises around 40% surgery, 40% outpatient clinics, and 20% work on the ward. Close working relationships and good communication skills are fundamental for patient care and involve a myriad of other specialties such as intensive care, renal, cardiology, medical, and radiology. On-call hours can be extremely taxing, but at the same time exciting with emergencies such as ruptured aneurysms, bleeding fistulas, and ischaemic limbs presenting frequently!

Extras

Research is essential and highly regarded as it is the basis from which surgery can progress. It also allows for one to make evidence-based decisions in the management of patient care. Life on-call can be very hard work and is analogous to the waves breaking on the shore of an idyllic island. Sometimes, the waves can seem incessant and almost insurmountable, whilst at other times, a sea of calm presides and you can sit back, sip your mocktail, and congratulate yourself on your professional choice. There are opportunities for private work for those interested.

For further information

Vascular Society: The Vascular Society for Great Britain and Ireland. Tel: 0207 205 7150. Web: https://www.vascularsociety.org.uk Email: admin@vascularsociety.org.uk Twitter: @VSGBI

07:45	Arrive at work. Change immediately into scrubs
08:00	Catch up on admin and emails. Coffee.
08:30	Ward round of sickest inpatients with junior team
08:55	Send for first patient, ensure high dependency unit bed booked. Theatre team briefing
09:15	First patient arrives—a fem-fem bypass. Confirm consent, side, etc. Hand over to anaesthetist to work their magic
09:45	Start surgery
13:30	Close up, write notes, and fill in audit sheets
13:45	Grab lunch over vascular multidisciplinary team meeting
14:30	Continue operating list, including debridement of diabetic foot. Last patient cancelled due to bed shortage
18:00	Mini-ward round of sick and postoperative patients
18:30	Home time unless having to deal with an emergency or postoperative complication

Myth	Fem-pop, fem flop, fem chop.
Reality	No one likes the smell of rotten flesh. Most patients do well—amputations are a last resort.
Personality	A positive 'never say die' attitude, determination, and ability to empathize are key, particularly when 9-hour complex bypass surgery fails and results in amputation.
Best aspects	Repairing a ruptured aneurysm and saving lives.
Worst aspects	Getting up close and personal with smelly feet.
Route	Core surgical training (CST) (p. 61), followed by specialty training in vascular surgery (ST3+). Exams: MRCS; FRCS.
Numbers	500 consultants, of whom 10% are women.
Locations	Hospital-based in large district general hospitals and teaching hospitals.

Life		Work
Quiet On-call		Busy On-call
Boredom		Burnout
Uncompetitive		Competitive
Low salary		High salary

▌ Virology

Clinical virology is a relatively new specialty that is rarely out of the news. There is a good mix of clinical work, laboratory liaison, and research and development. Clinical virologists concentrate on the diagnosis and management of patients with viral infections. Rapid diagnosis, using molecular-based tests, and monitoring resistance to antiviral drugs are key parts of this specialty. Interpreting and understanding the relevance of viral infections in a variety of clinical situations make the job both satisfying and rewarding, and the constant evolution of both diagnostics and pathogens makes work both intellectually challenging and exciting.

*That was written in 2019 before the Covid-19 pandemic further demonstrated that if you're interested in general medicine with a focus on infectious diseases, managing viral infections, a multidisciplinary approach, understanding laboratory methods, and involvement in local, regional, and/or national strategy, and research, this is a career for you.

The patients

Are individuals in hospital or the community with acute or chronic viral infections. This includes those who have travelled to areas where specific viral infections are endemic, those who need screening for infections that cause complications in pregnancy, and patients after organ transplantation who are at risk of latent viral infections that may reactivate.

The work

Many new and emerging infections are caused by SARS-CoV-2, Zika, Ebola, Nipah, hepatitis E, and influenza viruses. Clinical virologists advise and write guidance regarding viral diagnosis and management. They also spend more time on the wards and in clinics, seeing patients and advising clinical and laboratory colleagues on investigation and treatment. An increasing number of antiviral treatments are available, and ensuring antiviral drugs are prescribed and used appropriately is critical. Liaison with health protection teams and advising on public health issues, together with a clinical role acting as an interface between specialists and the laboratory, are key. Clinical virologists are part of the MDT and are involved in meetings and ward rounds, focusing on the management of immunocompromised patients.

The job

A clinical virologist's main role is to aid the diagnosis and management of individuals with infectious diseases. This involves a variety of clinical duties, but with additional laboratory-related activities e.g. management of diagnostic tests and interpretation of serological and molecular results. Clinical virology is increasingly clinically orientated, with opportunities to take part in ward-based activities and clinics. The multidisciplinary nature of the job involves daily contact with a variety of healthcare professionals, including hospital doctors, GPs, microbiologists, infection control nurses, clinical scientists, and public health doctors. On-call includes dealing with blood-borne viral exposure incidents e.g. needlestick injuries, rabies exposures, transplant donor screening results, and potential viral haemorrhagic fever infections in travellers returning home. Most of these can be handled over the telephone.

Extras

Clinical virology continues to be at the forefront of technological advances involving the evolution of laboratory techniques. Virologists can also be closely involved with public health on a local and national level and there is a lot of potential for carrying out research, attending conferences, and teaching and training in different settings. There is little, if any, private practice. Flexible training and working are well established.

For further information

The Royal College of Pathologists, London. Tel: 020 7451 6700. Web: https://www.rcp ath.org Email: info@rcpath.org Twitter: @RCPath

The UK Clinical Virology Network. Web: http://www.clinicalvirology.org

08:45	Handover from previous day, authorize and discuss test results where clinically relevant
10:30	Haemato-oncology multidisciplinary meeting
12:00	Review a bone marrow transplant recipient with an influenza virus infection
13:00	Lunch
13:45	Outpatient clinic, e.g. HIV, sexual health, viral hepatitis
16:00	Laboratory authorization, review molecular test results, and discuss with clinical teams
17:30	Go home; might be on-call overnight

* During the COVID-19 pandemic, jobs also included frequent discussions concerning patients and staff with COVID-19, and remote meetings on local, regional, and national basis, e.g. updating guidance, use of personal protective equipment (PPE), and clinical trials.

Myth	Stuck in laboratory, not interacting with staff or seeing patients.
Reality	It is changing rapidly from more laboratory-based to increasingly involved in multidisciplinary work and often seeing patients on the wards and in clinics.
Personality	Approachable, calm, meticulous, logical, good communicators, and inquisitive.
Best aspects	Job diversity; tend to get interesting questions in grey areas that you might not have considered previously.
Worst aspects	As with any job, there is a certain amount of routine work.
Route	Internal medicine training (IMT) (p. 44) or acute care common stem–acute medicine (ACCS-AM) (p. 37), followed by combined infection training (CIT) (p. 52), then 2 years of medical virology training (ST5+). Exams: MRCP; FRCPath.
Numbers	64 consultants, of whom 36% are female.
Locations	Teaching hospital or regional laboratory.

Life		Work
Quiet On-call		Busy On-call
Boredom		Burnout
Uncompetitive		Competitive
Low salary		High salary

▌ Voluntary service overseas (VSO)

Returned volunteers say that giving service overseas as a volunteer ranks among the best times in their professional and personal lives. Volunteers work somewhere that really needs their professional skills. The type of placement varies, depending on where the volunteer has reached in their career. They commonly provide a clinical service whilst training local doctors, and perhaps nurses, in clinical and/or educational skills. Since the volunteer's impact must be sustainable after leaving, it is insufficient merely to provide a clinical service. Volunteers don't make money but shouldn't be out of pocket after receiving a living allowance.

The patients

The poorest people in the world. They present with advanced disease, preventable disease, and conditions unseen in the UK. But common things are common, and so much that comes in is easily recognized. Many patients flock to each clinic session. They will have saved or borrowed small amounts of money to get healthcare, or there may be pre-payment mechanisms, credit schemes, or free state provision. Transport to the facility might be their greatest cost. Despite the costs, they are disproportionately grateful for what the doctor offers them.

The work

The major health problems of developing countries include high maternal mortality, high infant and child mortality, and deaths from infectious diseases, including HIV/AIDS and malaria. Clinical work is therefore most likely to address one or more of these issues and will be combined with teaching. Although a diploma in tropical medicine is valuable, it is by no means essential. In addition, volunteers may be asked to join meetings with the local health authorities that plan services around these problems.

The job

Although applications are for a specific placement, VSO staff are good at helping prospective volunteers find their most suitable role. Hospitals and other health facilities are much poorer with fewer supplies than a UK doctor is used to. It is always hard work. But most volunteers who can rise to challenges, seek adventure, and tolerate the unknown are very fulfilled. Generalists, paediatricians, obstetricians, gynaecologists, and infectious diseases and public health trainees and specialists are most needed in development work, which aims for long-term health improvements. In contrast, emergency medics, surgeons, and anaesthetists in aid work, often providing urgent care during crises. Many specialties allow time out of programme (p. 101) for trainees to volunteer.

Extras

VSO provides training at home before leaving and orientation after arrival in the country, as well as on-the-job support, including web-based information about the country and volunteering in general. Volunteers are infrequently stuck alone in the middle of nowhere and are more likely to have other volunteers around for support. They live in a completely different culture, really feel they're being useful, and can take opportunities to travel. Unlike 20 years ago, social media mean they aren't cut off from friends and family. Most returned volunteers really value the NHS!

For further information

Voluntary Service Overseas (VSO). Tel: 020 8780 7500. Web: https://www.vsointernatio nal.org Email: enquiry@vsoint.org Twitter: @VSO_Intl

---

A day in the life ...

(Note: varies greatly between days and volunteers!)

07:00 Early start to reduce paperwork and talk to colleagues before seeing patients

08:00 Ward round setting up patients' care for the day

09:30 Outpatients with lots of gross pathology and diagnostic puzzles. Little time for each patient

11:00 Teaching session with colleagues

12:00 Lunch break and a rest during the heat of the day

14:00 Meeting with provincial health department

15:30 Outpatients clinic: 15 patients. Again, little time for each

16:30 Timetable says to finish. In fact, catch up on everything postponed from earlier

18:00 Meet other volunteers for early-evening socializing

19:30 Prepare and eat food

21:00 Early to bed (it's dark!)

Myth	Isolated, altruistic do-gooders working from mud huts in the middle of nowhere.
Reality	Fun-loving, hard-working, team players with capacity to manage the unexpected and to temporize when faced with the unknown.
Personality	Reasonable self-confidence with low anxiety; an independent worker who is comfortable communicating with anyone and everyone.
Best aspects	New ways of being oneself—living differently, practising differently, and learning all the time.
Worst aspects	Watching children and adults dying unnecessarily. Too many people cannot be helped because investigations, drugs, and supplies are not available.
Route	ST3+ level in most specialties and some roles limited to consultants. Will require deanery and/or employer approval. Vacancies listed on VSO website.
Numbers	No limits.
Locations	Twenty-five of the poorest countries in Africa, Asia, and the Pacific Region. Usually working in a local hospital and maybe visiting outlying clinics.

Life						Work
Quiet On-call						Busy On-call
Boredom						Burnout
Uncompetitive						Competitive
Low salary						High salary

Index

A

academic career 23–5
academic clinical fellow xxi, 23
academic foundation programme 23
academic GPs 42, 174–5
academic medicine 110–11
academic surgery 112–13
academic training 87
Academy of Medical Royal Colleges 96
Accreditation of Transferable Competences
    Framework (ATCF) 22
acting up as a consultant 12
acute care common stem (ACCS) 37–8
acute internal medicine 114–15
acute medicine (ACCS) 37
addictions psychiatry 55
aid work 30
allergy 116–17
anaesthetics 37, 39–41, 118–19
annual review of competency progression
    (ARCP) xxi, 7, 95
Applied Knowledge Test (AKT) 43
Approved Programme 21
armed forces 26–7, 120–25
    Army 120–1
    bursaries/cadetships 26
    consultants 26
    foundation programme 26
    general duties medical officer 26
    GPs 26
    Royal Air Force Medical Officer 122–3
    Royal Navy Medical Officer 124–5
    specialty training 26
Army 120–1
associate specialist 19
audiovestibular medicine 126–7
audit 83, 85
aviation and space medicine 128–9
awards 83, 85

B

banding supplements 99
bariatric surgery 130–31
basic pay 99
basic training 36
biochemistry 52, 136–7
bullying 104
burnout 101–2

C

Calman, Sir Kenneth 92
cardiology 132–3
    paediatrics 49, 252–3
cardiothoracic surgery 134–5
career break
    future job prospects 101
    returning to work 105
career changes 22, 32–3
CASC 55, 56
case-based discussion (CBD) 5
Certificate of Completion of Training
    (CCT) xxi, 3, 7, 12, 36
Certificate of Eligibility for General Practice
    Registration (CEGPR) xxi, 13, 20, 21
Certificate of Eligibility for Specialist
    Registration (CESR) xxi, 12, 20, 21
Certificate of Experience 4
Champion of Flexible Training 98
chemical pathology 52, 136–7
child and adolescent psychiatry 55, 268–9
childcare 105
Clinical Assessment of Skills and
    Competencies (CASC) 55, 56
clinical benchmarking 87
clinical biochemistry 52, 136–7
clinical fellow 19–20, 72, 77
clinical genetics 138–9
clinical immunology 52, 196–7
clinical lectureship 23–4
clinical neurophysiology 140–1
clinical oncology 59, 60, 142–3
clinical pharmacology and
    therapeutics 144–5
clinical radiology 59, 282–3
Clinical Skills Assessment (CSA) 43
clinical station 75
clinical supervisor xxi, 95
clinical teaching skills 5
clinical virology 52, 316–17
Combined Infection Training (CIT) 53, 53
Combined Programme 21
community paediatrics 49, 258–9
conference abstracts and presentations 83,
    84, 85
consultant xxi, 3, 12
    acting up as a consultant 12
    armed forces 26
    Certificate of Eligibility for Specialist
        Registration (CESR) xxi, 12, 20, 21